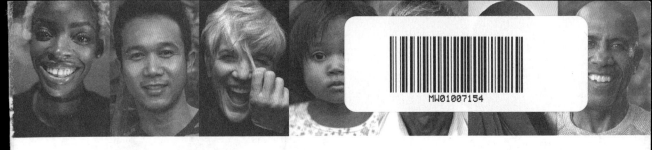

The Challenges of Health Disparities

Implications and Actions for Health Care Professionals

Darren Liu, DrPH, MHA, MS
Associate Professor
MHA/MPH Program
College of Health Sciences
Des Moines University
Des Moines, Iowa

Shartriya Collier-Stewart, EdD
Associate Dean
School of Education
Nevada State College
Las Vegas, Nevada

Betty Burston, PhD
Professor-in-Residence
Department of Health Care Administration and Policy
School of Community Health Sciences
University of Nevada, Las Vegas
Las Vegas, Nevada

Heidi H. Mulligan
Owner
A Woman of A Thousand Words
Health Care Consulting
Monterey, California

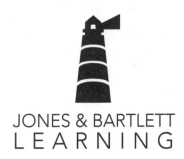

JONES & BARTLETT
LEARNING

World Headquarters
Jones & Bartlett Learning
5 Wall Street
Burlington, MA 01803
978-443-5000
info@jblearning.com
www.jblearning.com

Jones & Bartlett Learning books and products are available through most bookstores and online booksellers. To contact Jones & Bartlett Learning directly, call 800-832-0034, fax 978-443-8000, or visit our website, www.jblearning.com.

Production Credits

VP, Product Management: David D. Cella
Director of Product Management: Michael Brown
Product Manager: Sophie Fleck Teague
Product Specialist: Danielle Bessette
Associate Production Editor: Robert Furrier
Senior Marketing Manager: Susanne Walker
Production Services Manager: Colleen Lamy
Manufacturing and Inventory Control Supervisor: Amy Bacus
Composition: codeMantra U.S. LLC
Cover Design: Scott Moden
Text Design: Scott Moden
Rights & Media Specialist: Thais Miller
Media Development Editor: Shannon Sheehan
Cover Image: © EyeEm/Getty Images, © Hero Images/Getty Images, © pixelheadphoto digitalskillet/Shutterstock, © Westend61/Getty Images, © Tassii/Getty Images, © Andy Dean Photography/Shutterstock, © Photodisc/Getty Images, © artpixelgraphy Studio/Shutterstock, © pixelfusion3d/Getty Images, © janon kas/Shutterstock, © Marie Killen/Getty Images, © ImagesBazaar/Getty Images, © wavebreakmedia/Shutterstock
Printing and Binding: McNaughton & Gunn
Cover Printing: McNaughton & Gunn

Library of Congress Cataloging-in-Publication Data
Names: Liu, Darren, 1974- author. | Burston, Betty C., author. | Stewart, Shartriya C., author. | Mulligan, Heidi H., author.
Title: The challenges of health disparities: implications and actions for health care professionals / Darren Liu, Betty C. Burston, Shartriya C. Stewart, Heidi H. Mulligan.
Description: First edition. | Burlington, Massachusetts: Jones & Bartlett Learning, [2019] | Includes bibliographical references.
Identifiers: LCCN 2018024739 | ISBN 9781284156096 (paperback)
Subjects: | MESH: Healthcare Disparities | Health Facility Administrators | Data Collection | Research Design | Socioeconomic Factors | United States
Classification: LCC RA971 | NLM W 76 AA1 | DDC 362.1068—dc23
LC record available at https://lccn.loc.gov/2018024739

6048

Printed in the United States of America
22 21 20 19 18   10 9 8 7 6 5 4 3 2 1

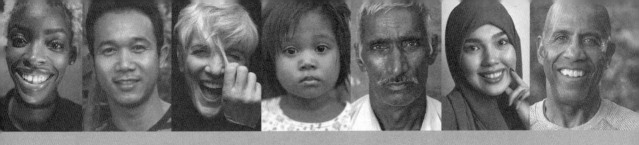

Contents

**PART III Disparities in Health
           Care   109**

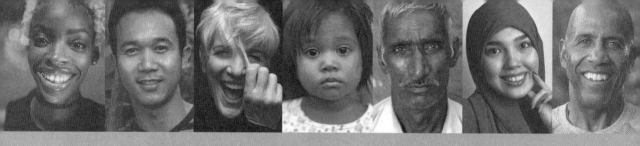

Preface

The purpose of this text is a highly ambitious one. Specifically, it is that of reconstructing the field of health disparities and, by doing so, stimulating change in the approaches used throughout the healthcare arena with regards to differences that characterize health outcomes and health care. For example, health and health care are academic disciplines, and they are rooted in fact and in the natural and computational disciplines. However, definitions of health disparities and approaches to solving disparities have become filled with innuendo. For example, Braveman and colleagues (2011), in a seminal article on health disparities, demonstrated the intrusion of intentional subjectivity rather than intentional objectivity into the study of this field through their summary of the definitions of health disparities that now dominate research and policy. This definition was introduced by a subcommittee that was organized by the U.S. Department of Health and Human Services (2008), Advisory Committee for Healthy People 2020. These authors assert that:

> Based on the subcommittee's work, we propose that health disparities are systematic, plausibly avoidable health differences adversely affecting socially disadvantaged groups; they may reflect social disadvantages, but causality need not be established. This definition, grounded in ethical and human

rights principles, focuses on the subset of health differences reflecting social injustice, distinguishing health disparities from other health differences also warranting concerted attention, and from health differences in general.

While other definitions of health disparities have been used, this definition defines the current framework that dominates scholarship and textbooks on this subject. Our argument is that this highly subjective definition of health disparities has been divisive and has adversely impacted the crafting of effective solutions that will advance the whole of humankind. Rather than supporting reductions in health disparities, this definition has supported the emergence of contemporary subtribalism, because, in many respects, the very definition separates individuals into "tribes" based on racial/ethnic, gender, geographic, and/or other commonalities. Rather, the described definition supports "excessive" loyalty to one's own self-defined group to the degree that loyalty to the holistic unit of humankind is subordinated. In other words, as currently defined, health disparities are not approached merely as a statistical concept that is inclusive of disproportionalities in health outcomes that can be empirically verified across any grouping. Thus, the dominant definition literally eliminates data mining processes that seek to identify inequalities in health outcomes or healthcare practices across all groupings. Accordingly, it has pitted the economically advantaged against the economically disadvantaged, females against males, nonwhite ethnic groups against whites, and so on.

Furthermore, the current definition uses emotionally charged language such as *social justice and injustice*, *equity versus nonequity*, and so on. Our argument is that this framework has generated an entire field of study that is supporting the emergence of a "we against them" battleground that is adversely affecting the growth of a unified humanity that can collectively utilize its strengths to ensure human survival. As we point out in various chapters, extraordinary disparities in life expectancy exist between regions and countries. Yet, the definitions used have precluded the identification of the fact that all humankind has also experienced very positive benefits over time.

However, it is not only healthcare researchers who have framed disparities in this way. Disparities in income, education, housing, and so on all support, rather than reduce, a divided humanity and, as a result, preclude the crafting of effective programs, policies, and initiatives to decrease existing disparities. For example, far more healthcare administrators oversee hospitals or clinical care groups that offer women's health clinics than men's health clinics. Yet, men die more often from nearly all major diseases. A healthcare administrator who is aware of this disparity can create one clinic that serves all family members, including those with specialized needs.

The prevailing definition of healthcare disparities also explicitly instructs those who would reduce remediable differences to not focus upon health inequalities in general nor on the causes of observed inequalities. In doing so, opportunities for maximizing economies of scale in solutions are lost. Moreover, a "shotgun" rather than a "rifle" approach is applied to the design of interventions. Yet, from a healthcare administrator's perspective, a sophisticated analysis of "causes" and the directing of dollars to these "causes" can improve outcomes and lower the costs of reducing remediable differences in health outcomes and in the care received by all subgroups.

This text seeks to demonstrate that humankind has participated in an upward spiral of unequally distributed benefits. Within this context, this text describes empirical data on the "causes" of disparities in health care and health outcomes and recommends strategies for addressing health disparities based not on justice or injustice, but rather on the nature of every remediable cause, whether it is provider based, patient based, environmentally based, or based on education, income, marital status, or other "social determinants."

Only by addressing each category of variables in the disparity chain can health disparities be remediated. This may require pediatricians to consult with parents on the educational progress of each child in their care given that education is a strong predictor of health disparities later in life. It may require that case managers be assigned to young patients, who can then link unemployed transition-age youth to college preparatory programs at open admissions colleges given that income is a strong predictor of health disparities later in life. It may also lead to healthcare administrators partnering with clinicians to improve prevention and individual disease self-management efforts by signing a statement of compliance/noncompliance that states the decreases in life expectancy that are associated with morbidity-related behavioral choices. Stated differently, this text can be used to explicitly shift the health disparities framework away from the current ". . . the glass is half empty" approach to one which documents that the glass from which humankind now sips is most certainly ". . . half full." Research and data clearly demonstrate that an upward trajectory for humankind requires cooperation and accommodation rather than division and conflict. It is a goal that can only be achieved when we recognize that for humankind, it is both the "best of times and the worst of times."

Accordingly, the objectives of this book are several. All societies have a division of labor. Within the United States, farmers and ranchers feed the world. Psychiatrists, psychologists, motivational speakers, and religious leaders serve as caretakers of the minds, emotions, and spirits of the residents of this country. Academic institutions, whether community colleges, universities, or research entities, have self-appointed themselves as the "factories" whose tasks include the training of minds and the production of new knowledge. Stated differently, academicians, freed from the burdens of existence in the trenches of lived life, have the leisure to overview reality and to serve as thought leaders. Thus, a primary objective of this book is that of examining health disparities and healthcare disparities through the lens of original thought and from a reflective rather than reactive perspective.

A second and related objective is that of prompting readers to examine, challenge, and synthesize the expressed ideas into even newer thinking that supports growth, solidarity, and the reunification of humankind.

A third aim of this book is to provide a tool on health disparities that is not only of use to students of healthcare administration and professional healthcare administrators but also to clinicians, public health professionals, educators, social scientists, policymakers, community leaders and advocates, and individuals and families. Thus, we have sought to include the dual objectives of preparing a textbook that is also an informational manual that will deliver value to consumers of healthcare services.

Finally, yet foremost, the objective of this book is enhancing the knowledge and skills of current and future healthcare administrators, public health professionals, and clinicians by

developing much-needed skills. In some respects, these occupations embody a tremendous amount of transformational capital. Despite a greater effort to integrate the preventative, we remain a curative-oriented world. Healthcare administrators and clinicians manage curative institutions. Thus, healthcare administrators are positioned to not only link sick or ill patients with diagnostics and treatment services, but those professionals and their staff can also use the occasion of non-freedom from illness or disease to promote wellness to the family members of the injured and/or the sick.

Toward this purpose, we introduce readers to novel views regarding health disparities as a concept. In addition, we shift the measurement of health disparities from the maximal rate difference currently used by the U.S. government to the use of difference analysis with reference groups as a more appropriate measurement tool.

This text also increases knowledge of key disparities in death rates in general as well as by various illnesses and diseases. The data presented have been carefully selected to only include key statistics that should be a part of the intellectual arsenal of any healthcare administrator, public health professional, and/or clinician. If a healthcare administrator is health disparity illiterate, it weakens his or her ability to understand the impact of patient mix upon the quality ratings of the different institutions that comprise the overall healthcare system. Thus, most chapters in this book are somewhat data heavy. Importantly, the text provides attention to multiple types of healthcare delivery institutions. Not only are traditional healthcare disparities in physician care, hospital care, and long-term care institutions reviewed, but disparities in other areas are also examined.

The text also identifies strategies to strengthen self-management and prevention as critical tools for incorporation into the services provided by every component of the healthcare system. More concretely, selected chapters review a number of preventable chronic diseases and discuss the breadth, depth, and nature of ongoing disparities.

This text is also based upon educational pedagogy and research that shows that the learning process embodies several different levels of learning. At the first level, it is important to know and recall new facts, concepts, and terms, as well as historical information. This type of learning is called level 1 learning. It is based on an approach from the field of education that was introduced by Benjamin Bloom and his colleagues in 1956. However, as a future healthcare administrator, public health professional, clinician, or policy analyst, knowing and remembering alone are insufficient. Data, concepts, historical facts, and so on are simply ingredients, much like the materials needed for building a house or baking a cake. Knowledge is the input into the human brain, which then allows us to analyze and apply it.

But, as humans, we analyze and apply knowledge by deconstructing and examining it, and then putting it back together to determine whether the information is logical. We then apply it to real-world situations in order to make it useful. These activities are considered to be *level 2 learning*. Finally, we evaluate knowledge and information by critiquing it and checking the premises (*level 3 learning*). The findings generated from these processes are then used to generate new knowledge and to plan and design solutions.

Such an approach is critical to the learning process. Roberson (2013) and other psychologists have suggested that ensuring that each learner understands the relevance of the materials to be learned supports the overall learning process. In addition, the competencies at each of these levels are so critical to the skills needed by future and current healthcare administrators, public health professionals, and clinicians that they are now embodied in the accreditation process.

But, competency-based knowledge is also important for another reason. In today's advanced society every person needs to know how to acquire new knowledge, analyze and apply that new knowledge, and use it innovatively to improve the human condition. We urge each reader to continue to explore, debate, and addend the overall theory that in spite of the need for additional progress, humankind has, indeed, continually improved the human condition.

Critical to our aim, the entirety of this text is designed to prompt readers to formulate their own analyses, strategies, and solutions to ongoing health and healthcare disparities. Through this journey, it is anticipated that current and future healthcare administrators, public health professionals, and clinicians will gain skills needed to accelerate positive change.

Darren Liu, DrPH, MHA, MS

Betty Burston, PhD

Heidi H. Mulligan

Shartriya Collier-Stewart, EdD

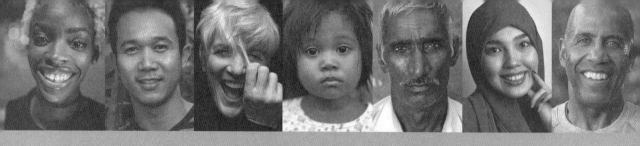

Acknowledgements

While lone individuals can accomplish much, human endeavors are exponentially advanced when a highly synchronized team brings together their unique skills to facilitate project completion. Accordingly, we are so very grateful to the team whose collective input allowed this text to manifest itself. First, we must thank Mike Brown, Robert Furrier, Danielle Bessette, and other Jones & Bartlett Learning staff who were willing to publish the first dialogic textbook. We also are grateful to the Jones & Bartlett Learning editors who supported this endeavor. Special thanks to George Mulligan, a good friend, who came out of retirement and spent countless hours on his new "hobby," which entailed checking the tables, figures, and numbers to ensure that they are accurate. Last, but not least, we would like to acknowledge the contributions of the following scholars who spent their precious time proofreading our work. This book could not have been accomplished without their help and insight:

Bernardo Ramirez, MD, MBA, Associate Professor of Health Management, and Informatics at University of Central Florida;

Denise Smart, MPH, DrPH, Associate Professor of College of Nursing at Washington State University, Spokane;

Dooyoung Lim, PhD, Assistant Professor of MHA Program at Des Moines University;

Ginny Garcia-Alexander, PhD, Associate Professor of Sociology at Portland State University;

Pi-Hua Liu, PhD, Assistant Professor of Clinical Informatics & Medical Statistics Research Center at Chang Gung University, Taiwan;

Simon Geletta, PhD, Professor of MPH program at Des Moines University;

Takashi Yamashita, MPH, PhD, Associate Professor of Sociology at The University of Maryland, Baltimore County;

Tami Swenson, PhD, Assistant Professor of MHA Program at Des Moines University, and

Thistle Elias, DrPH, Assistant Professor of School of Public Health at University of Pittsburgh.

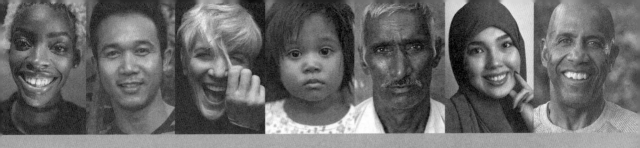

Foreword

In *The Challenges of Health Disparities: Implications and Actions for Healthcare Professionals*, Darren Liu, DrPH, MHA, MS; Betty Burston, PhD; Shartriya Collier-Stewart, EdD; and Heidi H. Mulligan seek to broaden and redefine current approaches to the study of health disparities. In doing so, the authors seek to encourage hands-on exploration of issues that in the past have often clouded discussions of remediable differentials in health and healthcare outcomes. In seeking to prepare readers to approach this much-discussed health issue, the authors query rather than tell, and analyze instead of describing, addressing queries such as "What are the implications of different definitions of disparities for research and policy?" and "How do data sources vary in quality and relevance for investigating different facets of health disparities?" The text will be useful for students seeking to confront one of the greatest challenges of health policy and public health in the United States.

After decades of research into the causes and consequences of health disparities in the United States, what is new, and what is likely to push this field forward? What have we learned that will allow us to reduce the avoidable mortality and morbidity that disproportionately affects vulnerable segments of the U.S. population?

One important line of inquiry comes from research examining the ratio of spending on social services and public health versus spending on medical care. In the United States, this ratio is often calculated as the sum of social service and public health spending divided by the sum of Medicare and Medicaid spending. States (and countries) with a higher ratio have better health outcomes by a number of indicators, including adult obesity; asthma; days with poor mental health; days with activity limitations; and mortality associated with lung cancer, acute myocardial infarction, and type 2 diabetes (Bradley et al., 2016). Thus, investing in health through social spending may be critical for reducing health disparities. A Brookings Institute study found that members of the Organization for Economic Co-operation and Development (OECD) spend, on average, about $1.70 on social services for every $1 on health services, whereas the United States spends just 56 cents (Butler, Matthew, & Cabello, 2017). This is more than a threefold difference.

A 2016 RAND study quantified the population health benefits of greater social spending in a multicountry study (Rubin et al., 2016). This study reported a positive relationship between social expenditures and life expectancy at birth, even after adjusting for gross domestic product (GDP). Increasing social expenditures as a percentage of GDP by 1% was associated with an additional 0.05 years (18 days) of life across populations. The study authors note,

> If we imagine for a moment that this is a direct causal effect, then increasing social expenditures by one percentage point in the United States would result in 16 million additional years of life across the entire U.S. population (320 million × 0.05).

Since this effect is largest for vulnerable populations, such as those with low incomes, this policy lever is likely to reduce health disparities.

On a clinical level, this approach can be buttressed with routine collection of data on "non-medical, health-related social needs" during patient encounters. A *National Academy of Medicine* review has identified key indicators for social needs that are in themselves not medical but that are highly related to health outcomes (Billioux, Verlander, Anthony, & Alley, 2017). Most centrally, these include housing quality and security (including utilities), access to healthy food, interpersonal safety, and access to transportation. A broader approach would add literacy, community support, and financial strain. Collecting this information routinely in clinical encounters would help the healthcare establishment recognize the significance of these health-related social needs for medical care. New efforts to link social services to medical care, such as HealthLeads, have emerged to provide wraparound services, but a more general connection at the level of policy and funding is needed.

The problem of health disparities persists, but these new lines of inquiry and evaluation suggest that we can close the gap and improve population health. A key question is whether changing social determinants of health, whether through increased social spending or specific targeting of health-related social needs, yields benefit in population health outcomes for the most vulnerable segments of society. This text seeks to advance these new approaches to the remediation of disparate health outcomes wherever they may exist.

Steven M. Albert, PhD
Professor and Chair, Department of
Behavioral and Community Health Sciences
Philip B. Hallen Endowed Chair in
Community Health and Social Justice
University of Pittsburgh, Pennsylvania

▶ References

Billioux, A., Verlander, K., Anthony, S., & Alley, D. (2017). Standardized screening for health-related social needs in clinical settings. The Accountable Health Communities Screening Tool. Discussion paper, National Academy of Medicine. Retrieved from https://nam.edu/standardized-screening-for-health-related-social-needs-in-clinical-settings-the-accountable-health-communities-screening-tool/

Bradley, E. H., Canavan, M., Rogan, E., Talbert-Slagle, K., Ndumele, C., Taylor, L., & Curry, L. A. (2016). Variation in health outcomes: The role of spending on social services, public health, and health care, 2000–09. *Health Affairs, 35*(5), 760–768.

Butler, S. M., Matthew, D. B., & Cabello, M. (2017). Re-balancing medical and social spending to promote health: Increasing state flexibility to improve health through housing. Brookings Institution, February 15. Retrieved from https://www.brookings.edu/blog/usc-brookings-schaeffer-on-health-policy/2017/02/15/re-balancing-medical-and-social-spending-to-promote-health-increasing-state-flexibility-to-improve-health-through-housing/

Rubin, J., Taylor, J., Krapels, J., Sutherland, A., Felician, M., Liu, J., Davis, L., & Rohr C. (2016). Are better health outcomes related to social expenditure? A cross-national empirical analysis of social expenditure and population health measures. RAND. Retrieved from https://www.rand.org/pubs/research_reports/RR1252.html

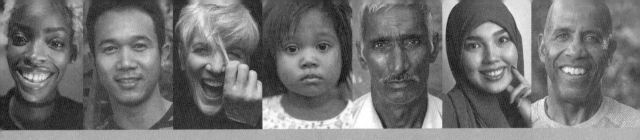

Contributors

Michelle Sotero, MPH, PhD
Assistant Professor
Department of Health Care Administration
    and Policy
School of Community Health Sciences
University of Nevada, Las Vegas
Las Vegas, Nevada

Xan Goodman, MLIS, AHIP
Health Sciences Librarian
Assistant Professor
Lied Library
University of Nevada, Las Vegas
Las Vegas, Nevada

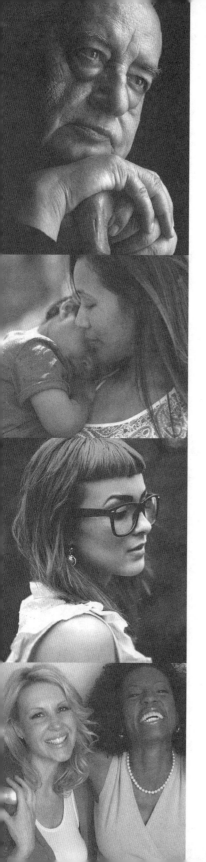

PART I

Fundamentals of Health Disparities

"Today the fate of humankind is even more crucially linked than ever before. The boundaries between the problems of 'others' and 'our' problems are being increasingly erased."

—**Janez Drnovšek**, past president of Slovenia, 59th Session of the General Assembly of the United Nations, September 21, 2004

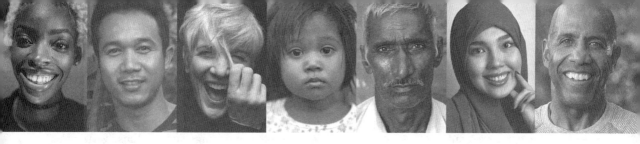

CHAPTER 1

Health Disparities: The Best of Times, the Worst of Times

"It was the best of times, it was the worst of times. . . ."

—**Charles Dickens** (1812-1870), author of A Tale of Two Cities

LEARNING OBJECTIVES

After completing this chapter, each learner will be able to:

- Summarize and critique the thesis that with regard to current health outcomes, the United States can be described within the framework of the present being the "best of times and the worst of times."
- Describe how the concept of health and health disparities extends beyond the area of health care and into the realms of history, sociology, philosophy, and other disciplines.
- Describe the historical circumstances that have shaped the emergence of health disparities.
- Define contemporary *tribalism,* and explore how the concept suggests the need for novel approaches to the field of health disparities.

▶ The Status of Humankind

Several famous lines from Charles Dickens' classic novel, *A Tale of Two Cities* (1859), are often used to denote the contradictory forces that simultaneously operate in any given historical period. In introducing a complex fictional plot regarding the prelude to the French Revolution, Dickens writes:

It was the best of times, it was the worst of times, it was the age of wisdom, it was the age of foolishness, it was the epoch of belief, it was the epoch of incredulity, it was the season of Light, it was the season of

Darkness, it was the spring of hope, it was the winter of despair. . . .

These much-quoted lines are extremely applicable to the present.

By virtually any measure of progress, for the whole of humankind, this is the "best of times." **BOX 1.1** lists a few reasons why this statement is true. Additional data can be cited to demonstrate that, when viewed as a whole, the present is indeed the "best of times" for humans worldwide.

However, as one considers these words, it becomes clear that they also can be applied to efforts to engage in dialogue regarding current inequalities in health outcomes within the United States. The contradictory nature of the health status of Americans becomes immediately apparent when one examines life expectancy. Yes, life expectancies have increased for

all of humankind. However, dramatic differences in life expectancy exist between various subgroups by race/ethnicity, sex, geographic area, sexual preference, income and education, or other groupings. Indeed, those variations are so severe that residents of Hong Kong have a life expectancy that is multiple decades higher than the citizens of Chad (CIA. World Factbook, 2017). Similarly, persons who live in Summit County, Colorado (86.83 years), have a life expectancy that is more than two decades longer than persons who live in Oglala Lakota County, South Dakota (66.8 years) (Institute for Health Metrics and Evaluation, 2017).

Over recent years, citations regarding inequalities such as these appear to have masked the tremendous growth in life expectancy that has occurred across all groups. However, life expectancy is not at the highest level in American history (e.g., the life

---

BOX 1.1   Why It Is the "Best of Times" for Humanity

- Both males and females worldwide are, on average, taller and heavier than at any other time in their approximately 1.8 to 2 million years on Earth as Homo ancestral and modern species (Will, Pablos, & Stock, 2017). These changes have occurred due to improvements in nutrition and health care, increased food availability and access, and the emergence of new technologies. Greater height and weight support the survival of humankind (University of Cambridge, 2017).
- Humans are living longer and, as a result, are able to improve the human condition through greater social, economic, and intellectual capital. Mean life expectancy at birth for people *in the world* as a whole has increased from 50 years in 1960 to approximately 71.5 years in 2015 (Zijdeman & da Silva, 2015).
- Humans have access to more technology than at any other point in history, and they use this technology to improve the human condition. Internet World Statistics (2017) estimated that as of June 2017, 51.7% of the world's population was able to use the Internet. Global communication strengthens the ability of humankind to share information to support survival and growth.
- Although it remains a problem, extreme global poverty has decreased, thereby allowing more of humankind to improve their condition in life. Roser and Ortiz-Ospina (2018) argue that increased access to material goods has been accompanied by improvements in health and education.
- According to Roser (2017), on average, deaths from violence have decreased over the history of humankind.

Internet World Statistics. (2017). Internet growth statistics: Today's road to e-commerce and global trade. Retrieved from www.internet.worldstats.com; Roser, M. (2017). Ethnographic and archaeological evidence on violent deaths. Our World in Data. Retrieved from https://ourworldindata.org /ethnographic-and-archaeological-evidence-on-violent-deaths; Roser, R., & Ortiz-Ospina, E. (2018). Global extreme poverty. Our World in Data. Retrieved from https://ourworlddata.org./extreme-poverty/; University of Cambridge (2017, November). Height and weight evolved at different speeds in the bodies of our ancestors. *Science Daily*. Retrieved from https://www.sciencedaily.com/releases/2017/11/10171108092241.htm; Will, M., Pablos, A., & Stock, J. T. (2017). Long-term patterns of body mass and stature evolution within the hominin lineage. *Royal Society Open Science, 4*. doi: 10.1098 /rsos.171339; Zijdeman, R., & Ribeiro da Silva, F. (2015). Life expectancy at birth (total). CLIO-INFRA UP TO 1949; UN Population Division for 1950 to 2015. IISH Dataverse. V1. Retrieved from http://hdl.handle.net/10622/LKYT53

expectancy of non-Hispanic white populations, dropped by 1 month from 2013 to 2014) (Arias, 2016). Yes, inequalities in life expectancies are abundant. Yet, drastic increases in life expectancy in the United States occurred from 1900 to 2015. **TABLE 1.1** provides data on the increases in life expectancy at birth for White and African American males and females for selected years from 1900 to 2014 (National Center for Health Statistics, 2017). As the data reveal, every single group listed has gained more than 30 additional years of life over this time period. Although data on life expectancy are not presented for all subgroups, Table 1.1 reveals that despite subgroup inequalities in life expectancy, it is literally the "best of times" in that people in the United States are now living much longer than in the distant past.

But, those who choose to view the present as the worst of times can also support their claim. For example, although Americans are no longer plagued by many of the infectious diseases that threatened the length of life in earlier historical periods, preferences for high-calorie foods and a sedentary lifestyle have elevated the prevalence and incidence of chronic illnesses such as obesity, diabetes mellitus, stroke, and heart disease.

The applicability of Dickens' paradigm of the contradictory is also observable in the fact that America's various subgroups have achieved legislated "freedoms" that were nonexistent during earlier periods. Free African American communities, working in partnership with advocates for humankind that spanned race/ethnicity, gender, and nationality (LaRoche, 2014), sought to address systemic inequalities as part of the underground railroad. Likewise, women suffrage leaders throughout the nineteenth century were also supported and assisted by males such as California's Aaron Sargent, a state senator, and others. Sexual minorities (Katz-Wise, Reisner, White et al., 2016), collectives of individuals in support of religious freedom (Curtis, 2016), and others have, over decades and centuries, generated an era of mature change that has resulted in new laws, regulations, and initiatives. Yet, in the present, tensions and subgroup loyalties appear to be subordinating a commitment to the common good as individuals and groups choose to primarily engage in dialogues about differences.

Again, however, data and research reveal another portrait. The United States, often described as a "melting pot of nations" (McDonald, 2007), is closer to an achievement of this

TABLE 1.1 Life Expectancy at Birth by Race and Sex: 1900, 1950, 2000, 2015

| Year | White | | African American | |
	Males	Females	Males	Females
1900	46.6	48.7	32.5	33.5
1950	66.5	72.2	59.1	62.9
2000	74.7	79.9	68.2	75.1
2015	76.6	81.3	72.2	78.5

National Center for Health Statistics. (2017). Health, United States, 2016: With chartbook on long-term trends in health. Table 15, Life expectancy at birth (years), at age 65, and at age 75, by sex, race, and Hispanic origin, selected years 1900–2015, pp. 116-7. Hyattsville, MD: NCHS.

status than ever before. In 1900, the American population included the descendants of Irish Catholics who had sought refuge from the ravages of famine beginning in the 1840s. It also included immigrants from Scandinavia, Germany, Spain, Italy, the Netherlands, Greece, Russia, and other countries from throughout Europe. As a result, approximately 66.8 million, or 88%, of the country's 75.9 million residents were of European descent (Gibson & Jung, 2002).

Today, the demographic composition of the United States is much different. According to the U.S. Bureau of the Census Population Clock, 327,591,527 persons lived in the United States as of April 22, 2018. One birth occurred every 8 seconds; one death every 11 seconds, and one immigrant, often from a different continent, entered the country every 28 seconds. With every 14-second interval of the Population Clock, there is a net gain in population of one resident. Today, persons of European descent alone who are not Hispanic or Latino now comprise 61.3% of the U.S. population (U.S. Census Bureau, 2017). **TABLE 1.2** provides a breakdown of the race/ethnicity of the population to whom healthcare administrators, public health professionals, physicians, nurses, allied health professionals, hospitals, laboratories, managed care and traditional insurance providers, long-term care facilities, the mental and behavioral healthcare infrastructure, dialysis centers, and other components of the health system deliver services to in the United States today.

While evidence exists that it is the "best of times" relative to life expectancy, a number of social indicators that affect health care also support this claim. The percentage of the U.S. population who are high school graduates is 87.0%—a historical high. Approximately 30.3% of U.S. residents have a college degree. As of 2016, the proportion of persons in poverty was 12.7%, a decrease from 14.8% in 2013 (U.S. Census Bureau, 2016). Indeed, as one reviews data across subgroups, it becomes clear that, on average, all American subgroups have achieved some share of the

TABLE 1.2 U.S. Population by Race/Ethnicity: 2016

Race/Ethnicity	% of U.S. Population
White alone, non-Hispanic or Latino	61.3
Hispanic/Latino	17.8
African American	13.3
Two or more races	2.6
Native Hawaiian and other Pacific Islander	0.2
American Indian and Alaskan Native	1.3
Asians alone	5.7
Foreign-born	13.2

U.S. Census Bureau. (2016). American FactFinder. Annual Estimates of the Resident Population by Sex, Age, Race, and Hispanic Origin for the United States, States and Counties: April 2010 to July 2016, 2016 Population Estimates. https://www.census.gov/data/tables/2017/demo/popest/nation-detail.html

highly sought after "American Dream." Nevertheless, the very concept of health disparities stimulates sentiments of division, images of one subgroup competing with another for scarce health resources, and a psychic and emotional uneasiness that can best be described as *contemporary subtribalism*.

▶ Contemporary Subtribalism

Under all circumstances, planning, organizing, directing, and assessing the delivery of healthcare services to diverse groups is far from simple. However, the administration of healthcare services has become even more complex because of underlying tensions that exist between subgroups. The concepts of *contemporary tribalism* and *contemporary subtribalism* provide a framework that can aid in understanding these emerging and growing tensions.

In developing an understanding of the concept of contemporary subtribalism, it is necessary to first ask, "What is a tribe?" Anthropologists' definitions of tribes have now been standardized in the English language through their inclusion in various dictionaries. The following are some definitions of **tribe** found in popular dictionaries:

- "A social group comprising numerous families, clans, or generations together with slaves, dependents, or adopted strangers" (*Merriam-Webster Dictionary*, n.d.).
- "A group of people that includes many families and relatives who have the same language, customs, and beliefs" (*Merriam-Webster Learners Dictionary*, n.d.).
- "A group of people, or a community with similar values or interests, a group with a common ancestor, or a common leader" (YourDictionary, n.d.).
- "A group of people, often of related families, who live together, sharing the same language, culture, and history, especially those who do not live in towns or cities" (*Cambridge Dictionary*, n.d.).
- "A large group of related families who live in the same area and share a common language, religion, and customs" (*Macmillan Dictionary*, n.d.).
- "A unit of sociopolitical organization consisting of a number of families, clans, or other groups who share a common ancestry and culture and among whom leadership is typically neither formalized nor permanent" (The Free Dictionary, n.d.).
- "A social division in a traditional society consisting of families or communities linked by social, economic, religious, or blood ties, with a common culture and dialect, typically having a recognized leader"; "A distinctive close-knit group" (derogatory); "A social division of (usually preliterate) people" (*Oxford Living Dictionary*, n.d.).
- "A traditional social group of people. Most tribes have existed much longer than existing states and countries" (Vocabulary.com, n.d.).
- "A group of people, or a community with similar values or interests, a group with a common ancestor, or a common leader" (*American Sign Language Dictionary*, n.d.).
- "A group of people who are linked by physical and societal factors such as place of residency or birth, ancestry, culture and customs, religious beliefs, economics, blood relations, common language, or other social constructs, who may or may not have a common ancestor or common leader" (*The Authors*).

The term **subtribe** can be defined as a subset of a larger tribe. In applying this terminology, the term seeks to bypass rather than support anthropological arguments regarding colonialism versus indigenous peoples (Robertson, 2016). Rather, this language is applied as a reference to subgroup loyalties that can mask the needs of the larger society and subordinate them to the interests of the subgroup. To distinguish the use of the word *subtribe*, the term *contemporary subtribalism* has been coined.

Contemporary subtribalism is defined as the emergence of values, beliefs, and attitudes that develop in defense and protection of any subgroup, (whether defined by race/ethnicity, sex, sexual preference, religion, geographic area, occupation, and/or any other grouping) when such feelings of loyalty become so intense as to mask solutions and strategies that generate win-win outcomes for all subgroups. This definition comprises the approach that frames the entirety of this text; that is, the data introduced, the research presented, and the strategies recommended are designed to introduce healthcare administrators, public health professionals, clinicians, researchers, policy makers, and consumers to win-win health disparity approaches that are mutually beneficial to each of the subgroups being served.

Contemporary subtribes compete for resources in general, including healthcare resources. When shifts in the number, nature, and socioeconomic and political power of contemporary subtribes occur, a redistribution of healthcare resources takes place. Healthcare administrators, public health professionals, and clinicians can play the role of a mediator by ensuring that the healthcare services provided by the institutions that they lead are not aligned in such a way that they provide more resources to any of these competing and oftentimes conflicting groups at the expense of other groups. Healthcare administrators and other influencers must be able to rise above contemporary subtribalism and understand that cooperation and accommodation are the tools of social interaction that will achieve a win-win solution for all people. In order to deliver optimal services, healthcare administrators, public health professionals, and clinicians must thoroughly understand the magnitude, causes, and remedies for disparities in those areas of the healthcare system that fall under their leadership.

This task is, however, made extremely difficult because subtribal differences also exist in the distribution of other, non-healthcare-related resources. Differences in the distribution of societal resources exist by race/ethnicity and sex. Within these subtribes, additional subtribes can be identified based on age, geographic area, socioeconomic status, religion and rates of religious participation, education and educational access, sexual preference and gender identification, and even by the distribution of the various types of intelligences that have been identified as characteristic of humankind (Gardner, 1993). These subtribes oftentimes see each other as the enemy and stand poised

to file lawsuits against healthcare institutions whose administrators allow persistent *preventable* disparities to characterize the services provided when patterned differences across such subgroups can be documented.

In some respects, the first subtribe into which humans are divided is the region of the world in which they live. Individuals self-describe, and often are described by others, as European, Asian, South American, African, and so on. Accordingly, one may first approach health disparities by comparing the status of people based on the geographic region where they were born.

▶ Disparities by Geographic Region: The First Subtribes of Humankind

The land on planet Earth is currently divided into 195+ geopolitical areas many of which have been labeled as *countries*. (Note, however, that some geographic areas are, for a number of reasons, not included within the term *country* as currently defined by the United Nations, the U.S. Department of State, and other authorities.) **TABLE 1.3** lists the world's populations according to each geographic region. **FIGURE 1.1** shows a map of these regions.

When the population that resides in each of these regions is aggregated, it reveals that approximately 7.5 billion persons now inhabit the earth (World Population Review, 2017). **FIGURE 1.2** shows the world population distribution by region as of 2017.

TABLE 1.4 breaks down by region the **gross domestic product (GDP) per capita**, an economic concept that is used to measure amount of dollars each resident would have based on the market value of all goods and services produced in that region.

As Table 1.4 indicates, significant differences exist in per capita wealth by region. As

TABLE 1.3 World Population Distribution by Region

Region	Number of Countries	% of Global Population
North America	2	4.8
Latin America and the Caribbean	33	8.6
Oceania	14	0.5
Europe	44	9.8
Asia	48	59.7
Africa	54	16.6

Constructed by authors from data found in the United Nations, Department of Economic and Social Affairs, Population Division (2017). World Population Prospects 2017 – Data Booklet (ST/ESA/SER.A/401).

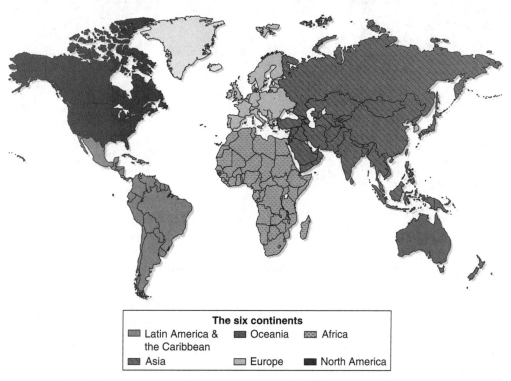

The six continents

- Latin America & the Caribbean
- Oceania
- Africa
- Asia
- Europe
- North America

FIGURE 1.1 Six world regions.

Map Source: Created by authors with mapchart.net.

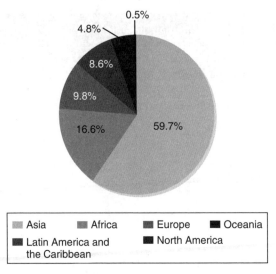

FIGURE 1.2 World population by region: 2017.

Data from Statista, 2017. Global Population Shares, https://www.statista.com/statitics/237584/distribution-of-the-world-population-by-continent, accessed December 26, 2017.34

TABLE 1.4 Gross Domestic Product (GDP) per Capita by Region, 2016

Region	GDP per Capita (U.S. dollars)	% of Difference
World average	$10,300	Reference
North America	$37,477	+263.85
Oceania	$35,087	+240.65
Europe	$25,851	+150.98
Latin America and the Caribbean	$8,520	−17.28
Asia	$5,635	−45.29
Africa	$1,809	−82.43

Data from World Atlas (2017). The continents of the world per capita GDP. These data were accessed by the authors on December 16, 2017.

indicated, the mean per capita GDP across all regions was $10,300 in 2016 (the latest date for which data were available at the time of each country's output) (World Atlas, 2017). However, individuals living in North America had a GDP that was 263.85% higher than the world's mean per capita GDP of $10,300. Oceania, which includes Australia, Guam, New Zealand, the Fiji Islands, and other areas, had a per capita income that was 240.65% higher. Europe had a GDP per capita that was 150.98% higher than the world average. Latin America and the Caribbean's GDP was 17.28% lower than the global mean. Asia's wealth per person was 45.29% lower than

BOX 1.2 A Sample of Differences in the Key Regions of the World by Distribution of Natural Resources

North America's Natural Resources
- The third largest land area, North America, includes highly fertile soil, an abundance of fresh water and forest, a range of climates which contribute to a varied ecosystem that allows a multitude of agricultural products to be provided, and other resources.
- The natural resources also include coal, iron, copper, gold, silver, and other resources.

Oceania
- This area includes gold, natural gas, copper, coal, iron ore, forests, uranium, and others.
- The land mass of Oceania is primarily underwater.

Europe
- This area has resources of oil, natural gas, gold, bauxite, natural gas, timber, zinc, and others.
- This is the second smallest land mass next to Australia.

Latin America and the Caribbean
- This region, with the fourth largest land mass, has some oil and natural gas deposits, rivers that can be navigated, a temperate climate with regular waterfalls that supports food production, forests, waterways for fishing, cork, freshwater, chromium, titanium, lead, minerals, and other resources.

Asia
- This region has the largest land mass of all regions. This land mass supports water, petroleum, fish, forests, natural gas, timber, tin, zinc, nickel, copper, and other resources.

Africa
- This region has the second largest land mass and has, according to some analysts, the largest supply of natural resources worldwide including gold, silver, petroleum, uranium, silver, diamonds, oil, gas, timber, and others.

Date from the Central Intelligence Agency, The World Factbook, 2017/2018. https://www.cia/.gov, accessed April 21, 2018.

the world average, and Africa's mean GDP per capita was 82.34% lower.

Why do the described differences in GDP per capita exist by region?

One of the earliest theorists to investigate differences in income and wealth across nations was the economist Adam Smith (1776). Adam Smith argued that the production, allocation, and distribution of goods and services through an institutional mechanism that allows each individual to make buying and selling decisions based upon their own self-interest would ultimately generate the greatest gross domestic product.

While the institutional mechanism used to make economic decisions is important, other researchers have identified a much broader range of variables that can "explain"

the described differences in total and per capita income between the described regions. First, each region differs in natural resources. **BOX 1.2** lists a few of these differences.

Resources alone, however, do not create differences in the gross domestic product of countries. Kruss, McGarth, Petersen, and Gastrow (2015) emphasize the highly critical role of education in general and higher education in particular. Sulaiman, Bala, Tijani et al., (2015) report on has similar findings. However, Suizzero and Tisdell (2016) assess theories that argue that the contemporary wealth of a region is actually traceable to the early development of humankind in various regions. Stated differently, some anthropologists suggest that the early development of tools and the timing of the shift away from hunting and gathering in a society also created a developmental

TABLE 1.5 Differences in Mean Life Expectancy at Birth by Gender and Region, 2015				
World Region	**Life Expectancy - Female**	**% of Difference**	**Life Expectancy - Male**	**% of Difference**
All regions	73.8	Reference	69.2	Reference
Africa	63.2	−14.36	59.8	−13.58
Asia	74.4	+0.81	70.5	+1.88
Europe	81.1	+9.89	74.3	+7.37
Latin America and the Caribbean	78.5	+6.37	71.9	+3.90
North America	81.8	+10.84	77.2	+11.56
Oceania	80.6	+9.21	76.2	+10.12

Data from 2015 found at the United Nations. Department of Economic and Social Affairs. Population Division 2017. Annex Table A1 – Selected mortality indicators in 2015. Life expectancy at birth (years) World Mortality 2017: Data Booklet, pp. 10-18, New York: United Nations. Accessed from http://www.un.org/en/development/desa/population/publications/mortality/world-mortality-cdrom-2017.shtml

chain that is still reflected in contemporary differentials in income and wealth by region. Whether these theorists are or are not accurate, a large body of research suggests that the described differences in per capita income across regions reflect a complex assortment of cultural, anthropological, economic, physical, and other psychological factors.

Is there a relationship between income or wealth inequality and health?

Existing research confirms that people living in those regions with greater income and wealth also have better health. This relationship is so significant that a now classic study by Byrne (2003) is entitled "Health Equals Wealth." Similarly, Cutler, Lleras-Munez, and Vogl (2010) demonstrated linkages between access to material resources and health. However, researchers have also discovered that *healthier individuals also create greater wealth for a nation* (Suhrcke, McKee, Arce, Tsolova, &

Mortenson, 2005). Accordingly, it becomes appropriate to ask, "Are there disparities in life outcomes between regions with higher and lower per capita income?"

Recent data indicate that there are differences in life expectancy between regions. However, these differences are not as severe as the disparities that exist by mean per capita GDP, as shown in **TABLE 1.5**.

The data in Table 1.5 reveal the numerous combinations and permutations that can exist as individuals begin to allocate loyalties by subgroup. Specifically, the data suggest that, at present, females have an advantage in terms of life expectancy, independent of the subgroup identities that may exist by region. However, it also reveals that Africa is the only area with life expectancies that fall below the mean for all regions for both males and females. Asian females have life expectancies that are .81% higher than the mean for females in all regions and 7.51% higher than the mean for all males.

▶ Subgroup Differences in Health Outcomes by Country/Nation

A particularly interesting pattern can be identified when disparate health outcomes are compared by country/nation. Thus, let's construct a portrait of how the health outcomes of U.S. residents compare with those of the top 10 countries with the "best" health outcomes and the top 10 countries with the "worst" health outcomes.

How does one measure the "best" health outcomes?

Claxton, Cox, Gonzales, Kamal, and Levitt (2015) describe the importance of health outcomes for individuals independent of their country of residency. They reiterate the fact that health care is, in some respects, the single most important good or service that consumers can "purchase." Given that healthcare status affects the very existence of humankind, most people, upon reflection, will agree that health services and the mechanisms for their delivery are highly critical components of any region, country, state, city, or community. Although many measures of the performance of a healthcare system exist, the one that has been selected for the purposes of this text is life expectancy. The reason for the use of this variable is a simple one. Before issues of quality of life can be examined, the energy that is sometimes called the "life force" must be preserved. Stated differently, the issue of quality of data is irrelevant if life itself is not preserved.

Table 1.5 provides data on life expectancy.

What was the data source for Table 1.5?

The data source used for Table 1.5 was the United Nations World Mortality Report Data Booklet (2017). This data source is utilized by researchers, professors, students, and other entities and is considered a premiere source of data on countries worldwide. It is not, however, a primary data source; rather, it is a respected secondary source that is compiled from data not easily accessible by the general public.

What are some other sources that have similar data on the world's countries?

The World Bank (n.d.) publishes data on life expectancy and other measures such as GDP and GDP per capita on an annual basis (see data.worldbank.org); The International Monetary Fund also provides data on overall population (http://www.imf.org/en/Data), GDP, GDP per capita, and other economic measures. The United Nations Global Indicator Database (n.d.) includes statistical data on country-level disparities in terms of gender, overall poverty, and other variables (see data.un.org). The data provided are not "raw" but have been processed into an index. An **index** is a single number that utilizes weights and other statistical processes to develop a single summary measure.

Other online sites also provide life expectancy measures. However, these sites normally obtain their data from *The World Factbook* (Central Intelligence Agency, 2017 and 2018), which is considered as being a reasonably accurate source of secondary data for use in this chapter. The CIA World Factbook is published annually and provides data for each country/independent state and other geopolitical areas in 10 areas that include people and society, government, economy, and others.

Are you saying that the data may not be 100% accurate?

The massive amount of data that exists across the various countries, territories, and other geographic world divisions places virtually all data collected into the category of data estimates. A data estimate is an approximate number and is based upon currently available information. Thus, the data on life expectancy for countries worldwide are "guesses" in that they reflect the most accurate information available.

TABLE 1.6 Country Rankings Based on Life Expectancy, 2017

Rank	Country	World Region	Life Expectancy	% of Difference
32	United States	North America	80.0	Reference
1	Monaco	Europe	89.4	+11.75
2	Japan	Asia	85.3	+6.63
3	Singapore	Asia	85.2	+6.50
4	Macau	Asia	84.6	+5.75
5	San Marino	Europe	83.3	+4.13
6	Iceland	Europe	83.1	+3.88
7	Hong Kong	Asia	83.0	+3.75
8	Andorra	Europe	82.9	+3.63
9	Guernsey	Europe	82.6	+3.25
10	Switzerland	Europe	82.6	+3.25

Data from CIA World Factbook, 2017-2018. Accessed at https://www.cia.gov/library/publications/the-world-factbook/geos/et.html

Which 10 countries have the "best" health outcomes, as measured by life expectancy?

TABLE 1.6 lists the countries/independent states with the "best" healthcare outcomes as measured by life expectancy. Note that the United States is not among the top 10 countries.

Table 1.6 shows that the United States does *not* *have the best health outcomes in the world as measured by life expectancy. But, isn't the United States the most affluent country in the world, and doesn't it spend the greatest proportion of its GDP on health care?*

Despite its affluence, the United States is not in the top 10 with regard to health outcomes. **TABLE 1.7** lists the GDP of the 10 countries with the highest life expectancy and the percentage of GDP spent on health care. Although the percentage of GDP spent on health care could not be identified for each of these countries, Table 1.7 clearly demonstrates that the United States spends the greatest percentage of GDP on health care relative to those countries for which data were available. Table 1.7 contains data for 2014 (the last year that all the data in the table were available). In 2014, the United States ranked thirty-second in terms of life expectancy and, as of July 2017, the ranking was 43rd (CIA World Factbook, 2017).

What do the data in Table 1.7 reveal?

The data reveal that in 2014, the most recent data that were available for each of the countries, the United States spent 17.1% of its GDP on health care; in contrast, Monaco spent only 4.3%. Thus, the United States spent 297.67% more of its GDP on health

TABLE 1.7 Percentage of GDP Spent on Health Care of The Countries of Top 10 Life Expectancy, 2014

Rank	Country	World Region	Life Expectancy	Total GDP (Billion U.S. Dollars)	% GDP Spent on Health Care	% GDP Spent on Health Care U.S. vs. Comparison
1	Monaco	Europe	89.57	$7.27	4.3%	297.67% more
2	Macau	Asia	84.48	$82.09	N/A	—
3	Japan	Asia	84.46	$4,807.00	10.2%	67.64% more
4	Singapore	Asia	84.38	$462.60	4.9%	248.97% more
5	San Marino	Europe	83.18	$1.96	6.1%	180.33% more
6	Hong Kong	Asia	82.78	$405.00	N/A	—
7	Andorra	Europe	82.65	$3.36	8.1%	111.11% more
8	Switzerland	Europe	82.39	$478.30	11.7%	46.15% more
9	Guernsey	Europe	82.39	$3.45	N/A	—
10	Australia	Oceania	82.07	$1,454.00	9.4%	81.91% more
43[a]	United States	North America	79.56	$17,520.00	17.1%	—

[a]This number is U.S.'s ranking using all 267 geopolitical areas. However, when using all the 195 countries/independent states, the ranking is 32. The percent differences were calculated by the authors.
Central Intelligence Agency. (2017-2018). The world factbook. Retrieved from https://www.cia.gov/library/publications /the-world-factbook
Central Intelligence Agency. (2017). The world factbook.
Central Intelligence Agency. (2016). The world factbook.

care than did Monaco. Triple digit differences in the percent of GDP spent on health care also occurred between the United States and Singapore (248.97%), San Marino (180.37%), and Andorra (111.11%).

Why is there such a huge difference in health-care spending?

The differences in spending occur for several reasons. First, cultural values differ across these countries and the United States. Cultural values in the United States do not necessarily support maximum life expectancy. For example, while the cultures of some countries/independent states focus upon prevention, American culture remains centered around the enjoyment of pleasure and the use of health care to cure or abate symptoms when illness and/or disease occurs. This unspoken attitude is even observable among healthcare administrators, public health professionals, and clinicians. Although the percentage of GDP spent on health care could not be identified for each of these countries, Table 1.7 clearly demonstrates that the United States spends the greatest percentage of GDP on health care compared to those countries for which data are available.

These dollars are disproportionately spent on health resources needed to support the treatment of illness and disease.

Thus, the United States has the most comprehensive curative healthcare system in the world. This system consists of approximately 951,061 physicians (Kaiser Family Foundation, 2017a), 4,153,657 nurses (Kaiser Family Foundation, 2017b), 5,627 hospitals (American Hospital Association, 2018), 61,594 pharmacies (SK&A, 2017), 15,600 nursing homes (Harris-Kojetin et al, 2016), 274 managed care organizations (Kaiser Family Foundation, 2017c), and a vast array of other personnel and organizational systems that are available to address illness and disease once they occur.

Chambers (2015) cites data which reveal that in 2013, approximately $3.3 billion was spent by visitors from other countries who came to the United States to access the health resources in this country. In 2003, patients from other countries only spent $1.6 billion.

But I thought that many Americans also go abroad to purchase health care services?

The publication, Patients Beyond Borders (2017), includes Costa Rica, India, Israel, Malaysia, Mexico, Singapore, South Korea, Taiwan, Thailand, Turkey, and the United States as being "top destinations" in the medical tourism industry. However, while patients seek cosmetic surgery, dentistry, weight loss solutions, and, in some cases, curative medical solutions for late-stage cancer, and/or cardiovascular disease in these other countries, the American trade surplus for medical services are generally for highly complex curative solutions for which the United States' medical system is considered as a world leader. Moreover, many of the physicians who deliver services in other popular medical tourism regions were trained in the United States (Chen & Wilson, 2013).

Even if medical tourism is bypassed, discussions of the disparities in the percent of domestic product spent by the United States and other countries on health care require contexting by: (1) holding constant the severity of the illnesses/diseases treated in the United States relative to the other countries listed in Table 1.7; (2) characterizing the health problems of the residents of these other countries versus the American population; (3) comparing the distribution of each country's population by age, gender, education, and marital status; (4) identifying environmental differences between residents of the United States and residents of those countries who rank in the top ten in terms of life expectancy; and, (5) assessing other factors. However, the completion of such an analysis with such factors is beyond the range of topics for this text. Nevertheless, such data cannot be used to support an argument that the U.S. healthcare system is one that functions poorly and/or only "moderately well" without additional analysis.

However, the data presented reveal that the United States is nowhere close to being at the top of all countries in life expectancy rankings. However, additional statistical analysis is required in order to interpret the meaning of such a disparity.

Is there a full ranking of all countries?

A full ranking of all countries is available through the CIA's World Factbooks.

Infant mortality is often used to assess the functioning of a health care system.

Does the United States have the lowest infant mortality rate? The United States does not have the lowest infant mortality rate.

According to *The World Factbook* (Central Intelligence Agency, 2017), many countries and/or geopolitical areas have lower infant mortality rates than the United States. Indeed, countries such as Latvia, Taiwan, Israel, and Bosnia and Herzegovina have lower infant mortality rates than the United States. The United States currently ranks 57th in terms of infant mortality. But, such data cannot be immediately used to support the thesis that the U.S. healthcare system functions poorly and/or is only moderately efficient without the use of a robust statistical analysis. For example, Ahrens, Thoma, Rosen et al. (2017), using data obtained from the National Center for Health Statistics, found that from 2000–2010, multiple births infants were at higher risk of infant mortality due to unintentional injury and homicide. These are not, of course, factors that suggest a failure of the health care system. Matthews and MacDorman (2013) found that twins and other infants who are multiple births have an infant mortality rate that is 500% higher than single births. Medical technology in the United States that enhances maternal fertility through multiple births is advanced. Disparities in infant mortality rates in the United States are also associated with maternal age, maternal health status, marital status, education, and other variables. Thus, infant mortality rates may be higher in the United States because of the increase in the population of women over age 35 who can now, because of medical advances, select to give birth. However, at age 35, females in the United States are also more likely to be diabetic, hypertensive, and/or overweight. Thus, variables such as these must be held constant across countries in order to argue that higher infant mortality rates in the United States should be viewed as a "symptom" of a "flawed" American healthcare system.

So, are you saying that although the United States has the highest level of healthcare expenditures, both absolutely and relatively, but not the highest life expectancy nor the lowest infant mortality rate this data does not *suggest that health administrators and other healthcare personnel are failing in the maximization of outcomes from the healthcare resources available to them?*

This is the exact argument that is being made. An abundance of researchers use such data as a source for criticizing healthcare outcomes in the United States (Guyatt et al., 2007; Institute of Medicine and National Research Council, 2013; Preston & Ho, 2009). This conclusion is one that can, should be, and is, being challenged in this text. As mentioned, data on the American value structure suggest that the American public, on average, endorses, upholds, and revels in a lifestyle characterized by behaviors that do not support the maximum length and quality of life (Loprinzi et al., 2016). Moreover, a number of studies have confirmed that, overall, Americans are satisfied with the quality of the health care that they receive within the United States.

Huerta, Harle, Ford, Diana, and Menachemi (2016), utilizing data from the American Hospital Association's Annual Survey of Hospitals, as well as data from Medicare's Hospital Compare and other sources, discovered that, for hospitals, the higher costs of health care were directly associated with greater levels of patient satisfaction. Similarly, Joshi, McCormick, Sully, Garvan, and Plastaras (2016) found that 80.43% to 88.13% of workers were satisfied with the medical care that they received for their injuries.

Medicare's Hospital Compare for the year 2015 reported that approximately 80% of the participating hospitals received a satisfaction rating of 3 and above (Centers for Medicare and Medicaid Services, n.d.a). *Numerous other studies exist that reveal that, in general, Americans are satisfied with the U.S. healthcare system.*

Why, then, do comparisons in health care by country reveal that the United States healthcare system is ranked unfavorably compared with other countries? For example, the World Health Organization (2000), in their last healthcare ranking on efficiency by country placed the United States at thirty-seventh. This ranking was far behind Germany (5th), Canada (10th), Great Britain (1st), Japan (10th), and other countries based upon differences in costs, access, and outcomes. More recently, the Commonwealth Fund in a 2014 report which compared 11 countries, placed the United States last in terms of healthcare system performance (Davis, Stremkis, Squires et al., 2014).

Such comparisons are reminiscent of the stereotypical apples-to-oranges measure for the simple reason that a healthcare system and its administrators must maximize healthcare outcomes within the *framework of the existent culture and/or subcultures within each country.* Anthropologists have characterized American culture as valuing materialism, competition, personal and institutional freedom, equality, and other elements (Hofstede, 1991).

A number of other sources have also documented the importance of each country's values. For example, Roinen, LäHteenmaki, and Tvorila (1999) characterized some of these variables for residents of Finland—one of the countries that exceeds the United States in life expectancy. Their study identified three health-related factors (general health interest, light product interest, and natural product interest) and three taste-related factors (craving for sweet foods, using food as a reward, pleasure) that could be used to best describe the framework of a country's culture.

When this framework is applied to the American lifestyle, it appears that Americans are willing to trade off a few additional years of life in order to maintain the freedom to eat whatever is desired, to engage or not engage in physical activity, and to take part in other morbific activities of their choice. Thus, healthcare systems maximize healthcare outcomes but are constrained by the chosen lifestyles of a country's residents. The Mayo Clinic published a study that found 97.3% of the participating adults did not have healthy lifestyles. The parameters of the study included exercise, diet, smoker status, and body fat percentage (Loprinzi et al., 2016). Another study conducted by Li et al., (2017) found that Americans who choose to live according to a healthy lifestyle could expect to have a greater life expectancy compared to their counterparts who did not have healthy habits.

Do the data suggest that the U.S. healthcare system should not be harshly judged based on the fact that the United States spends the greatest proportion of its GDP on health care but does not have the highest life expectancy?

Yes, life expectancy is highest in Europe and the Far East. However, when life expectancy and those countries with the highest GDP are examined, an interesting portrait emerges. We direct the reader to the preliminary data and subsequent calculations that will support this argument. Consider a tool from statistics called the Pearson correlation coefficient. The **Pearson correlation coefficient (r)** is used to assess whether two or more variables are associated. This value provides a quantitative measure of the correlation between two variables ($-1 < r < 1$). Two variables can be positively correlated ($r > 0$), negatively correlated ($r < 0$), or uncorrelated ($r = 0$).

Because life expectancy and the percentage of GDP spent on health care are both quantitative variables, a Pearson correlation coefficient can be calculated in which life expectancy is the dependent variable and the percentage of GDP spent on health care is the independent variable. The Pearson correlation coefficient can be calculated using most standard statistics packages (e.g., SAS, SPSS, STATA, R) (Weaver & Wuensch, 2013). Importantly, for persons who are not statisticians, online statistical calculators now exist that require no advanced knowledge of statistics in order to use.

TABLE 1.8 shows life expectancy and percentage of GDP spending on health care for eight countries including the United States. It is important to remember that the Department of State, the United Nations, the CIA, and other authorities have varied listings regarding the number of and names for countries, independent states and other geopolitical areas. For our analyses, data were used from the CIA World Factbooks for the years 2014 and 2017. We have, however, provided information on the highest life expectancies, the commonly listed countries/independent states, and geopolitical areas. For example, the complete listing from the source does not include Vatican City (Holy See), Cabo Verde (Cape Verde), South Sudan, Nepal, Kosovo, Taiwan, Montenegro, or Palestine, nor a number of other island and/or other geopolitical entities. The table below includes the data used as a basis for the calculation of the Pearson correlation coefficient for the top 10 countries/independent states with the highest life expectancy in 2014. The year 2014 was used because correlation coefficient calculations require data for the same time period.

Pearson correlation:

$$r = -0.6409 \quad p = 0.12089$$

$$r^2 = .4108 \qquad n = 7$$

Based on these data, the Pearson correlation coefficient (r) is -0.6409. The p-value is 0.12089. Thus, the relationship between mean life expectancy and the percentage of GDP

TABLE 1.8 Data Used to Generate Pearson Correlation Coefficient		
Country	**Life Expectancy**	**% GDP Spent on Health Care**
Monaco	89.57	4.3%
Japan	84.46	10.2%
Singapore	84.38	4.9%
San Marino	83.18	6.1%
Andorra	82.65	8.1%
Switzerland	82.39	11.7%
Australia	82.07	9.4%
United States	79.56	17.1%

Source: CIA Constructed with country-specific data found in *The World Factbook* 2017-2018. https://www.cia.gov/library/publications/the-world-factbook /geos/et.html and CIA World Factbook 2017, and the CIA World Factbook 2016.

spent on healthcare expenditures is negative, of moderate strength and non-significant.

More specifically, there is a moderate and strong *negative* relationship between life expectancy and the percentage of GDP spent on health care. That is, for the top 7 countries for which data were available, the higher the percentage of GDP spent on health care, the lower the life expectancy. How might this be possible?

As can be seen, this simple analysis reveals that there is no basis for an analyst to claim that the American healthcare system is flawed because it spends the higher percent of GDP on health care but does not have the highest life expectancy. Yet, so many healthcare researchers explicitly assume that the relationship between the percentage of gross domestic product spent on health care is and/or ought to be positively related to life expectancy.

Papanicolas, Woskie, and Jha (2018) state that, "In 2016, the United States spent nearly twice as much as 10 high-income countries on medical care and performed less well on many population health outcomes," (pg. 1024). Jones and Kantarkian (2015) state, "The United States is the richest nation in the world, and we spend more on health care than any other nation (18% of our gross domestic product; two to three times more than other advanced nations). Yet, we rank poorly in objective measures of health care outcomes," (pg. 2194). Numerous similar statements could be cited. However, this often-repeated refrain is based upon the implicit assumption that these healthcare dollars are expended for preventive medicine and not for curative medicine. The negative correlation between the percentage of gross domestic product spent on health care and life expectancy directly validates such a statement. In effect, findings for the seven sets of countries with the highest life expectancy suggests that countries with populations who are culturally and personally oriented toward healthy living will spend a smaller percentage of gross domestic product on health care because residents have

less illnesses and diseases. Stated differently, logic suggests that sicker individuals and nations spend larger percentages of their income on health care than do healthier individuals and/or nations.

Another way to untangle this relationship is to examine the **coefficient of determination** r^2, which is a statistical tool that is used to determine the proportion of the variance in the dependent variable that can be predicted from the independent variable. It can be used to measure the percentage of the variation in life expectancy that is associated with the percentage of GDP that these countries spent on health care. In statistical packages, the value is usually presented as r^2 ($0 < r^2 < 1$). In this case, the r^2 was 0.4108. This value can be thought of as how strong the estimate is when x (i.e., percentage of GDP spent on health care) is used to predict y (i.e., life expectancy). In this case, 41.08% of the change in life expectancy is associated with the change in the percentage of GDP that these countries spend on health care. Moreover, as mentioned earlier, this association is a negative one (see **FIGURE 1.3**).

What does this exercise tell us?

This exercise suggests that current and future healthcare administrators, public health professionals, clinicians, researchers, and policy analysts may wish to eliminate the use of the statement, "The United States is the wealthiest nation in the world and spends the greatest proportion of its GDP on health care but has only moderate health outcomes!" As this simple exercise reveals, the assumption of a positive relationship between life expectancy and the percentage of GDP spent on health care is not accurate.

Furthermore, claims that the United States is the wealthiest nation on earth are also not correct. First, it becomes clear that the claim that the United States is the richest country in the world is incorrect. It is true that the United States has the highest GDP. For the year 2017, with all quarters reporting, the U.S. Department of Commerce, Bureau of

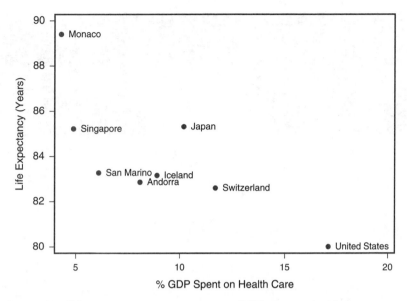

FIGURE 1.3 Scatterplot of life expectancy versus percentage of GDP spent on health care.

Economic Analysis (2018) estimated that the nation's GDP was $19,736.5 trillion. However, when GDP is modified by family size, a better estimate of wealth is revealed. When the U.S. GDP is converted to per capita income by dividing it by the total population, it can be seen that the United States barely ranks among the top 10 nations in the world in terms of income. Thus, while the United States does have the highest gross domestic product on the planet, it absolutely does not have the highest per capita income. **TABLE 1.9** below lists the nations with the highest life expectancy by per capita income.

As Table 1.9 reveals, of the top ten countries with the higher life expectancy, seven are significantly wealthier than the United States when per capita income is used as the measure of material affluence. Monaco, for example, is 98.90% wealthier than the United States while Macau is 148.08% wealthier. Singapore has a per capita income that is 51.8% higher and Australia's per capita income is 17.85% higher. Accordingly, it becomes important to apply a simple tool such as a correlation coefficient to ask, "What is the relationship between life expectancy and per capita income?"

In order to better understand whether an association exists between *life expectancy* and *per capita income* in the world today, an online calculator was used to estimate the correlation coefficient between per capita income and life expectancy using the data in the Table 1.8. The specific Pearson correlation coefficient that was used is available at Social Science Statistics (http://www.socscistatistics .com/tests/pearson/). The findings from the calculator indicate that the Pearson correlation coefficient of the relationship between life expectancy and per capita income was $r = 0.06028$. This Pearson correlation coefficient calculation indicates that there is a moderately strong and positive association between per capita income and life expectancy for the countries with the longest mean lifespans. However, this relationship is only marginally significant (0.065095). The coefficient of determination was 0.3634. This revealed that the percentage of the change in life expectancy that occurred with a percentage change in per capita income was 36.34%. **FIGURE 1.4** is the scatterplot of the relationship.

Thus, based on the argument that this is the "best of times" for humanity, it is not

TABLE 1.9 Per Capita Income of The Countries of Top 10 Life Expectancy and The United States, 2014

Rank	Country	Life Expectancy	Per Capita Income in U.S. Dollars	% Difference
32	United States	79.56	54,900	Reference
1	Monaco	89.57	109,200	+98.91
2	Macau	84.48	129,100	+135.15
3	Japan	84.46	37,800	−31.14
4	Singapore	84.38	84,600	+54.10
5	San Marino	83.18	63,300	+15.30
6	Hong Kong	82.78	55,700	+1.45
7	Andorra	82.65	51,300	−6.55
8	Switzerland	82.39	58,800	+7.10
9	Guernsey	82.39	52,300	−4.74
10	Australia	82.07	64,700	+17.85
$r = 0.6028$ $r^2 = 0.3634$ $n = 10$ $p = 0.065095$				

Constructed by authors with data from the CIA Factbook 2017-2018, CIA Factbook 2017 and CIA Factbook 2016.

merely healthcare expenditures that determine life expectancy. Higher *per capita income* correlates with multiple determinants of health outcomes. McGovern, Miller, and Hughes-Cromwick (2014) raise the possibility that investments are not merely needed in health care but in the other equally and/or more powerful determinants of health outcomes such as housing, family support services, education, employment, and so on. A higher per capita income allows expenditures

on non-healthcare-related determinants of health care to be made.

How did you calculate the Pearson correlation coefficient?

The data used to generate the Pearson correlation coefficient have been taken from information displayed in this chapter. Elsewhere, information will be provided on how to input data into various online statistical calculators in order to "harvest" information about

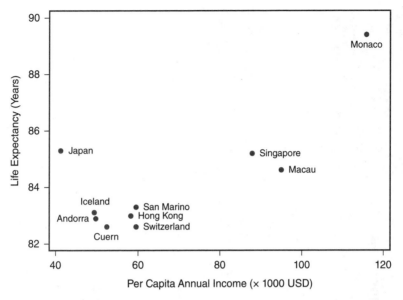

FIGURE 1.4 Scatterplot of life expectancy versus per capita income.

health disparities in communities and health-care institutions.

The Best and Worst of All Times

TABLE 1.10 shows that vast disparities exist between both life expectancies and per capita income for the 10 countries in the world with the highest life expectancies and the 10 countries in the world with the lowest life expectancies.

The data in Table 1.10 reveal that, for humans in the world in general, it is both the best of times and the worst of times. First, despite the existence of the observed disparities, individuals throughout the globe have experienced increases in life expectancy. For example, data from the 1998 CIA World Factbook reveal that in 1998, residents of Chad had a mean life expectancy of 48.22 years relative to 49.44 years in 2014 and 50.66 years in 2017. Likewise, persons who live in the United States had a life expectancy of 76.13 years in 1998 rather than the 79.56 years for 2014 and the 80.00 years in 2017 (CIA World Factbook, 1998; CIA World Factbook, 2017). Simultaneously, the vast disparities in life expectancy and

income can generate improvements for all of humankind.

What else do the data in Table 1.10 reveal?

The data in Table 1.10 also reveal that:

■ A resident of Monaco, the country with the highest life expectancy, could expect to live 81.16% longer than those who live in Chad, the country with the lowest life expectancy.

■ Persons living in Japan, on average, live 69.36% longer than those who live in Guinea-Bissau.

■ Those who lived in Singapore in 2014 can expect to have a life expectancy that is 67.12% longer than those who live in Afghanistan.

■ The population of Macau had a 2014 life expectancy that was 70.46% higher than those residing in South Africa.

■ San Marino's residents, on average, lived 64.58% longer than those who lived in Zambia in 2014.

■ Those who lived in Hong Kong in 2014 could expect to, on average, experience "lived life" 61.2% longer than those who live in the Central African Republic.

TABLE 1.10 Percentage Differences in Life Expectancy and Per Capita Income Between The Countries of Top 10 Highest vs. Lowest Life Expectancy, 2014

Rank	Country	Life Expectancy	% Difference (Life Expectancy)	Per Capita Income (U.S. Dollars)	% Difference (Per Capita Income)
1	Monaco	89.57	81.16% higher than Chad	$109,200	+3,944.44
192	Chad	49.44	Reference	$2,700	Reference
2	Macau	84.48	70.46% higher	$129,100	+878.03
191	South Africa	49.56	Reference	$13,200	Reference
3	Japan	84.46	69.36% higher	$37,800	+2,420
190	Guinea-Bissau	49.87	Reference	$1,500	Reference
4	Singapore	84.38	67.12% higher	$84,600	+4,130.00
189	Afghanistan	50.49	Reference	$2,000	Reference
5	San Marino	83.18	64.58% higher	$63,300	+653.57
188	Swaziland	50.54	Reference	$8,400	Reference

6	Hong Kong	82.78	61.20% higher	$55,700	+9,183.33
187	Central African Republic	51.35		$600	
7	Andorra	82.65	60.23% higher	$51,300	+12,725.00
186	Somalia	51.58		$400	
8	Switzerland	82.39	58.96% higher	$58,800	+1,447.37
185	Zambia	51.83		$3,800	
9	Guernsey	82.39	58.90% higher	$52,500	+377.27
184	Namibia	51.85		$11,000	
10	Australia	82.07	57.64% higher	$64,700	+255.49
183	Gabon	52.06		$18,200	

Central Intelligence Agency. (2017). *The World Factbook*. https://www.cia.gov/library/publications/the-world-factbook/geos/et.html

- Residents of Andorra could expect to, on average, inhabit earth 60.23% longer than those who lived in Somalia.
- Persons who lived in Guernsey had a life expectancy at birth that was 58,90% higher than those who lived in Namibia.
- Those who lived in Switzerland had a mean life expectancy that was 58.90% higher than residents of Zambia.

In addition, the quality of day-to-day life in countries that are characterized by the lowest life expectancies is very different from those of their higher-income counterparts. This is because of the vast differences in per capita income. Yet, when such comparisons are left unsaid and unacknowledged, even those who live in the world's poorest nations also live in the best of times.

How can this be the case?

It is the "best of times" for all humans who inhabit planet Earth, because each region and country discussed in this chapter has achieved the longest life expectancy and the greatest per capita income in its known history.

Does this mean that higher per capita income "causes" life expectancy to be higher in the top 10 countries?

Not quite. It simply suggests that enough evidence exists for a more sophisticated analysis to be conducted to determine whether this relationship is causal.

Why would a healthcare administrator, public health professional, clinician, or other healthcare professional need to know this information?

It will enable healthcare administrators and other personnel to better manage their organization by allowing them to quickly and simply understand whether a strong association exists between their various operational policies and procedures and healthcare outcomes.

The collection of knowledge is just one of the many skills that health care administrators and other personnel need in order to address health disparities. **BOX 1.3** includes a listing of other important required skills.

BOX 1.3   Helping Healthcare Administrators to Manage the Delivery of Win-Win Disparity-Reducing Services to All Consumers: The Needed Skills

- Skill #1: Know the primary sources of national, state, and local data that can be used to summarize health disparities.
- Skill #2: Know the sources of national, state, and local data for selected components of the U.S. healthcare system.
- Skill #3: Know general public health data regarding the health and illness areas in which disparities are most prevalent.
- Skill #4: Know how to read and apply univariate and bivariate analysis to data to determine whether healthcare disparities exist.
- Skill #5: Know the language needed in order to assign a statistician the task of analyzing internal data to determine whether any observed disparities are justifiable by factors over which they have no control.
- Skill #6: Apply evidence-based health disparities reduction strategies.
- Skill #7: Analyze theories of organizational change and write a win-win health disparities reduction plan that does not lead to "losses" by one subgroup in order for another subgroup to improve.
- Skill #8: Be able to appraise, assess, and dilute the operation of conscious and/or unconscious "tribalistic" attitudes, beliefs, and opinions that contribute or could contribute to avoidable health disparities in their current or targeted segment of the healthcare system.

Chapter Summary

What is the topic of this text? How will that subject matter be approached? Does this health disparities book differ in any respect from those already in the marketplace? Whether latent and/or made explicit, these key questions are attached to every new book that becomes part of the world's knowledge base. This chapter provided an orientation to the subject of health disparities from the perspective of a group of authors from different backgrounds and experiences. It is our hope that this team, which includes three professors of healthcare administration, a professor of education who brings new views to the field, a healthcare consultant with intensive experience advising health administrators in the real world, and a professor with a background in library science, will provide fresh and new insights into a field that will necessarily grow in importance over future years.

Review Questions and Problems

1. Based on the discussion in this chapter, do you believe that individuals adopt fads and fashions in their thinking about health and health-related subjects in the same way as they do with their clothing?
2. Select, read, and cite three articles regarding health disparities. Write a critique (250 to 350 words) regarding whether each article reflects similar thinking regarding the subject matter.
3. Do you accept the concept of contemporary subtribes? If so, which subtribes have your greatest degree of loyalty?
4. Are there additional skills that you would like to obtain from reading a text on health disparities?
5. Do you view the present as the "best of times" or the "worst of times" relative to health care?
6. Will using simple online statistical calculators encourage you to more frequently analyze data to explore whether previously undiscussed relationships exist?
7. How do institutionalized definitions of *tribe* differ from the definition of *contemporary subtribalism*?
8. How does gross domestic product differ from gross domestic product per capita?

Key Terms and Concepts

coefficient of determination (R^2) A statistical tool that is used to determine the proportion of the variance in the dependent variable that can be predicted from the independent variable.

contemporary subtribalism The emergence of values, beliefs, and attitudes that develop in defense and protection of any subgroup, whether defined by race/ethnicity, sex, sexual preference, religion, geographic area, occupation, and/or any other grouping when such feelings of loyalty become so intense as to mask solutions and strategies that generate win-win outcomes for all subgroups.

gross domestic product (GDP) per capita An economic concept that is used to measure the amount of dollars each resident would have based on the market value of all goods and services produced in a country.

index A single number that utilizes weights and other statistical processes to develop a single summary measure.

Pearson correlation coefficient (r) Statistical tool used to assess whether two or more variables are associated.

tribe "A group of people who are linked by physical and societal factors such as place of residency or birth, ancestry, culture and customs, religious beliefs, economics, blood relations, common language, or other social constructs, who may or may not have a common ancestor or common leader."

subtribe A tribe or subdivision within a tribe.

References

Ahrens, K. A., Thoma, M. E., Rossen, L. M. Warner, M. & Simon, A. E. (2017). Plurality of birth and infant mortality due to external causes in the United States, 2000-2010. *American Journal of Epidemiology 185*(5), 335–344. Doi: 10.1003/aje/kww/119.

American Hospital Association. (2018). Fast facts on U.S. hospitals, 2018. Retrieved from http://www.aha.org/research/rc/stat-studies/fast-facts.shtml

American Sign Language Dictionary. (n.d.). Tribe. Retrieved from https://www.handspeak.com/word/search/index.php?id=1616

Arias, E. (2016). Changes in life expectancy by race and Hispanic origin in the United States, 2013–2014. NCHS Data Brief, No. 244. Hyattsville, MD: National Center for Health Statistics.

Bloom, B., Englehart, M., Furst, E., Hill, W., & Krathwohl, D. (1956). *Taxonomy of educational objectives: The classification of educational goals*. New York: Longman, pp. 201–207.

Braveman, P. A., Kumanyika, S., Fielding, J., LaVeist, T., Borrell, L. N., Manderscheid, R., & Troutman, A. (2011). Health disparities and health equity: The issues is justice. *American Journal of Public Health*, 101(Suppl 1), S149–S155. doi:10.2105/AjPH2010300062

Byrne, D. (2003). *Health equals wealth*. Bod Gastein, Austria: European Health Forum.

Cambridge Dictionary. (n.d.). Tribe. Retrieved from https://dictionary.cambridge.org/us/dictionary/english/tribe

Centers for Medicare and Medicaid Services. (n.d.a). Hospital Consumer Assessment of Healthcare Providers and Systems (HCAHPS). Retrieved from http://www.hcahpsonline.org

Centers for Medicare and Medicaid Services. (n.d.b). National health expenditures 2016 highlights. Retrieved from https://www.cms.gov/Research-Statistics-Data-and-Systems/Statistics-Trends-and-Reports/NationalHealthExpendData/Downloads/highlights.pdf

Central Intelligence Agency. (2017). *The world factbook*. Retrieved from https://www.cia.gov/library/publications/the-world-factbook

Chambers, A. (2015). Trends in U.S. health travel services trade. USITC Executive Briefing on Trade, Office of Industries.

Chen, L. H., & Wilson, M. E. (2013). The globalization of healthcare: Implications of medical tourism for the infectious disease clinician. *Clinical Infectious Diseases*, 57(12), 1752-1759. https://doi.org/1.1093/cid/cit540.

Claxton, G., Cox, C., Gonzales, S., Kamal, R., & Levitt, L. (2015). Measuring the quality of healthcare in the U.S. Peterson-Kaiser Health System Tracker. Retrieved from https://www.healthsystemtracker

Curtis, F. (2016). The production of American religious freedom. (New York: New York University Press) 2016. *Journal of American History* 104(2), 469–470. https://doi.org/10.1093/jahist/jax184.

Cutler, D., Lleras-Munez, A., & Vogl, T. (2010). Socioeconomic status and health: Dimensions and mechanisms. In: Glied, S., & Smith, P.C. (eds.), *The Oxford handbook of health economics* (pp. 124–163). Oxford: Oxford University Press.

Davis, K., Stremkis, K., Squires, D., & Schoen, C. (2014). Mirror, mirror on the wall: How the performance of the U.S. health-care system compares internationally. 2014 update. The Commonwealth Fund. Pub. No. 175, pg. 13.

Dickens, C. J. H. (1859). *A tale of two cities*. London: Chapman Hall.

Free Dictionary. (n.d.). Tribe. Retrieved from https://www.thefreedictionary.com/tribe

Gardner, H. (1993). *Frames of mind: The theory of multiple intelligences*. New York: Basic Books.

Gibson, C., & Jung, K. (2002). *Historical census statistics on population totals by race, 1790 to 1990, and by Hispanic origin, 1790 to 1990, for the United States, regions, divisions, and states*. Washington, DC: U.S. Census Bureau.

Guyatt, G., Devereaux, P. J., Lexchin, J., Stone, C., Yalnizyan, A., Himmelstein, D., ... Bhatnagaret, N. (2007). A systematic review of studies comparing health outcomes in Canada and the United States. *Open Medicine*, 1(1).

Harris-Kojetin, L., Sengupta, M., Park-Lee, E., Valverde, R., Caffrey, C., Rome, V., & Lendon, J. (2016). Long-term care providers and services users in the United States: Data from the National Study of Long-Term Care Providers, 2013–2014. National Center for Health Statistics. *Vital Health Stat, 3*(38). Retrieved from https://www.cdc.gov/nchs/fastats/nursing-home-care.htm

Hofstede, G. (1991). *Cultures and organizations: Software of the mind, intellectual cooperation and its importance for survival*. New York: Harper Collins.

Huerta, T. R., Harle, C. A., Ford, E. W., Diana, M. L., & Menachemi, N. (2016). Measuring patient satisfaction's relationship to hospital cost efficiency: Can administrators make a difference? *Health Care Management Review*, 41(1), 56–63.

Institute for Health Metrics and Evaluation. Growing Gap between longest and shortest lifespans in the U.S. emphasizes the need for policy action. See http://www.healthdata.org/news-release/growing-gap-between-longest-and-shortest-lifespans-us-emphasizes-need-policy-action.

Institute of Medicine and National Research Council. (2013). *U.S. Health in International Perspective: Shorter Lives, Poorer Health*. Washington, DC: The National Academies Press. https://doi.org/10.17226/13497

Jones, G. H., & Kantarjian, H. (2015). Health care in the United States – basic human right or entitlement? *Annals of Oncology 26*(10), 2193-2195. https://doi.org/10.1093/annonc/mdv321.

Joshi, A. B., McCormick, Z. L., Sully, K., Garvan, C., & Plastaras, C. T. (2016). Factors that predict satisfaction with medical care: Data from 27,212 injured workers surveyed for 14 Years. *Journal of Occupational and Environmental Medicine, 58*(1), 101–107.

Kaiser Family Foundation. (2017a, October). Professionally active physicians. Retrieved from http://kff.org/other/state-indicator/total-active-physicians/

Kaiser Family Foundation. (2017b, October). Total number of professionally active nurses. Retrieved from http://kff.org/other/state-indicator/total-registered-nurses/

Kaiser Family Foundation. (2017c, September). State health facts: Total Medicaid MCOs. Retrieved from http://kff.org/other/state-indicator/total-medicaid-mcos/

Katz-Wise, S.L., Reisner, S.L., White, J.M., & Keo-Meier, C.L. (2016). Differences in sexual orientation diversity and sexual fluidity in attractions. Among gender minority adults in Massachusetts. *Journal of Sex Research 53*(1), 74–84. doi:10.108/ 00224499.2014.1003028.

Kruss, G., McGrath, S., Petersen, I., & Gastrow, M. (2015). Higher education and economic development: the importance of building technological capabilities. *International Journal of Educational Development, 43*(1), 22–31.

LaRoche, C. J. (2014). Free black communities and the underground railroad: The geography of resistance. *Journal of American History, 101*(4), 1264–1265, https://doi.org/10.1093/jahist/jax066

Loprinzi, P. D., Branscum, A., Hanks, J. & Smit, E. Healthy Lifestyle Characteristics and Their Joint Association With Cardiovascular Disease Biomarkers in US Adults. Mayo Clinic Proceedings, 2016; DOI: 10.1016/j.mayocp.2016.01.009

Macmillan Dictionary. (n.d.). Tribe. Retrieved from https://www.macmillandictionary.com/us/dictionary/american/tribe

Matthews, T. J., & MacDorman, M. F. (2013). Infant mortality statistics from the 2010 period linked birth/infant death dataset. *National Vital Statistics Report 62*(8), 1–26.

McDonald, J. J. (2007). *American ethnic history: Themes and perspectives.* Edinburgh: Edinburgh University Press.

McGovern, L., Miller, G., & Hughes-Cromwick, P. (2014). Health policy brief: The relative contribution of multiple determinants to health outcomes, health affairs. Retrieved from https://www.healthaffairs.org.doi:1377/hpb2014082/904487

Merriam-Webster Dictionary. (n.d.). Tribe. Retrieved from https://www.merriam-webster.com/dictionary/tribe

Merriam-Webster Learners Dictionary. (n.d.). Tribe. Retrieved from http://www.learnersdictionary.com/definition/tribe

National Center for Health Statistics. (2017). Health, United States, 2016: With chartbook on long-term trends in health. Table 15, Life expectancy at birth at age 65, and at age 75, by sex, race, and Hispanic origin, selected years 1900–2015. Hyattsville, MD: NCHS.

Oxford Living Dictionary. (n.d.). Tribe. Retrieved from https://en.oxforddictionaries.com/definition/tribe/

Papanicolas, J., Woskie, L. R., & Jha, A. K., (2018). Health care spending in the United States and other high-income countries. *Journal of the American Medical Association 219*(10), 1024–1039. Doi:10.1001/jama.2018.11.1150.

Patients Beyond Borders (2017). Medical tourism statistics and facts. www.patientbeyondborders,com. Accessed April 22, 2018.

Preston, S. H., & Ho, J. Y. (2009). Low life expectancy in the United States: Is the health care system at fault? NBER working paper, no. 15213. Washington, DC: National Bureau of Economic Research.

Roberson, R. (2013, September). Helping students find relevance: Teaching the relevance of course content can help students develop into engaged, motivated and self-regulated learners. Psychology Teacher Network. Retrieved from http://www.apa.org/ed/precollege/ptn/2013/09/students-relevance.aspx

Robertson, D. L. (2016). Decolonizing the academy with subversive acts of indigenous research: A review of *Yakama Rising* and *Bad Indians. Sociology of Race and Ethnicity, 2*(2), 248–252.

Roinen, K., LäHteenmakim, L., & Tvorila, H. (1999). Quantification of consumer attitudes to health and hedonic characteristics of foods. *Appetite, 33*(1), 71–88. https://doi.org/10.1006/appe/1999.0232

SK&A. (2017, April). National pharmacy market summary: Market insights report. Retrieved from http://www.skainfo.com/reports/most-powerful-pharmacies

Smith, A. (1776). An inquiry into the nature and causes of the wealth of nations, *1 (1 ed.).* London: W. Strahan. Retrieved 2018-04-07., volume 2 via Google Books.

Statista. (2017). Global population shares. Retrieved from https://www.statista.com/statitics/237584/distribution-of-the-world-population-by-continent

Suhrcke, M., McKee, M., Arce, R. S., Tsolova, S., & Mortenson, J. (2005). *The contribution of health to the economy in the European Union.* Luxembourg: Office for Official Publications of the European Communities.

Sulaiman, C., Bala, U., Tijani, B. A., Waziri, S. I., & Maji, I. K. (2015). Human capital, technology, and economic growth: Evidence from Nigeria. *Sage Open Journal.* 10.1177/2158244015615166.

Svizzero, S., & Tisdell, C. A. (2016). Economic evolution, diversity of societies and stages of economic development: A critique of theories applied to hunters and gatherers and their successors. *Cogent Economics & Finance. 4*(1), doi:10.1080/23322039.2016.1161322.

U.S. Census Bureau. (2016, July 1). QuickFacts. Retrieved from https://www.census.gov/quickfacts/fact/table/US/PST045216

U.S. Census Bureau. (2018). Population clock. Retrieved from https://www.census.gov/popclock/

U.S. Department of Commerce, Bureau of Economic Analysis. (2018, February 28). National income and product accounts. Gross domestic product: Fourth quarter and annual 2017 (second estimate). Retrieved from https://www.bea.gov/scb/2018/02 -february/0218-gdp-and-the-economy.htm

U.S. Department of Health and Human Services. (2008). The Secretary's Advisory Committee on National Health Promotion and Disease Prevention Objectives for 2020. Phase I report: Recommendations for the framework and format of Healthy People 2020. Retrieved from http:// www.healthypeople.gov/sites/default/files/PhaseI_0.pdf

U.S. Department of Health and Human Resources. (2017). NHE fact sheet, 2016. Retrieved from https://www.cms .gov/research-statistics-data-and-systems/statistics -trends-and-reports/nationalhealthexpenddata/nhe -fact-sheet.html

United Nations. (n.d.). Global Indicator Database. Retrieved from data.un.org

United Nations, Department of Economic and Social Affairs, Population Division (2017). World Mortality 2017: Data Booklet.

Vocabulary.com. (n.d.). Tribe. Retrieved from https:// www.vocabulary.com/dictionary/tribe

Weaver, B., & Wuensch, K. L. (2013). SPSS and SAS programs for comparing Pearson correlations and OLS regression coefficients. *Behavior Research Methods*, *45*(3), 880–895.

World Atlas. (n.d.). The continents of the world per capita GDP. Retrieved from https://www.worldatlas.com

World Bank. (n.d.). World Bank Open Data. Retrieved from https://data.worldbank.org

World Health Organization. (n.d.). NHA indicators. Global Health Expenditure Database. Retrieved from http://apps.who.int/nha/database/ViewData /Indicators/en

World Health Organization. (2000). *The World Health Report 2000: Health systems: improving performance.* Geneva: World Health Organization.

World Population Review. (2017). Continent and region populations, 2017. Retrieved from world population .com/continents

Worldometers. (n.d.). Retrieved from www.worldometers .info

Yanping, L., Pan, A., Wand, D. D., Liu, X., Dhana, K., Franco, O., . . . Hu, F. B. Abstract 20397: The impact of healthy lifestyle on life expectancy in the U.S. population. *Circulation*, 2017;136:A20397.

Your Dictionary. (n.d.). Tribe. Retrieved from http://www .yourdictionary.com/tribe

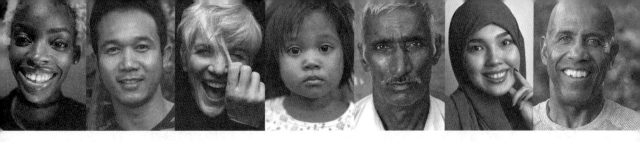

CHAPTER 2

What Are Health Disparities?

"People with disabilities…experience health care disparities, such as lower rates of screening and more difficulty accessing services, compared to people without disabilities."

—**Lisa Lezzoni**, Director, Mongan Institute for Health Policy, Massachusetts General Hospital

LEARNING OBJECTIVES

After completing this chapter, each learner will be able to:

- Compare and contrast alternative definitions of *health disparities*.
- List the determinants of health, and identify how society has contributed to different health outcomes.
- Support or critique the hypothesis that social stratification and health outcomes are linked.
- Match one of the three approaches to social stratification (structural functionalism, conflict theory, or hybrid approach) with your belief system.
- Analyze the thesis that healthcare administrators, like public health professionals and clinicians, must to be involved in preventive and other areas of patient health care to improve present and future health outcomes.

▶ Introduction

A variety of definitions of health disparities have been put forward. Consider some of those offered by various government agencies:

- "Differences in access to or availability of facilities and services" (National Institutes of Health, U.S. National Library of Medicine, n.d.).

- "A particular type of health difference that is closely linked with social, economic, and/or environmental disadvantage. Health disparities adversely affect groups of people who have systematically experienced greater obstacles to health based on their racial or ethnic group" (U.S. Department of Health and Human Services, 2011).
- "Health inequalities that are considered unnecessary, avoidable, and unfair/unjust" (World Health Organization, 2008).

A primary purpose of this text is to broaden the definition of health disparities so that those working in health care can better address the needs of all subgroups with unique health needs and/or differential health outcomes. Healthcare administrators and other healthcare professionals are uniquely positioned to participate in a growing movement that seeks to advance life outcomes for the whole of humankind. This movement requires maximum health outcomes for all.

Dehlendorf, Bryant, Huddleston, Jacoby, and Fujimoto (2010) provide an excellent summary of current approaches to the field of health disparities. Specifically, these authors address the counter intuitive approach currently used in defining health disparities. They say, "A central aspect of the most accepted definitions is that not all differences in health status between groups are considered to be disparities, but rather only differences which systematically and negatively impact less advantaged groups are classified as disparities," (pg. 212).

We believe that these current approaches must change if health disparities is to become a field of study that supports advancement in the whole of humankind. While the term *disparities* simply means "differences," the field of health disparities has been constructed on an inherently subtribalistic definition. This is because health disparities have been both explicitly and implicitly defined in a way that is exclusive of differences in health outcomes that randomly occur. Rather, the focus is only upon those differential outcomes that are the result of systems of social stratification within a country. This chapter examines social stratification and its effects on health outcomes.

▶ Systems of Social Stratification

What do we mean by the phrase *systems of social stratification*? In this text, **systems of social stratification** are those societal

mechanisms whereby people are positioned in a hierarchy based on their wealth, status, power, prestige, gender, race/ethnicity, and other identifying characteristics.

Social stratification is the basis for a caste or class society in which specific subgroups of people are grouped into categories based on certain characteristics. For example, in the United States, one common example of social stratification is the division of the populace by wealth. **FIGURE 2.1** illustrates the three major "classes" of Americans according to their earning power. **TABLE 2.1** includes the income ranges for each "class".

The field of health disparities emerged in the United States as the study of racial/ethnic differences in health outcomes and, over time, expanded to include other demographic factors such as socioeconomic status, sex, age, rural/urban populations, and most recently, gender identification. The concept underlying the field of health disparities, as currently constructed, is that the observed differences in health outcomes are the result of the maltreatment of selected subgroups in a society by other subgroups.

But aren't health disparities a thing of the past? It sounds like the field of health disparities is a type of affirmative action program based on health issues.

This is definitely not the case. Health disparities as a field emerged because differential outcomes that occur in health are directly related not only to historic behaviors of individuals and social systems but to current ones as well.

▶ How Society Has Contributed to Differential Health Outcomes

Penner et al. (2010), in a study of physicians, found that a number of these practitioners embodied and acknowledged bias against

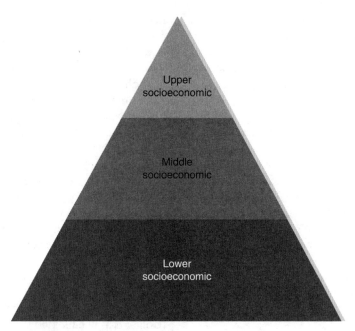

FIGURE 2.1 Social stratification of Americans by income.

TABLE 2.1 Social Stratification of Americans By Income (2014)

- Upper income class: >$124,925 per year for a family of three
- Middle income class: $41,641 to $124,925 for a family of three
- Lower income class: <$41,641 for a family of three

Data From: CIA Factbook 2017–2018, CIA Factbook 2017 and CIA Factbook 2016.

African American patients and that this attitude affected treatment and treatment outcomes. Hu, Schreiber, Jordan, George, and Nerenz (2017), in a study of 22 primary care sites, found that income, education, race/ethnicity, gender, etc., were associated with 25% to 50% of differences in patient outcomes for persons with diabetes and hypertension. James (2017) completed a literature review which revealed that in the recent past, as well as today, physicians of European descent attributed lower intelligence and other negative traits to persons of Spanish and Indian descent, as well as to persons of African descent.

The continuing impact of adverse experiences based on race/ethnicity transcends direct experiences with healthcare professionals. Ong, Cerrada, Lee, and Williams (2017) conducted research with 152 first-year Asian American college students. They found that even today, diverse responses to the students' ethnicity had such a severe impact on the students that the length and quality of their sleep were impaired. And, as is known, the duration and quality of sleep intermediate health outcomes. Steptoe, Peacey, and Wardle (2006), in a study of 17,465 students of higher education from 27 universities worldwide, found that the odds of poor health were 46% higher for students who slept 6 hours per night versus 7 to 8 hours. For those students who slept less than 6 hours, the odds of poor health was 99% higher.

Howard (2016) reported that Jewish American, African American, East Indian, and other physicians encountered patients who chose to place their personal health at risk rather than be served by a physician of a different race, ethnicity, or religion. These are just a few examples of how race, religion, income, and other factors across virtually all of America's systems and institutions continue to influence the health status of various subgroups. Thus, the field of health disparities has been established to identify, decrease, and ultimately eliminate remediable disparities in health outcomes that reflect individual behaviors and systemic practices that are a part of a sequence of events that may result in lower life expectancies and a greater burden of illness and disease among various subgroups.

Emergence of Systems of Social Stratification

Systems of social stratification appear to be a natural phenomenon in the evolution of humankind. This social phenomenon seems to emerge in response to the distribution of power in a society and/or other social unit. Tattersall (2003), Gibbons (2006), and other researchers have found anthropological evidence that early modern humans, that is *Homo sapiens*, emerged in Africa. Similarly, Ao, Dekkers, Wei, Qiang, and Xiao (2013) have identified the presence of early hominids in the northern regions of China. Yet, some people are reluctant to accept that either Africa and/or Asia were early sites of *Homo sapiens*. The refusal to accept anthropological evidence is a direct reflection of the cumulative impact of ethnocentrism and other forms of social stratification. Similarly, various beliefs and attitudes based upon tribalism and sub tribalism exist regarding gender and other variables. For example, Streed, McCarthy, and Haas (2017), using data from the Centers for Disease Control and Prevention (CDC), determined

that both personal and institutional forces in present and past American society are associated with higher rates of unemployment and lower income among U.S. residents who do not adhere to traditional gender norms. Similarly, transgender, lesbian, bisexual, gay and other sexual minorities have less access to high-quality health care (Albuquerque et al., 2016). Societal factors interact in such a way that health outcomes are disproportionately more likely to be reported as poor or fair among affected populations. Disparities also occur based on sex, independent of gender identification. Because more power has been allocated to males historically, females are oftentimes included as a population that experiences health disparities. Yet, bilateral differentials exist between the two sexes that can lead to men experiencing health disparities (Collier & Williams, 1981).

What do you mean by "bilateral"?

The term "bilateral" is derived from the Latin language and is made up from the two words *bi* meaning "two", and *lateralis* meaning "pertaining to the side." Thus, anything labeled bilateral has two sides. The term "bilateral differentials" is defined as unequal outcomes that affect two sides. Health disparities are currently viewed as a unilateral phenomenon. The continuing theme in this text is that as members of humankind, it is important to identify sub group disparities wherever they exist.

For example, the observation is frequently made that although white females live longer than white males, white females experience illness and disease at higher rates than white males. However, if both males and females were surveyed, it might be expected that not merely a plurality, but a majority would select a longer life expectancy accompanied by greater illness over a lower life expectancy. Thus, an altered definition of health disparities is needed that addresses health outcome differentials by sex in general. For example, Alexandre et al. (2018) demonstrate the criticality of the inclusion of males and females in disparity research. Their analysis of 1,413 seniors revealed that while some symptoms of frailty are more common in women, others are more common in men. However, the historic placement of women in a lower level within the system of social stratification of all nations has led to this group's identification as a health disparity population under the prevailing definition.

How did systems of social stratification develop in the United States and worldwide that initially subordinated individuals by sex first and then by race/ethnicity?

Anthropological evidence reveals that the lifestyle and culture of early humans was based upon hunting and gathering. In hunting and gathering societies, the smaller stature and weight of females, in combination with women's role as child-bearers, initiated the establishment of **patriarchy**, or male-dominant societies (Hooks, 2004).

However, the skills and competencies needed for the survival of humankind are no longer predominantly linked with physical strength. Indeed, the human assets needed to ensure the future survival of humankind are distributed across all individuals and subgroups. This fact alone suggests a highly critical need for a restructuring of sociocultural beliefs, values, folkways, laws, institutions, and other sociocultural components so that an **axiology**, or value structure, is created that is supportive of human survival, growth, and development. Such an outcome requires the diminution of beliefs, attitudes, and behaviors that create dysfunctions associated with sex or gender.

Are you saying that focusing on health disparities that are primarily based on historical circumstances that have adversely impacted certain groups is dysfunctional to humankind's current and future needs?

That is exactly the argument that this text makes. This text seeks to alter the field of health disparities so that it will better serve humanity by focusing on addressing all remediable subgroup differences—wherever they are identified. The argument is also made that anger regarding past disharmonious relationships among subgroups generates a chain of actions that moves humankind toward greater division, rather than the unity needed for future survival.

What are some of the factors associated with inequalities by race/ethnicity?

In order to understand racial/ethnic inequalities, we must begin with the concept of ethnocentrism. **Ethnocentrism** refers to the tendency of people to view their own subgroup as superior and to reject subgroups with different physical, cultural, behavioral, and/or other characteristics. Ethnocentrism is often based upon visible differences, such as skin color or other physical features, whereas in-group/outgroup alliances are not based on permanent, unalterable differences. The term *ethnocentrism* has its origins in psychology, sociology, anthropology, and the other social sciences. Initially attributed to the psychologist, William Graham Sumner (1906), more recent evidence has revealed that Sumner did not originate this concept but merely popularized the term to describe this highly critical aspect of human behavior (Bizumic, 2014). Bizumic (2014) traces the use of the term *ethnocentric* to scholars before Sumner. Sumner did, however, add to our understanding of current levels of tribalism by originating the terms *in-group* and *outgroup*.

What do you mean by "in-group" and "outgroup"?

An **in-group** is any group with which an individual identifies. This identification is not necessarily based upon race/ethnicity, culture, gender, etc. Nevertheless, once self-identification takes place, it commands the loyalty of its members. An **outgroup** is a group with which an individual does not identify and is often accompanied by hostility toward that group.

From Ethnocentrism to Racism

Ethnocentrism has long been associated with wars and military conflict throughout human history. Early in human history, conditions in hunting and gathering societies were such that it did not make sense to keep one's "enemies" alive and enter them into slavery. As human society became more complex, and the means of survival shifted from hunting and gathering to agriculture, the enslavement of enemies became functional to the survival of the emerging societies. Schiedel (2007) demonstrates this tendency through the growth in the use of slaves in ancient Egypt, Rome, and other societies. Interestingly, although ethnocentric beliefs allowed enemies captured in war to be enslaved, slavery was not accompanied by an ontology that defined the enslaved as being less than human. **Ontology** is a useful framework by which to examine society, as it is the study of the nature of existence, including the nature of things in relationship to each other (Schiedel, 2007).

How did the enslaved come to be characterized as having subhuman status?

The ontology changed from one in which slavery was the natural outcome of losses associated with war to one in which the enslaved were considered as innately inferior to their masters through the influence of the Catholic Church after Christianity became the religion of Rome.

Are you saying that Christianity helped redefine slaves as subhumans?

Yes, that is the case. Saint Thomas Aquinas in his *Summa Theologica* (circa 1270) is credited with arguing that some groups are "naturally" slaves. A litany of biblical scriptures defined an inherently natural order between slaves and masters, with slaves being subservient to their masters. Even those Church philosophers and officials who eventually began to oppose slavery imposed a new hierarchy that legitimized it as a system of social stratification by those who were not a part of the subtribe of people who practiced Christianity. Accordingly, the nature of slavery as a human phenomenon was transformed, thereby leading to the institutionalization of these new beliefs in the very core of Western philosophy.

Shouldn't the field of health disparities primarily address the consequences of this "ontology" upon health outcomes?

The beliefs, values, and other norms and social systems and structures needed to continue to propel humanity forward in one era may be totally unsuitable in a different time period. During periods when various clusters of humankind were spatially and communicatively isolated, ethnocentrism and other forms of tribalism and subtribalism actually enhanced human survival. An excellent example of this is the current debate regarding the constitutional right to guns. During America's early period, when agrarian life created a multiplicity of threats and the criminal justice system was underdeveloped, home-based access to guns was critical. However, in a highly urbanized society populated by individuals with extremely large permutations and combinations of values and beliefs regarding when these objects should and ought to be used, easy access to guns generates highly volatile circumstances that generate a health risk for all. But, let's focus on our primary argument, which is that early tribalism was helpful to the survival of humankind.

For most of human history, strangers were a threat to survival. Tribal units were required to address core human survival needs. **Philosophical anthropology** is a rather controversial area of study that uses philosophy (which focuses on the nature of all that is in existence) to study humankind, including intrapersonal, interpersonal, and all aspects of people as humans (Pihlstrom, 2003). While its validity has been challenged by some thinkers, it nevertheless serves as a framework that can be used to examine humankind.

Arjoon, Turriago-Hoyos, and Thoene (2015) argue that every single aspect of the behavior of humans as individuals and/or as parts of organizations can better support the "common good" when a conceptual framework is applied that enhances harmony among humans. Because current and future healthcare administrators, public health professionals, and clinicians are managers of healthcare institutions, they are thus positioned to adopt and use such a framework.

▸ Redefining Health Disparities

As one considers the definitions of health disparities that were introduced at the beginning of this chapter, it becomes clear that key premises largely left unsaid are embedded within them. The following makes explicit several of these premises.

Premise 1: The American Belief That "All Humans Are Created Equal"

From early childhood, Americans are acculturated into the concept that "all humans are created as equals" (Armitage, 2007). Attributed to Thomas Jefferson and the immortal document that is held sacred to all Americans, the U.S. Declaration of Independence, this concept of equality was introduced into American culture as a *literal* rather than a *symbolic* truth. Moreover, the premise of literal equality has now diffused from the United States and into both the legal documents as well as the consciousness of other countries (Hillier, 1997). Indeed, this principle has been so widely adopted that it is now incorporated into the preamble to the United Nations' Universal Declaration of Human Rights (UN General Assembly, 1948).

This philosophical foundation, when applied as a premise underlying health disparities, suggests that because person A is equal to person B, who is equal to person C, then their health outcomes, as measured by rates of mortality and morbidity, will be roughly equal. Thus, persons using this definition conclude that the absence of equal outcomes indicates that health disparities exist. This premise also indicates that the measurement of health disparities occurs at an individual level; that is, that all Americans "should" have roughly the same life expectancy and the same distribution of illness and disease.

What's wrong with this premise?

This premise, however, is far too literal and too narrow. Even at birth, inequalities occur by race/ethnicity, gender, and other variables in the distribution of congenital conditions. For example, African Americans are more likely to have encephalocele and trisomy 18 than are non-Hispanic Caucasians. Similarly, Hispanics are more likely to experience anencephaly and anotia/microtia than are Caucasians. They are also less likely to experience hypospadias. **BOX 2.1** describes common inequalities that occur at birth for non-Hispanic whites relative to other ethnicities. **BOX 2.2** outlines birth defects that are more common in American Indian/Alaskan Native children relative to white children.

Why did you introduce these data on birth defects?

The data presented in Boxes 2.1 and 2.2 reveal that health disparities cannot be defined based upon the philosophical principle of the equality of all humans. The data on birth defects demonstrate two trends. First, individuals are *innately* characterized by differences in health outcomes. It also demonstrates that health disparities can never be defined by comparing individual outcomes. Rather, the concept must be based upon groups of individuals; that is, the concept of health disparities only exists as a

BOX 2.1   Birth Defects with Higher Rates of Occurrence in Non-Hispanic Whites

Birth Defects More Common Among Caucasians Than American Indians/Alaskan Natives

- Hypospadias is a birth defect that is specific to males. It is a condition in which the urinary opening is not at the usual location on the head of the penis.

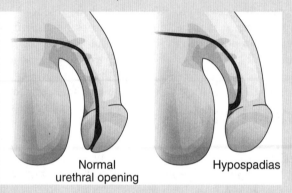

Normal
urethral opening   Hypospadias

Birth Defects More Common Among Caucasians Than Asian Americans

- Spina bifida without anencephaly is characterized by a defect in the neural tube. Anatomically speaking, the neural tube is hollow at birth but serves as the structure that ultimately allows the brain and the spinal cord to develop. With spina bifida, the formation of the brain, spinal cord, and/ or meninges is incomplete at birth.
- Truncus arteriosus is a congenital heart disease that is characterized by the dislocation of a blood vessel known as the truncus arteriosus. In truncus arteriosus, the vessel is sourced in the right and left ventricles. Normally, two vessels (pulmonary artery and aorta) are attached to this blood vessel.

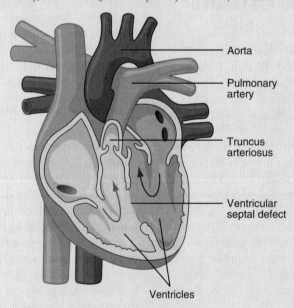

Aorta

Pulmonary
artery

Truncus
arteriosus

Ventricular
septal defect

Ventricles

- Aortic valve stenosis involves a narrowed aortic valve. As a result, the flow from the heart's lower left chamber (ventricle) into the aorta and to the body is reduced or completely eliminated. Because the valve does not properly open, the heart must overexert itself as it pumps blood through the valve.

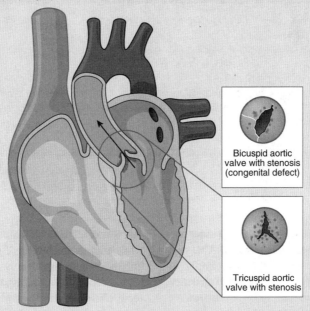

Bicuspid aortic valve with stenosis (congenital defect)

Tricuspid aortic valve with stenosis

- Hypoplastic left heart syndrome is a rare congenital birth defect in which the left side of the heart is less than fully developed.
- Coarctation of the aorta is another congenital birth defect that is disparately associated with white children. The aorta in this case is undersized. Thus, insufficient oxygen is delivered throughout the body.

Birth Defects More Common Among Caucasians Than African Americans

- Aortic valve stenosis.
- Cleft lip with or without cleft palate occurs when the lip does not fully close during fetal development.

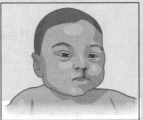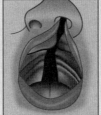

- Pyloric stenosis is a congenital condition that prevents an infant's food from moving into the small intestine.
- Gastroschisis is a birth defect of the abdominal (belly) wall that results in the baby's intestines being located outside of the body.

BOX 2.2 Birth Defects More Common Among American Indians/Alaskan Natives Than Caucasians

- Encephalocele is a neural tube defect where the brain as well as the associated membranes protrude from the skull.
- Anotia is a congenital deformity where the pinna (external ear) does not develop. Microtia is a similar condition where the pinna is underdeveloped.
- Cleft lip with or without cleft palate.
- Limb deficiency, which involves missing, incomplete, or other abnormalities involved in the development of any limb at birth. With upper limb deficiency, the upper limbs are unformed or partially formed. With lower limb deficiency, the lower parts of the legs are unformed or partially formed.
- Trisomy 18, or Edwards syndrome, is a condition that causes severe developmental delays due to an extra chromosome 18.

Mayo Foundation for Medical Education and Research, http://www.mayoclinic.org/

measurement of differences in health outcomes across various "tribes and subtribes." This suggests that another premise is also implicitly operative in the discussion of health disparities.

Premise 2: Health Disparities as a Mathematical Concept

In the second premise that undergirds the concept of health disparities, the notion of equality becomes more than just a philosophical construct and ventures into the realm of mathematics. More specifically, the definition of equality that is embodied in this unstated approach to health disparities is based upon the mathematical concept of equivalence. Mathematically, **equivalence** refers to relationships between numbers that, although different, are equal in value, effect, force, and/or significance:

$5 = 5$ is an equality.

$1 + 4 = 2 + 3$ is an equivalent relationship.

Consistent with this definition, the distribution of illness and disease across various American subgroups would not be considered problematic by policy makers or citizens if the outcomes were equivalent as measured by mortality rates and/or overall health quality. Stated differently, if one individual had the co-occurring

diseases of diabetes mellitus and hypertension while another experienced obesity and asthma, but the length and quality of life were equal, the existence of health disparities would simply require current and future healthcare administrators, public health professionals, and clinicians to understand how to best provide prevention and treatment services that are congruent with the clinical conditions of the consumers whom they serve. Utilizing this premise, healthcare administrators, policy makers, researchers, and scholars would exhibit indifference as to whether the unit of analysis is the individual and/or his or her unique tribe or subtribe.

Premise 3: Health Disparities as a Statistical Concept

The third premise that underlies the concept of health disparities is based upon **nonequivalent inequalities** that are not only observable at the individual level but at the group level as well. As mentioned, equivalent inequalities would have no differential impact upon life expectancy. In contrast, nonequivalent inequalities will result in differential life expectancies. Indeed, each of the definitions of health disparities provided are based on this concept. When deconstructed, it becomes clear that whereas the first premise was based upon a philosophical concept and the second is grounded in mathematics, the third approach is based upon the statistical concept of a normal curve.

What is a normal curve?

The normal curve incorporates the notion of the simultaneity of equality within inequality. Specifically, the construct of a normal curve requires values of a phenomenon for various groups. The premise is that it is unrealistic to expect perfect equality within the universe. However, we can reasonably expect an *equal distribution of inequalities*. This distribution results in a bell-shaped **normal curve** (**FIGURE 2.2**). With a normal curve, approximately 68.21% of all values fall plus or minus one standard deviation from the mean. Approximately 27.18% of values fall plus or minus two standard deviations from the mean. Finally, an estimated 4.3% of values fall plus or minus three standard deviations from the mean, and 0.2% of values fall plus or minus four standard deviations from the mean. Consider the following additional definitions to enhance your understanding of this concept:

■ "A symmetrical bell-shaped curve representing the probability density function of a normal distribution. The area of a vertical section of the curve represents the probability that the random variable lies between the values which delimit the section" (FreeDictionary.com, n.d.).

■ "A bell-shaped curve showing a particular distribution of probability over the values of a random variable" (Dictionary.com, n.d.).

One can empirically confirm such a statement by simply observing the belled shape of trees and/or the belled shape of mountains. When applied to health disparities, the implication is that while various individuals with similar human characteristics may have differences in health outcomes as measured by both illness and disease and mortality, *the common origins of humankind would suggest that an equal distribution of inequalities will be observable across subgroups.*

This premise, although most often left implicit rather than made explicit, dominates the study of health disparities. But other premises also co-occur with the statistical approach to health disparities.

Premise 4: Health Disparities as a Sociological Concept

An abundance of well-known data confirms that health disparities are not equally distributed across various groups and subgroups. As a result, several sociological premises have become embedded in the concept of health disparities. As mentioned earlier in the chapter, when systematic asymmetric outcomes occur within a society, sociologists define these skewed patterns as *systems of social*

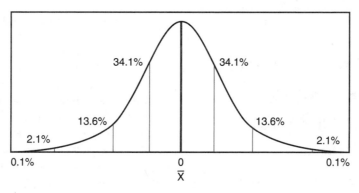

FIGURE 2.2 Normal curve.

stratification. Systems of social stratification may be reflective of differences in the universe from which the subpopulations are drawn (i.e., biological, genetic factors, etc.). In contrast, socioeconomic inequalities may represent the outcome of sociocultural and/or other factors in the physical environment.

While sociologists have, for more than a century, sought to document the causes and correlates of socioeconomic inequalities, it is only relatively recently that a comparable body of research has emerged in the area of health. Known as **health disparities research**, this emerging field seeks to identify those areas of health that are characterized by sustained differences in mortality and morbidity across subgroups. Interestingly, despite the fact that highly significant differences exist in death rates and the incidence of major illness by race/ethnicity, gender, income, education, disability, geography, sexual preferences, religion, and even personality type, many healthcare administrators, public health professionals, and clinicians are unaware of the magnitude of these differences. Indeed, most healthcare personnel would, if queried regarding these trends, probably be unable to cite accurate data descriptive of the nature of currently prevailing health disparities. Even those populations that are at risk of early death and/or avoidable illness and disease are often unaware of the potential impact of their own behaviors upon the quality and length of their lives. Rather, an implicit worldview has been adopted that does not fully hold individuals accountable for their own contributions to health disparities.

▶ Choosing a Worldview for the Analysis of Data on Health Disparities

The importance assigned to health disparities by a healthcare administrator, public health professional, and/or clinician is directly responsive to his or her ontological and axiological perspective regarding the nature of systems of social stratification.

Could you refresh our memory of what you mean by ontology and axiology?

Consider the following definitions of *ontology*:

- "A particular theory about the nature of being or the kinds of things that have existence" (*Merriam-Webster*, n.d.).
- "The branch of metaphysics that studies the nature of existence or being as such" (Dictionary.com, n.d.).
- "A set of concepts and categories in a subject area or domain that shows their properties and the relations between them" (*Oxford Dictionaries*, n.d.).

Based on these definitions, it becomes clear that all individuals have an ontology. Because a healthcare administrator, public health professional, and/or clinician has been granted the authority and the power to serve as an agent of change, it becomes important for his or her ontology and axiology regarding social stratification to be made explicit.

Recall that axiology is a value structure. It can be defined as "The study of the nature, types, and criteria of values and of value judgments especially in ethics" (*Merriam-Webster*, n.d.). An alternative definition is that it is "The branch of philosophy dealing with values, as those of ethics, aesthetics, or religion" (Dictionary.com, n.d.).

Take the brief survey in **BOX 2.3** to better understand your own philosophical beliefs regarding inequality. Based on your answers to the questions in Box 2.3, you will find that your beliefs regarding the nature of inequalities will fall within one of three approaches to social stratification: structural functionalism, conflict theory, or a hybrid approach. Simply count your answers in each category to determine whether you embrace the beliefs of functionalism, conflict theory, or whether your beliefs are hybrid.

BOX 2.3 Uncovering Your Beliefs Regarding Unequal Distributions of Inequality

Directions: Please answer each question below as quickly as possible. Be as honest as possible regarding your values, beliefs, and opinions. (There are no right or wrong answers.)

1.	Society has many parts, and these parts work together to generate a stable and functional society. (Structural functionalism)	T ☐ or F ☐
2.	Inequality in society is equivalent to the functioning of the human body. In order for the body to function, it has various types of organs, muscles, bones, etc. Although human roles and positions differ in responsibility and reward, these differences support the welfare of the whole society. (Structural functionalism)	T ☐ or F ☐
3.	The basic building block of a healthy functioning society is the family. When families lose strength, it reverberates throughout the larger society. (Structural functionalism)	T ☐ or F ☐
4.	Human nature itself is divided between the desire to reward only self and a desire to assist others. (Conflict theory)	T ☐ or F ☐
5.	Continuous conflict exists and always exists in society over the distribution of resources. (Conflict theory)	T ☐ or F ☐
6.	Persons who are physically, emotionally, and/or socially or militarily stronger acquire disproportionate shares of a society's resources and use these resources to their advantage. Therefore, government intervention is needed to ensure that all humans have the basic resources needed for survival. (Conflict theory)	T ☐ or F ☐
7.	Stated differently, the stronger and/or more powerful groups in a society will dominate if the weaker groups do not take social action. (Conflict theory)	T ☐ or F ☐
8.	It is impossible for health and other resources to be distributed in such a way that everybody is better off. In order for one group to be better off, another group or subgroup will become worse off. (Conflict theory)	T ☐ or F ☐
9.	Independent of the odds, individuals can always choose to improve their position in life whether it is their health or their income. (Hybrid)	T ☐ or F ☐
10.	Through investments in the three primary forms of human capital—education, health, and social capital—health disparities can be reduced and everyone can be made better off. (Hybrid)	T ☐ or F ☐

Developed by Talcott Parsons (1951) through the integration of theoretical perspectives from a number of philosophers, **structural functionalism** is now seen as a highly partisan approach to systems of social stratification that is supportive of the status quo.

In contrast, the views that appear to dominate scholarly work in the area of health disparities are based on conflict theory. **Conflict theory** assumes that competition and conflict over scarce resources are natural forces between groups and subgroups. Whether the discussion surrounds health outcomes regarding race/ethnicity, gender, and/or other features, the framework used has a subtext that suggests the application of conflict theory. Conflict theory has its origins in the work of Karl Marx (Lenski, 1984). However, contemporary sociologists apply this framework in the analysis of subgroup disparities (Sears, 2005). The question becomes, "*Which of these theoretical frameworks appear to be most descriptive of differential health outcomes by subgroups within the United States?*"

▶ Healthcare Disparities Versus Health Disparities

Health disparities are population and subpopulation differences in outcomes. **Healthcare disparities** are the differential processes and outcomes that occur within the operation of various components of the healthcare system. The emphasis thus far has been upon a redefinition of health disparities. However, it can be argued that current job descriptions of healthcare administrators *do not necessarily give them intervention power over health disparities nor healthcare disparities.*

How do you draw this conclusion?

BOX 2.4 provides summary statements from a number of healthcare administrator job descriptions. However, it is interesting that the duties and responsibilities of a healthcare administrator as described or implied in

---

BOX 2.4 Sample Position Descriptions for Healthcare Administrators

Position Description 1

The healthcare administrator will be expected to oversee the day-to-day operation of the family clinic while ensuring the cohesiveness of all services provided. Specific duties include but are not limited to:

- Serving as a liaison on any governing boards with other medical staff and departments heads
- Ensuring that all policies set by the governing board are properly followed
- The recruitment, hiring, and evaluation of other personnel
- Planning and advising on department budgets
- Co-developing quality assurance procedures
- Participating in fundraising (if applicable) and community health planning
- Remaining current on recent healthcare laws and regulations
- Remaining current on healthcare-related technological and other advances
- Mentoring other staff
- Other duties

Position Description 2

The healthcare administrator will manage and coordinate health/medical services at the facility. This personnel will be tasked with the day-to-day management of all healthcare services provided to our clients. Specifically, this personnel's responsibilities will include the following:

- Overseeing at least 20 personnel. (This management directive includes interviewing, hiring, firing, and evaluating prospective and current employees.)
- Co-designing and organizing trainings for new hires
- Maintaining a personnel calendar to conduct scheduling
- Overseeing and managing the health information management systems
- Ensuring that all policies and procedures are current and in-line with federal, state, and local laws and regulations
- Interfacing with accounting as needed to manage fiscal operations (i.e., budget planning, service rate determination, etc.)
- Serving as a liaison between department heads, medical staff, and governing boards, etc.
- Attending all required meetings (i.e., board, interdepartmental, community or other external entity, etc.)
- Co-developing facility objectives and providing input on the evaluation of these objectives
- Conducting regular productivity surveys to monitor the effectiveness of facility resources and assess the staffing and resource needs
- Other

Position Description 3

The health administrator will oversee clinical and administrative operations on a day-to-day basis. Responsibilities will include:

- Supervising all clinic workers
- Performing staffing and department coordination
- Working with the accounting/finance department on budgets and expenditure reports
- Keeping up-to-date with federal, state, and local laws and regulations and ensuring their inclusion into the clinic's policies and procedures
- Serving as a liaison to the board, other department heads, community stakeholders, and others as needed
- Other

scholarly articles differ from those published by employers. **BOX 2.5** describes findings from just a few of the numerous articles on the duties and responsibilities of healthcare administrators.

Is this text directed toward all three occupational areas, that is, healthcare administrators, public health professionals, and clinicians?

Yes, it is. Researchers with similar views as those noted in Box 2.5 could also be cited that support the thesis that healthcare administrators have the power and authority to not merely reduce or prevent remediable differences in outcomes across subgroups in terms of the healthcare services which they oversee, but in the disparities in health outcomes in general

as well. However, a collective effort across the disciplines—healthcare administrators, public health professionals, and clinicians— is required if remediable differences in health outcomes are to be diminished in such a way that all humankind experiences improved health outcomes. Thus, this text is directed toward all health professionals in health care.

Why would you argue that healthcare administrators, public health professionals, and clinicians can use their positions to reduce remediable differences in healthcare and health outcomes?

Potter (2018) argues that the time has arrived for nurse administrators to address all complementary areas of health and health care by becoming *involved in partnerships* that

---

BOX 2.5 Duties and Responsibilities of Healthcare Administrators: The View of Scholars

- Parand, Dopson, Renz, and Vincent (2014) provide a detailed description of healthcare administrators' duties. These duties include ensuring the quality of the clinical services provided through a given healthcare institution. Because differential healthcare delivery processes and outcomes across, between, and within subgroups are considered as a measurement of quality, healthcare disparities management is, indeed, a duty of healthcare administrators.
- Brennan (2016) emphasizes the fact that all healthcare professionals have a duty to use their skills for the maximization of all patient outcomes. Again, this charge is implicitly inclusive of not delivering any unwarranted differential care via clinical practice, medical education, biomedical research, and/or healthcare administration.
- Suarez-Balcazar, Mirza, and Garcia-Ramirez (2018) describe how all healthcare professionals can partner to not merely prevent or reduce healthcare disparities but community-based health disparities as well.

---

support change in the overall way that health care is perceived and delivered. Leng and Partridge (2018) describe the importance of data in quality improvement. This research suggests that healthcare administrators, public health professionals, and clinicians must be able to utilize the large datasets generated by their institutions for quality improvements. These quality improvements may include not just the care that was delivered. Specifically, each of these categories of healthcare professionals has opportunities to improve disparities by refusing to miss opportunities to deliver the highest-quality services in their respective areas.

I still don't understand why healthcare professionals would want to partner to assume duties related to health disparities!

The reason is that existing research reveals that health care determines only 10% to 20% of one's health outcomes! This suggests that if remediable health disparities are to be reduced and/or eliminated, each of these groups of professionals must serve as participants in addressing the other determinants of health outcomes as well. The next section discusses the major determinants of health that must be targeted in order to address disparities in health.

▶ The Determinants of Health Outcomes in the United States

Population health is generally defined as a study of nonclinical and clinical variables that determine the health outcomes of various groups or subgroups of individuals. As one reviews data on health outcomes in the United States, it becomes clear that addressing health disparities is made far more complex by the fact that health care is only a small contributor to health outcomes. Specifically, researchers have discovered that health outcomes by race/ethnicity, socioeconomic status (Braveman & Gottlieb, 2014), gender, geography, and other variables are influenced by five primary factors: (1) modifiable individual behaviors, (2) socioeconomic environment, (3) physical environment, (4) genetics, and (5) health care (McGovern, Miller, & Hughes-Cromwick, 2014).

Researchers have been actively engaged in seeking to quantify these relationships for several decades. For example, as early as 1982, Hadley analyzed data on adults aged 18 to 64 years and discovered that medical care explained a much lower proportion of negative health outcomes than previously believed. Subsequent analyses have had similar findings. McGovern et al. (2014) report that in 1990, approximately 5% of all U.S. deaths were attributed to alcohol use (categorized as a behavioral determinant of health) whereas in 2000, this percentage had decreased to 3.5%. Moreover, in 1990 approximately 4% of all deaths were due to microbial agents and 3% were due to toxic agents (both categorized as environmental determinants of health). However, in 2000 these percentages had dropped to 3.1% and 2.3%, respectively. Additionally, researchers have also identified the health care social determinants of health as being linked to positive health outcomes. For example, Starfield, Shi, and Macinko (2005) discuss the positive relationship between primary care and more positive health outcomes.

In contrast, lifestyle, a variable that is heavily influenced by one's position in the system of social stratification but yet is individually modifiable, plays a highly significant role in health outcomes. Østbye and Taylor (2004), for example, reconfirmed the loss of life years associated with the lifestyle variable tobacco use. Similarly, McGovern et al. (2014) compiled research that empirically measured the contributions of acknowledged determinants of health outcomes into a single table. While the estimates of the percentage contribution of each of the determinants of health outcomes differed, the data suggest that partnerships are not only needed within the arena of healthcare providers and professionals but with persons from other disciplines as well. For example, one study estimated that 50% of all deaths in the United States in 1977 were directly related to modifiable lifestyle factors (U.S. Department of Health and Human Services, 1980). Another study found that lifestyle/behavior contributed 36% to health outcomes (Danaei et al., 2009). Researchers also confirm that each subgroup's position in the system of social stratification intermediates their individual choices and behaviors. Thus, a greater inclusion of social circumstance is present in more recent research on the determinants of health outcomes. Booske et al. (2010), for example, applied empirical analysis and credited social stratification as the source of 40% of health outcomes. Independent of the precise contributions of each variable to health outcomes, empirical data support the conclusion that reductions in health and healthcare disparities require facilitated change in every single area of the determinants of health outcomes.

If 36% to 50% of health outcomes are associated with health behaviors, then why doesn't the United States spend that proportion of health expenditures on behavioral and/or mental health preventions and interventions to change behavior?

Several factors are at play here. First, the public health framework has not defined failure to change an unhealthy behavior as a mental and/or behavioral health problem. Second, it has not identified the processes required to transition the American public's knowledge of what constitutes "healthy" behaviors into behavioral health change.

But isn't it a mental and/or behavioral health problem when people know how to prevent illness and diseases but do not change their nonhealthy behaviors?

It is, indeed. Healthcare administrators, public health personnel, clinicians, and others are uniquely positioned to treat nonadherence to "healthy" behaviors as a behavioral and/or mental health problem and design cognitive behavioral prevention and intervention programs for families that begin with the birth of a child and continue until behavioral change actually occurs. We, the authors, define addictions to unhealthy foods despite knowledge of the impact of such choices on human health as a mental and behavioral health problem that is fully equivalent to a substance use disorder. We define physical activity aversion as a mental and behavioral risk problem.

Are you saying that successful programs of behavioral change can do much to improve health disparities by not mandating change, but rather by supporting individuals in reversing past choosing behaviors that generate positive health outcomes?

Yes, this is one of the implications of this discussion.

But aren't there prevention and intervention programs that have already been implemented by public health professionals?

Yes. However, the failure of an individual to adopt behaviors that support longer life expectancy and wellness over their life span has not yet been defined by American society as a form of behavior that is so irrational as to comprise a mental and/or behavioral health dysfunction. Yet, such a definition is necessary in order to make these behaviors eligible for "treatment" using mental and behavioral health dollars.

But the research indicates that social determinants of health are also major determinants of health outcomes, including health disparities. Right?

Yes. The determinants of health outcomes imply that healthcare administrators and other personnel must partner with schools and other educational systems to assist children, youth, and their parents in accumulating educational capital. Educational capital is needed to support financial investments so that families have non-labor-based income streams. Other information is also needed regarding accumulating income and gaining financial literacy because deficiencies in these areas can lead to families' residency in neighborhoods characterized by smokestacks, landfills, food deserts, medication deserts, and other conditions that adversely impact human health.

Are you saying that the position descriptions of healthcare administrators require broadening in order to link the healthcare sector with appropriate partners to better address health disparities and not merely healthcare disparities?

Yes, indeed.

Chapter Summary

Health and healthcare disparities cannot be viewed from the perspective of a single discipline. Examination of disparities involves philosophy, mathematics, statistics, and history. Before a healthcare administrator, public health professional, or clinician can begin to provide leadership in crafting policies, programs, and initiatives to ensure that their organizational entity does not explicitly or implicitly support avoidable disparities, reflection is required. The purpose of this chapter has been that of stimulating original thought leadership regarding an area in the field of health that is rapidly becoming populated by intellectual clichés. In this regard, this chapter began with a discussion and comparison of alternative definitions of health disparities. It then provided a historical overview that provides an understanding of how current asymmetries in health outcomes emerged. It then introduced concepts from sociology to support the discussion of current definitions of health disparities. Finally, the chapter emphasized the importance of addressing every single determinant of health so that remediable health disparities can be ultimately reduced or eliminated.

Review Questions and Problems

1. Several definitions of health disparities that have been adopted by thought leaders in the field have been introduced in this chapter. Do these definitions have subtle differences in meaning, or do they all have equivalent meanings?

2. If you heard a speaker at a conference make the statement, "These subgroups are blaming others for their health outcomes when they should be blaming themselves!," how would you respond?

3. Do you find yourself leaning more toward structural functionalism or conflict theory? Explain.

4. Review three or more articles about structural functionalism and conflict

theory. Blend both theories together into a new one that can be used to explain health disparities.

5. Were you surprised to discover that health care contributes such a small proportion to health outcomes? Why or why not?

6. Define *health disparities* in your own words.

7. What is the origin of the concept that "All men are created equal"?

8. How does mathematical equality differ from mathematical equivalence?

9. Describe the normal curve.

10. Define *ontology* and *axiology*. How do they differ?

11. Who is considered the "father" of structural functionality? Of conflict theory?

12. List the five determinants of health.

13. Select two studies that examine a determinant of health outcome, such as unhealthy nutrition practices, alcohol consumption, tobacco use, etc. Compare the studies (250 to 350 words).

Key Terms and Concepts

axiology The study of the nature of value and valuation, and of the kinds of things that are valuable (Oxford Dictionary).

conflict theory Assumes that competition and conflict over scarce resources are natural forces between groups and subgroups.

equivalence Relationships between numbers that, although different, are equal in value, effect, force, and/or significance.

ethnocentrism Tendency of people to view their own subgroup as superior and to reject subgroups with different physical, cultural, behavioral, and/or other characteristics.

health disparities Population and subpopulation differences in health outcomes.

health disparities research Emerging field that seeks to identify those areas of health that are characterized by sustained differences in mortality and morbidity across subgroups.

healthcare disparities The differential processes and outcomes that occur within the operation of various components of the healthcare system.

in-group Any group with which an individual identifies; identification is not necessarily based upon race/ethnicity, culture, gender, etc.

nonequivalent inequalities This term references relationships that are mathematically different that do not equate to the same sum. For example, if an individual with hypertension had the same life expectancy as one with out diabetes, it would be an equivalent inequality. If these differences are associated with different life expectancies, it becomes a nonequivalent inequality.

normal curve A bell-shaped curve that shows the probability distribution of a continuous random variable.

ontology The study of the nature of existence, including the nature of things in relationship to each other.

outgroup A group with which an individual does not identify; often accompanied by hostility toward that group.

patriarchy Male-dominant societies.

philosophical anthropology Controversial area of study that uses philosophy (which focuses on the nature of all that is in existence) to study humankind, including intrapersonal and interpersonal relationships and all aspects of people as humans.

population health The study of nonclinical and clinical variables that determine the health outcomes of various groups or subgroups of individuals.

social stratification Basis for a caste or class society in which specific subgroups of people are grouped into categories based on certain characteristics.

structural functionalism A highly partisan approach to systems of social stratification that is supportive of the status quo.

systems of social stratification Societal mechanisms whereby people are positioned in a hierarchy based on their wealth, status, power, prestige, gender, race/ethnicity, and other identifying characteristics.

References

Albuquerque, G. A., de Lima Garcia, C., da Silva Quirino. G., Alves, M. J. H., Belém, J. M., dos Santos Figueiredo, F. W., & Adami, F. (2016). Access to health services by lesbian, gay, bisexual, and transgender persons: Systematic literature review. *BMC International Health and Human Rights*, *16*(2). doi: 10.1186/5/2014-015-0072-9

Alexandre, T. D. S., Corona, L. P., Brito, T. R. P., Santos, J. L. F., Duarte, Y. A. O., & Lebrão, M. L. (2018). Gender differences in the incidence and determinants of components of the frailty phenotype among older adults: Findings from the SABE study. *Journal of Aging and Health*, *30*(2), 190–212.

Ao, H., Dekkers, M. J., Wei, Q., Qiang, C., & Xiao, G. (2013). New evidence for early presence of hominids in North China. *Scientific Reports*, *3*. doi: 10.1038/srep02403

Aquinas, Saint Thomas. (1265–1274 [2007]). Summa theologica. Charleston, SC: Bibliobazaar.

Arjoon, S., Turriago-Hoyos, A., & Thoene, U. (2018). Virtuousness and the common good as a conceptual framework for harmonizing the goals of the individual, organizations, and the economy. *Journal of Business Ethics*, *147*(1), 143–163.

Armitage, D. (2007). *The Declaration of Independence: A global history*. Cambridge, MA: Harvard University Press.

Bizumic, B. (2014). Who coined the concept of ethnocentrism? A brief report. *Journal of Social and Political Psychology*, *2*(1). doi: 10.5964/jspp.v214.264

Booske, B. C., Athens, J. K., Kindig, D. A., Park, H., & Remington, P. L. (2010). Different perspectives for assigning weights to determinants of health. Working paper. University of Wisconsin Population Health Institute, Madison, WI.

Braveman, C. P., & Gottlieb, L. (2014). The social determinants of health. It's time to consider the causes of the causes. *Public Health Reports*, *129*(1), 19–31.

Collier, B. J., & Williams, L. N. (1981). Towards a bilateral model of sexism. *Human Relations*, *34*(2), 127–139.

Danaei, G., Ding, E. L., Mozaffarian, D., Taylor, B., Rehm, J., Murray, C. J., & Ezzati, M. (2009). The preventable causes of death in the United States: Comparative risk assessment of dietary, lifestyle, and metabolic risk factors. *PLoS Med*, *6*(4), 4e1000058b.

Dehlendorf, C., Bryant, A. S., Huddleston, H. G., Jacoby, V. L., & Fujimoto, V. Y. (2010). Health disparities: Definitions and measurements. *American Journal of Obstetrics and Gynecology*, *202*(3), 212, 213.

Dictionary.com. (n.d.). Axiology. Retrieved from http://www.dictionary.com/browse/axiology

Dictionary.com. (n.d.). Normal curve. Retrieved from http://www.dictionary.com/browse/normal-curve

Dictionary.com. (n.d.). Ontology. Retrieved from http://www.dictionary.com/browse/ontology

FreeDictionary. (n.d.). Normal curve. Retrieved from http://www.thefreedictionary.com/normal+curve

Gibbons, A. (2006). *The first human: The race to discover our earliest ancestors*. New York: Doubleday.

Hadley, J. (1982). *More medical care, better health?: An economic analysis of mortality rates*. Washington, DC: Urban Institute Press.

Hillier, T. (1997*). Sourcebook on public international law*. London & Sydney: Cavendish Publishing.

Hooks, B. (2004). *The will to change: Men, masculinity, and love*. New York: Washington Square Press.

Howard, J. (2016, October 26). Racism in medicine: An 'open secret'. Retrieved from https://www.cnn.com/2016/10/26/health/doctors-discrimination-racism/index.html

Hu, J., Schreiber, M., Jordan J., George, D. L., & Nerenz, D. (2017). Associations between community sociodemographics and performance in HEDIS quality measures: A study of 22 medical centers in a primary care network. *American Journal of Medical Quality*, *33*(1), 5–13.

James, S. A. (2017). The strangest of all encounters: Racial and ethnic discrimination in U.S. health care. *Cadernos de saúde pública*, *33*(Suppl 1). doi: 10.1590/0102-3113X00104416

Leng, G., & Partridge, G. (2018). Achieving high-quality care: A view from NICE (The National Institute for Health and Care Excellence). *Heart*, *104*(1), 10–15.

Lenski, G. E. (1984). *Power and privilege: A theory of social stratification*. Chapel Hill: University of North Carolina Press.

McGovern, L., Miller, G., & Hughes-Cromwick, P. (2014). The relative contribution of multiple determinants to health outcomes. Health Policy Brief. Retrieved from https://www.rwjf.org/en/library/research/2014/08/the-relative-contribution-of-multiple-determinants-to-health-out.html

Merriam-Webster. (n.d.). Axiology. Retrieved from http://www.merriam-webster.com/dictionary/axiology

Merriam-Webster. (n.d.). Ontology. Retrieved from http://www.merriam-webster.com/dictionary/ontology

Ong, A. D., Cerrada, C. J., Lee, R. A., & Williams, D. R. (2017). Stigma consciousness, racial microaggression, and sleep disturbance among Asian Americans. *Asian American Journal of Psychology*, *8*(1), 72–81.

Østbye, T., & Taylor, D. H. (2004). The effect of smoking on years of healthy life (YHL) lost among middle-aged and older Americans. *Health Services Research*, *39*(3), 532–551.

Oxford Dictionaries. (n.d.). Ontology. Retrieved from http://www.oxforddictionaries.com/us/definition/american_english/ontology

Parsons, T. (1951). *The social system*. London: Routledge.

Penner, L. A., Dovidio, J. F., West, T. V., Gaertner, S. L., Albrecht, T. C., Dailey, R. K., & Mankova, T. (2010). Aversive racism and medical interactions with Black patients: A field study. *Journal of Experimental Social Psychology, 46*(2), 436–440.

Pihlstrom, S. (2003). On the concept of philosophical anthropology. *Journal of Philosophical Research, 28*(1), 259–286.

Potter, T. (2018). Shifting the paradigm: Educating nurse administrators to be full partners. *Journal of Nursing Administration, 1*, 1–2.

Scheidel, W. (2007). The Roman slave supply. Princeton /Stanford Working Papers in Classics. Retrieved from https://www.princeton.edu/~pswpc/pdfs/scheidel /050704.pdf

Sears, A. (2005). *A good book, in theory: A guide to theoretical thinking.* Peterborough, ON: Broadview Press.

Starfield, B., Shi, L., & Macinko, J. (2005) Contribution of primary care to health systems and health. *Milbank Q.* Sep *83*(3), 457–502.

Steptoe, A., Peacey, V., & Wardle, J. (2006). Sleep duration and health in young adults. *Archives of Internal Medicine, 166*(16), 1689–1692.

Streed, C. B., McCarthy, E. P., & Haas, J. S. (2017). Association between gender minority status and self-reported physical and mental health status in the United States. *JAMA Internal Medicine, 177*(8), 1210–1212.

Suarez-Balcazar, Y., Mirza, M. P., & Garcia-Ramirez, M. (2018). Health disparities: Understanding and promoting healthy communities. *Journal of Prevention and Intervention in the Community, 48*, 1–6.

Sumner, W. G. (1906). *Folkways: A study of the sociological importance of usages, manners, customers, mores and morals.* Boston: The Athenæum Press.

Tattersall, I. (1997). Out of Africa again ... and again? *Scientific American, 276*(4), 60–67.

U.S. Department of Health and Human Services, Office of Minority Health, National Partnership for Action to End Health Disparities. (2011). Glossary of terms. Retrieved from https://minorityhealth.hhs.gov/npa/

U.S. Department of Health and Human Services, Public Health Service. (1980). Ten leading causes of death in the United States. Atlanta: Bureau of State Services.

U.S. National Library of Medicine. (n.d.). Health disparities. Retrieved from https://www.nlm.nih.gov /hsrinfo/disparities.html

United Nations General Assembly. (1948). Universal Declaration of Human Rights. Retrieved from http:// www.un.org/en/universal-declaration-human-rights/

World Health Organization. (2008). *Closing the gap in a generation: Health equity through action on the social determinants of health. Final report of the Commission on Social Determinants of Health.* Geneva: World Health Organization.

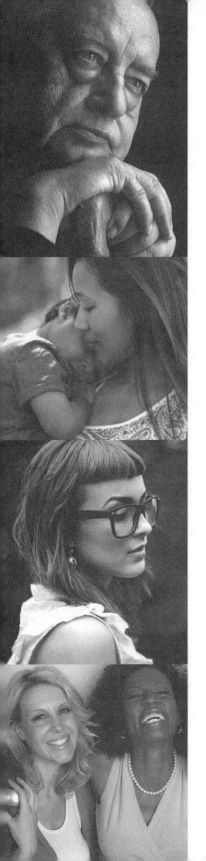

PART II

Researching and Assessing Health Disparities

"Research is creating new knowledge."

—**Neil Armstrong** (1930-2012), Apollo 11 Astronaut

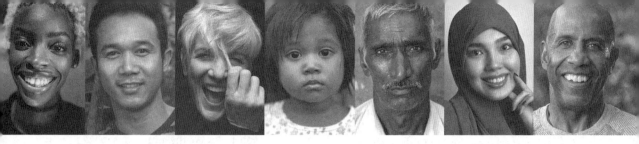

CHAPTER 3

How to Conduct Research on Health Disparities

"Research is to see what everybody else has seen, and to think what nobody else has thought."

—**Albert Szent-Gyorgyi** (1893-1986), a winnner of the Nobel Prize in Physiology or Medicine in 1937

Xan Goodman

LEARNING OBJECTIVES

After completing this chapter, each learner will be able to:

- Describe the value of working with a librarian who has been trained in public health, health science, or education.
- Summarize why excellent research skills are needed in order to access information that can be integrated into original thought in the area of health and healthcare disparities.
- Describe and use resources, tips, and tricks that will allow you to quickly access the health disparities information that you are seeking.
- Differentiate informational resources that are available for free on the web from those that must be accessed via a library affiliated with a college/university.
- Cite and use key databases that allow access to classic as well as the most recent academic articles, books, and government publications in the area of health disparities. We urge the reader to have access to a computer to be able to follow the directions to get the most from this chapter.

▶ Introduction

The field of health and healthcare disparities is, indeed, one that requires both a breadth and depth of knowledge that includes, but is not limited to, traditional disciplinary boundaries. While such a statement is, in some respects, applicable to all fields of study, it is particularly important when the goal of the inquiry is that of repositioning thought and scholarship in a field so that humankind can be better served.

▶ The Criticality of Access to a Librarian Trained in Health Science or Medicine for Health and Healthcare Disparity Research

Health and education are two highly critical areas of "investment" that have, in the past, advanced humankind. When searching for areas in which customized strategies are needed in order to prevent, intervene, screen and diagnose, treat, and administer programs that promote improvements in the length and quality of life of all humankind, the "ingredients" used are highly critical. Thus, access is needed to the best possible research.

Accordingly, the goal of this chapter is to help you, as a learner, discover resources, tips, and tricks to facilitate your research processes as you seek to develop your own views regarding health and healthcare disparities. Of course, you already know how to conduct research, but do you *really* know how to complete research? Are you guilty of relying on single-box searching (i.e., Google), using keywords and the single search box to locate scholarly articles? Be truthful! You probably think that the use of the single search box and keywords is perfectly fine. Do you already know how to "massage" the single search box to retrieve results related to your topic? Although you may be familiar with a few of the resources that are available freely on the web, have you accessed the numerous books and articles on health disparities that are available from your affiliated library? Are you familiar with the many subscription-based databases that are paid for by academic libraries to support the research of faculty and students at your institution? Did you know that your library offers a wide array of hidden resources that are not readily discoverable using a tool such as Google or Google Scholar? If you answered "no" to any one of these questions, you now understand the importance of this chapter.

But how do we learn about these resources?

Your best option with research is to contact a *trained librarian*. To emphasize this point, allow us for a moment to pull the veil off the "librarian mystique." In addition to training in library and information science, some librarians have earned disciplinary degrees in public health, science, education, and/or other related fields. Librarians at research universities will have completed a terminal degree in library and information science and will know about indexes and taxonomies and have specialized skills related to research inquiry that enable these individuals to assist researchers at all levels. Health science or medical librarians are frequently members of the Academy of Health Information Professionals (AHIP) and, as is true for public health practitioners, must annually complete up to eight continuing education credits each year. Thus, these types of librarians are a foundational resource for any researcher seeking to delve into the literature on health and healthcare disparities.

How can I arrange to work with these types of librarians?

First, at your home university, identify the name of the research librarian. Then make an appointment to learn about library resources on your campus. Librarians are frequently available for individual research consultations, to teach workshops related to resources, or to aid in serving as an advocate for the addition of needed journals or article databases that will support your work in health disparities. Now that we have pulled the veil off of librarianship, let's take a look at some freely available web-based resources to aid you in your health disparities research.

▶ Government Resources

This section presents government-based resources that are free and accessible using any Internet browser. Throughout this chapter, we will sprinkle quick search tips to help you better utilize single search boxes in your research process. Please note that you will get the most from this chapter if you are sitting at a computer and able to apply concepts as they are presented.

The National Library of Medicine

The **National Library of Medicine** (https://www.nlm.nih.gov) provides a variety of tools that can assist health and healthcare disparities researchers in their efforts. One well-known tool produced and maintained by the National Library of Medicine is **PubMed**. **MEDLINE** is the underlying database that "seeds" PubMed. You will see MEDLINE in some other paid article databases because the MEDLINE data are freely available from the National Library of Medicine for developers to create different applications using the data.

PubMed is the standard go-to resource for researchers searching biomedical literature. However, PubMed might not always be the best choice when searching for health disparities literature due to the sociobehavioral dimensions of health disparities questions.

How can I use PubMed?

PubMed (https://www.ncbi.nlm.nih.gov/pubmed/) indexes articles based on **Medical Subject Headings (MeSH)**. Biomedical literature indexed in PubMed is allocated to MeSH subject headings to aid in the discovery of their content (U.S. National Library

of Medicine, 2017b). As of January 2018, more than 28 million citations were indexed in PubMed (U.S. National Library of Medicine, 2017c). One thing to remember about PubMed is that there are no **full-texts** (i.e., the complete article) in the database. Users are provided links to freely available full-text articles or linked back to their home university library to obtain full-text material.

Another National Library of Medicine tool you may select to use is **Topic-Specific Queries** (https://www.nlm.nih.gov/bsd/special_queries.html). Topic-Specific Queries provide links to specific subsets of topics and will link you to a range of health disparity–related topics, such as queries specific to AIDS research, Healthy People 2020, health disparities, health literacy, and other health services research (HSR) queries (U.S. National Library of Medicine, 2016).

Can you provide an example?

Yes. Let's take a look at two types of resources linked through the National Library of Medicine: Minority Information Health Outreach and Health Services Research & Public Health.

U.S. Department of Health and Human Services Minority Information Health Outreach

FIGURE 3.1 shows the main screen for the National Library of Medicine web portal (https://www.nlm.nih.gov/). From the main page, click "Resources For You" drop-down menu, you will see six options; click "For Healthcare Professionals." It will take you to a page as shown in **FIGURE 3.2**. Click "Explore NLM" at the top, and then select "Health information." Under the "Specific Populations" heading, you will see a link to "Minority Health Information Outreach." Click that link and you will have access to resources covering the topic of minority health for four specific populations: African American, Alaska Native, American Indian, and Hispanic American

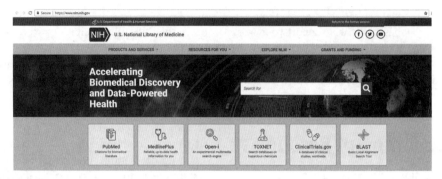

FIGURE 3.1 National Library of Medicine web portal.

Courtesy of National Library of Medicine.

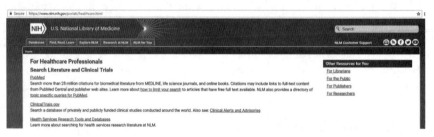

FIGURE 3.2 For Health Professionals web portal.

Courtesy of National Library of Medicine.

(see **FIGURE 3.3**). Each set of items will vary in content. You will find links to previous studies and reports about communities, ongoing studies, as well as other details. This content will change and be updated over time.

Health Services Research & Public Health

Back to the page as shown in Figure 3.2, click "Research at NLM," select the heading "Health Services Research & Public Health." You will land on the following page: Health Services Research & Public Health Information Programs (https://www.nlm.nih.gov/hsrph.html). This page is divided into six sections: (1) Collaborative Projects, (2) Databases, (3) Queries/Searches, (4) Outreach and Training, (5) Publications, and (6) Informatics. **FIGURE 3.4** shows the top part of the screen you will see.

A trove of resources related to health disparities can be found on this page. Here, we will highlight the Health Disparities link and then explore additional links in another section of this chapter. To view health disparities as a topic, look under the heading "Collaborative Projects," and then select "HSR Information Central: A Health Services Research Portal." Two lists of topics appear on this page: "HSR General Resources" and "HSR Topics." Under the heading "HSR Topics," select "Health Disparities." After you select "Health Disparities," you will see the screen shown in **FIGURE 3.5**. We recommend bookmarking this page with your preferred Internet browser. If you wish to receive content updates about health disparities, submit your e-mail for e-mail updates from the upper right box (Email Updates).

What do I do now?

On the same page of Health Disparities, you will see ten bullet points in a purple box. Select the first one, "Search Queries Using NLM Resources: Health Disparities," which will have two subsections below it. Clicking on

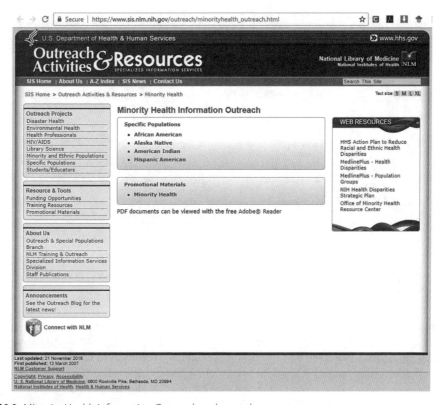

FIGURE 3.3 Minority Health information Outreach web portal.
Courtesy of US Department of Health and Human Services.

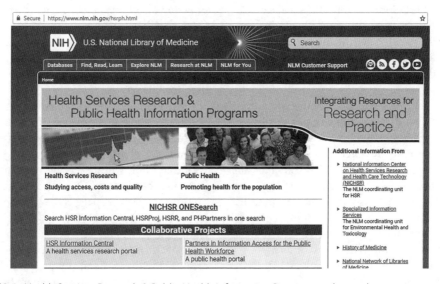

FIGURE 3.4 Health Services Research & Public Health Information Programs web portal.
Courtesy of National Library of Medicine.

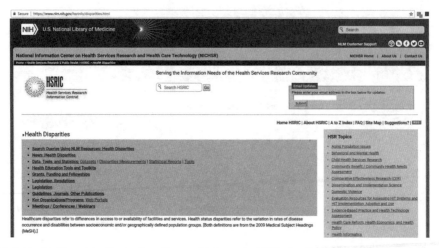

FIGURE 3.5 Health Disparities Topics from National Information Center on Health Services Research Information Central.

Courtesy of National Library of Medicine.

the first subsection - "HSRProj (Health Services Research Projects in Progress): Projects on Health Disparities" will take you to results based on the following queries:

> "Health disparities" OR "healthcare disparities" OR "health status disparities" OR inequality OR inequalities OR inquiries OR inequity OR inequitable OR inequitably OR "socioeconomic factors" OR "minority groups" OR "social determinants of health" OR racism OR exist OR ages OR "ethnic groups"

As you can see, this query includes terminology related to the topic of health disparities. It will compile a list of current and past health disparity research projects, as well as those in progress. The items will include the title, investigator, organization, agency, and country. You can also view the resulting list of projects from different funding agencies, such as American Cancer Society, the National Institutes of Health (NIH), and others.

The second subsection is - "MEDLINE®/ PubMed® Search and Health Disparities & Minority Health Information Resources."

This link will take you to a list of resources that provide health information on several minority communities. What is most helpful to a researcher on this page is the MEDLINE/ PubMed health disparities Search. **FIGURE 3.6** shows you the top part of this page.

When you are brainstorming terms related to minority health and healthcare disparities, the search strategy just described will provide you with synonyms and other related terms to enhance your search strategy. To view the full search strategy, visit "see the details of the search strategy" as shown in Figure 3.6, where you can find a list of terms that were used for this search.

At this point, let us return to Figure 3.5 and take a look at the "Data, Tools, and Statistics: Datasets | Disparities Measurements | Statistical Reports | Tools." Clicking on "Datasets" link will direct you to many publicly available datasets. One of the most useful links on the Dataset page is the Compendium of Publicly Available Datasets and Other Data-Related Resources.

Specifically, there is a PDF document created by the Federal Interagency Health Equity Team (FIHET) and lists more than 100 different publicly available datasets or data

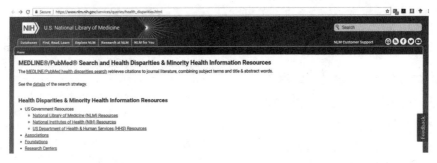

FIGURE 3.6 MEDLINE®/PubMed® Search and Health Disparities & Minority Health Information Resources.
Courtesy of National Library of Medicine.

resources from federal agencies, including the U.S. Census Bureau.

While I'm following you, this may be complicated for some of my classmates. Can you offer any tips?

Yes, I can do that for you. Check out **QUICK TIP 3.1**.

QUICK TIP 3.1

If you are searching at PubMed.gov (https://www.ncbi.nlm.nih.gov/pubmed/), a data-related search option is available. To use it, enter your query into the search box and click search button. On the right of the screen, you will see a box called "Find related data," as shown below.

Now, from the drop-down menu select a type of related data. Next, search and retrieve the results.

Let's continue with a review of the resources shown in Figure 3.5. Under the "Guidelines, Journals, Other Publications" link, you will find both **legacy** (i.e., old documents) and recent reports on health disparity topics. You now have access to more research than you can possibly use. Let's review some other sources now.

HealthReach: Health Information in Many Languages

HealthReach (https://healthreach.nlm.nih.gov) provides patient information in more than 60 languages but not all topics are in every language. Topics related to health disparities cover stress management, weight management, addiction, and more. Information is available for providers to learn cultural background information and other tools.

U.S. Department of Health and Human Services Office of Minority Health

The Office of Minority Health (https://minorityhealth.hhs.gov/) has been in existence since the mid-1980s and was responsible for publishing the seminal Heckler Report, also known as *Secretary's Task Force Report on Black Minority Health* (U.S. Department of Health and Human Services, Office of Minority Health, n.d.). Numerous reports, widgets, datasets, and other resources are linked from the Office of Minority Health website. You may also locate information on standards for cultural competency via links to the Center for Linguistic and Cultural Competency in Health Care.

The U.S. Department of Health and Human Services provides minority health information for four population groups: African Americans, Alaska Natives, American Indians, and Hispanic

Americans. You can learn more about these minority health resources at https://sis.nlm.nih.gov/outreach/minorityhealth_outreach.html.

American Indian and Alaska Native Health Portal and the Arctic Health Portal

Two significant portals of health information are the American Indian and Alaska Native Health (https://americanindianhealth.nlm.nih.gov/) and the Arctic Health (https://arctichealth.nlm.nih.gov/). Each of these portals provides a central source for information about the health and well-being of these populations.

Minority Health and Equity Archive

The Minority Health and Equity Archive (http://health-equity.lib.umd.edu/) hosted by the University of Maryland was first published in 2002. The archive has an emphasis on health equity for all populations. Five broad topics are available to search using advanced or basic search: Minority Health, Health, Practice, Research and Teaching. Documents include special collections focused on populations who have experienced health disparities and links to government publications related to health equity.

This is all very helpful! Any other tips?

This would be a good time to check out **QUICK TIP 3.2**.

> ### QUICK TIP 3.2
>
> Did you know that databases will sometimes have a thesaurus specific to that resource? Try using an available thesaurus to expand your search vocabulary. We recommend accessing AgeLine (https://health.ebsco.com/products/ageline) and EMBASE (https://www.elsevier.com/solutions/embase-biomedical-research) as examples.

▶ Article Databases

Article databases provide indexing, abstracts, and sometimes the full-text content. The following databases require a library subscription and are not freely available on the Internet. They form part of the "hidden web" of content that is unable to be discovered using an Internet search engine. The following article databases are available by subscription through your university library (the databases discussed here were accessed from the authors' affiliated university library websites):

- *AgeLine* covers social gerontological issues for populations older than 50 years. If you are particularly interested in long-term care disparities, for example, you might choose to use this resource.
- *EMBASE* is useful for health disparities research because of the international perspective and wide range of coverage, including biomedical, allied health, and medical content. EMBASE content is indexed using the EMTREE taxonomy. This is different from MeSH but similar in that EMTREE is the indexing thesaurus that undergirds the EMBASE content.
- *Ethnic Newswatch* (https://www.proquest.com/products-services/ethnic_newswatch.html) offers minority, ethnic, and native global perspectives. It also offers multidisciplinary coverage of magazines, newspapers, and scholarly journals for these populations.
- *Global Health* published by CABI (https://www.cabi.org/publishing-products/online-information-resources/global-health/) is one of the only dedicated public health databases. Global Health indexes journals, books, and reports and also can help you locate conference literature.
- *PsycINFO* (http://www.apa.org/pubs/databases/psycinfo/index.aspx) is a database produced by the American Psychological Association (APA). It dates back to the 19th century and contains a

mixture of books, book chapters, scholarly articles, and dissertations. If your health disparities topic has a psychological component, select PsycINFO to retrieve materials. As the role of behavioral change elevates in importance in the health disparity field, PsycINFO will become even more valued.

- *Web of Science* (https://clarivate.com/products/web-of-science/), formerly known as Web of Knowledge, covers the sciences and social sciences with its indexed content. Web of Science is an excellent choice to examine sociobehavioral aspects of health disparities. One particularly useful feature to assist you with tracking the literature is "Times Cited." You can use Times Cited to track how frequently a paper is cited and to view additional indexing and abstracting details for papers citing the tracked scholarly article.

Any more Quick Tips?

Check out **QUICK TIP 3.3** for information on interfaces.

QUICK TIP 3.3

As you search university library databases, you will frequently see different interfaces for each database. These interfaces represent the various vendors and their branding. Each vendor will offer tutorials, search tips, and other help pages to guide you through their interface. EBSCOhost is frequently the interface platform available at academic libraries. This tool offers a specialized thesaurus for indexing scholarly journals, books, and dissertations.

▶ Google and Google Scholar

We mentioned earlier that many students live in a single-search-box world. Two of the most widely used single search boxes are those on

Google and Google Scholar-an online resource that allows users to access scholarly articles, books, papers, and other materials, etc. To get the most out of either of these widely used tools, you should learn the tips that can help you to retrieve better and more relevant results. Google and Google Scholar offer much more beyond the single search box.

Researchers frequently start a search with either Google or Google Scholar. Consider the following example. Perhaps you have an interest in health disparities among persons treated by Nigerian traditional healers. How would you find information on these healers? Sometimes, reports generated in the country of interest or global reports by agencies such as the World Health Organization will contain relevant information. Scholarly articles move through the publication pipeline slowly. Moreover, the interval to the time of publication of scholarly materials means that one may not find details about the topic in the academic literature.

A search on Google or Google Scholar using the syntax for "filetype" can help you locate reports not found in the scholarly literature. For example, a filetype syntax search such as "health care disparities Asian filetype pdf" will retrieve publications in a PDF format (see **FIGURE 3.7**).

Sometimes unpublished information on a topic will be available as a PowerPoint. A similar search using the syntax "filetype ppt" will retrieve PowerPoint presentations (see **FIGURE 3.8**). Syntax searches in Google or Google Scholar are extremely effective in extracting unpublished information.

Strategies are also available to find published data or charts using Google. For example, to find images of charts and other data related to your topic, you would perform the search in google and then click "images" under the search bar or simply do it in https://images.google.com/. When you get to the results page with all associated images, you can also select "Tools" to view more options such as size, color, or time to narrow down your search (see **FIGURE 3.9**). Then, navigate to

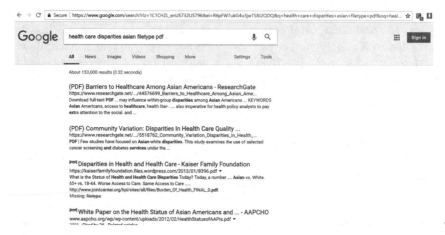

FIGURE 3.7 Google filetype pdf syntax search.

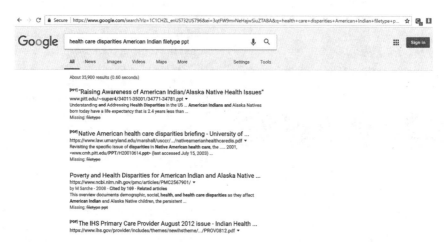

FIGURE 3.8 Google filetype ppt syntax search.

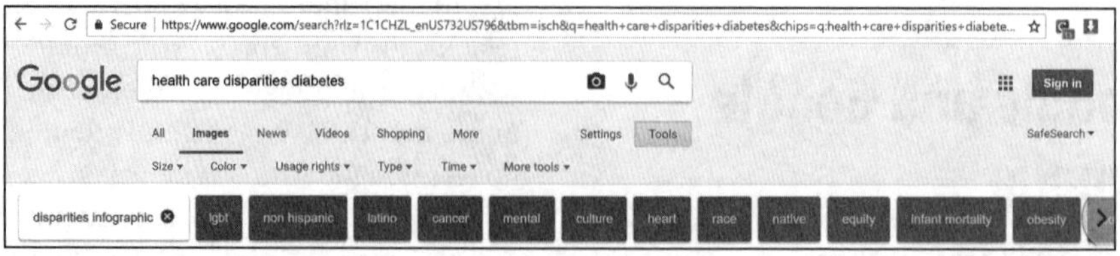

FIGURE 3.9 Google Image Search.

any image to view the source. This is a particularly useful tip for identifying data on challenging topics.

Google In Site Search

Have you ever tried a Google in site search? As you know, retrieving information from government websites such as the Centers for Disease Control and Prevention (CDC; https://www.cdc.gov) can sometimes be unwieldy. One way to refine a search (if you know the information you will need) within a particular website is to perform an **in site search**. To perform this search, you must have a website in mind. Here is an example. Say that you are interested in stress and health disparities in site: www.cdc.gov (see **FIGURE 3.10**). This search will retrieve information which mentioned the keywords you searched from within the CDC website. An in site search can be applied to any website.

Google Scholar Linking

As you are aware, Google Scholar is an excellent tool to retrieve scholarly literature on the open Internet. However, you can run into a "paywall." We are sure you are familiar with finding a perfect article and then being asked to pay money to access it. This set of circumstances comprises a **paywall**. If you are a faculty member, student, or staff person at a university, your university library will offer a borrowing service for a small fee, or the library will offer a free service that allows you to request articles from other libraries. This service is often referred to as an *interlibrary loan* (ILL).

Another way to discover content that your affiliated institution subscribes to is to use *Library Linking* in Google Scholar. University libraries provide their IP addresses to Google, and this facilitates a linking process to identify affiliated faculty, staff, and students of an institution. To setup Library Linking, you must login to your Google Scholar account. Look for the three bars in the upper left-hand corner of the screen; click these bars to view the other options. (You will also need the gear icon Settings option; see **FIGURE 3.11**.) Select the Settings icon, and then look for "Library Links" (see **FIGURE 3.12**).

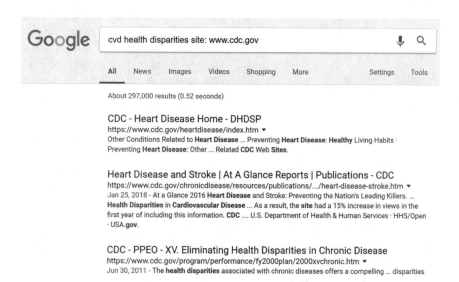

FIGURE 3.10 Google in site search results from the CDC.

Click the "Library Links" hyperlink. A window will open to a screen with a search box. Now enter your university library name in the search box. If your institution has shared its information with Google, you will see your institution's name and a checkbox. Check the box next to your institution's name and save your settings. Once you have done this, when searching Google Scholar away from your campus you will see links to your institution in your search results.

Google Scholar Advanced Search

Google Scholar has an Advanced Search option. Most research begins at the top of the funnel. That is, it begins with the broad results and tries to capture as much information about a topic as necessary. However, there are times when a search requires specificity. The fields available in Advanced Search are self-explanatory (see **FIGURE 3.13**). Hopefully, you can see how the options will deliver the specificity that your unique health disparity research may require.

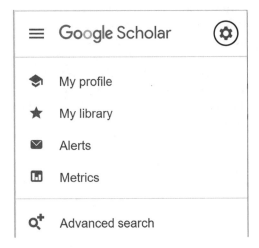

FIGURE 3.11 Google Scholar settings.

Chapter Summary

In this chapter, you were encouraged to learn the name of your health science or medical librarian and meet with this individual. Health science librarians are trained in information science and sometimes have disciplinary credentials. They may be available for one-on-one meetings and can advocate for the addition of information sources to your institution. This chapter also covered free resources available from the U.S. National Library of Medicine and information resources from other agencies that focus on issues of health equity and health disparities. Your search bandwidth should increase now that you can move beyond a single search box to use specialized thesauruses found in subscription article databases or PubMed. This chapter also described six licensed databases that can be used to find health disparity research. An explanation of syntax searching was provided to retrieve better results from Google and Google Scholar. You learned how to utilize settings in Google Scholar to make licensed hidden content discoverable off-campus. Last, you moved beyond the single box of Google

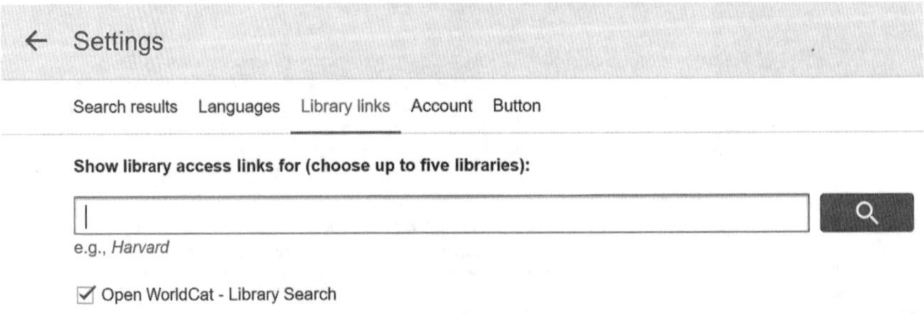

← Settings

Search results Languages Library links Account Button

Show library access links for (choose up to five libraries):

e.g., *Harvard*

☑ Open WorldCat - Library Search

FIGURE 3.12 Google Scholar library links.

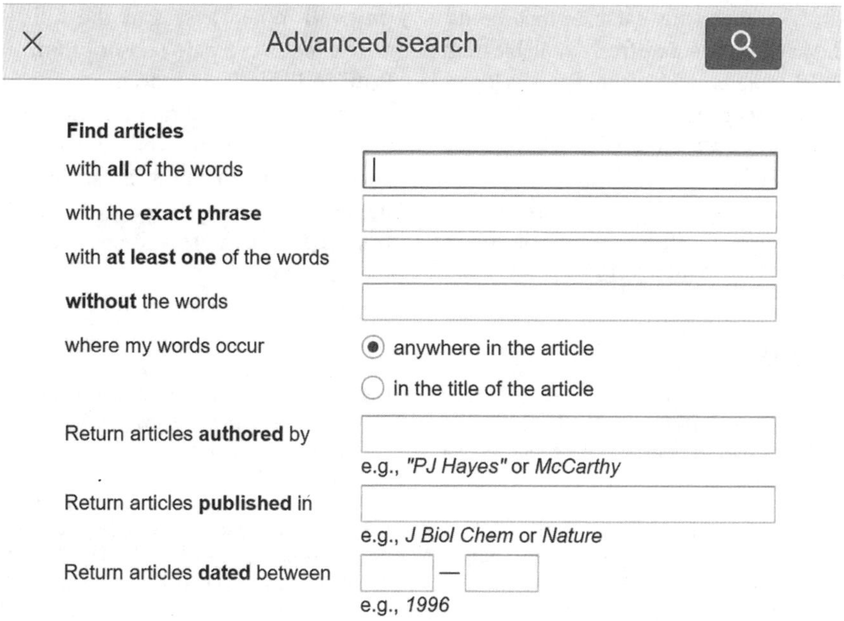

FIGURE 3.13 Google Scholar advanced search features.

Scholar to the Advanced Search option. These new tools in your toolbox will now allow you to break free from the single search box and find health disparity research that meets your informational needs and supports you in the formulation of original thought on the various case subjects.

Review Questions and Problems

1. Conduct a search for articles on one of the following topics:
   - The history of tribal conflict in _____ (any country of your choice).
   - Disparities in maternal health by income in _____ (any country of your choice).
   - Any topic of your choice.

2. Utilizing the strategies described in this chapter, create a file with abstracts of the articles you have selected. Now answer the questions below regarding the search process.

   a. Did you find it difficult to follow the direction in this chapter? Why or why not?
   b. Do you plan to utilize these research strategies in other classes?
   c. Can you read and understand these abstracts?

3. List three search engines where you commonly use "single-box" search strategies.

4. Perform an "in site" search on Google.

Key Terms and Concepts

full-text Access to the complete text of an article in a database.

in site search Google search strategy that enables the user to limit a search to a particular website.

legacy Older documents on health disparity topics.

Medical Subject Headings (MeSH) Syntax by which PubMed indexes articles to aid in the discovery of their content.

MEDLINE The underlying database that "seeds" PubMed. MEDLINE data are freely available from the National Library of Medicine for developers to create different applications using the data.

National Library of Medicine The federal agency responsible for many of the free tools that health and healthcare disparities researchers can use in their research efforts. Among its many offerings, it provides MEDLINE/PubMed.

paywall When access to the full text of an article requires a paid subscription.

PubMed The free search engine supported by the National Library of Medicine that is based on the MEDLINE database of references and abstracts on life sciences and biomedical topics.

topic-specific queries Provide links to specific subsets of topics.

References

U.S. Department of Health and Human Services, Office of Minority Health. (n.d.). About OMH. (August 23, 2016). Retrieved from https://minorityhealth.hhs.gov /omh/browse.aspx?lvl=2&lvlid=1

U.S. National Library of Medicine. (2016). Directory of topic-specific PubMed queries. Retrieved from https://www.nlm.nih.gov/bsd/special_queries.html

U.S. National Library of Medicine. (2017a). MEDLINE /PubMed health disparities and minority health search strategy. Retrieved from https://www.nlm.nih .gov/services/queries/health_disparities_details.html

U.S. National Library of Medicine. (2017b). MESH. Retrieved from https://www.nlm.nih.gov/pubs /factsheets/mesh.html

U.S. National Library of Medicine. (2017c). PubMed. Retrieved from https://www.ncbi.nlm.nih.gov/pubmed/

U.S. National Library of Medicine. (2017d). Fact sheet: PubMed, MEDLINE retrieval on the World Wide Web. Retrieved from https://www.nlm.nih.gov/pubs /factsheets/pubmed.html

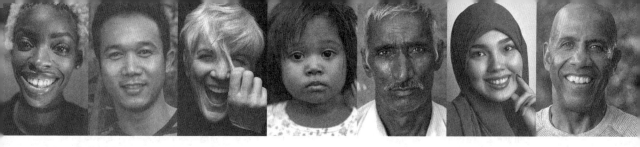

CHAPTER 4

Data Sources to Study Health and Healthcare Disparities

"Statistics is the grammar of science."

—**Karl Pearson** (1857–1936), an English mathematician and biostatistician

▶ Introduction

Unequal outcomes exist across various subgroups in American society specifically and in the global society in general. Moreover, these disparate outcomes may reflect differences in the characteristics of the groups and subgroups that are related to health. In order for healthcare administrators, public health workers, clinicians, policy makers, and other professionals to understand the causes of these disparities, key sets of data are needed. In addition, various statistical tools must be applied to these sets of data in order to allow the data to "tell the story." Accordingly, this chapter introduces a number of datasets and demonstrates very simple statistical methodologies that will allow a future or current healthcare administrator, public health professional, clinician, or other professional to extract information from the data available from these sources.

▶ Primary Versus Secondary Data

National datasets are typically used to gain information on *health* disparities. In contrast, analysis of *healthcare* disparities requires the use of data collected by each unique component of the healthcare delivery system, such as medical practices and/or medical systems, hospitals, nursing homes, organ transplant programs, etc. Thus, the identification of health disparities begins with the assembly and/or collection of data. Two types of data can be used. These data (and yes, the word *data* is plural) are primary data and secondary data.

Primary data can be defined as information that a researcher collects directly from an original source in order to answer one or more research questions. Healthcare organizations generate primary data that can be used to assess healthcare disparities.

Secondary data reference the use of data that was collected by someone else for their own purpose but that also can be used for other research purposes. In order to identify health disparities between various population groups or subgroups at the national level, secondary data collected by the public sector is oftentimes used.

Could you provide some examples?

If a current or prospective healthcare administrator decided to collect data on the cultural and individual values of every consumer served in order to relate their values, attitudes, and beliefs to their individual health outcomes, the data compiled comprises primary data. In contrast, if data from the Census Bureau were used to analyze the characteristics of the persons from whom a community-based health center's patients were drawn, the information used would be classified as secondary data.

Both types of data have their advantages and disadvantages. The greatest disadvantages to the collection of primary data are the costs involved and the risk that the data have a low probability of truly reflecting the universe from which it is drawn because of poor sampling strategies. As a result, most efforts to identify health disparities begin with the identification of secondary datasets. Strict guidelines are applied to the process of collecting secondary data in order to ensure that the data used are of high quality. As such, we recommend: *(1) do not use secondary sources of secondary data, and (2) only use primary sources of secondary data.*

Excuse me?

We mean whether seeking to identify healthcare disparities and/or engaging in inquiry regarding another issue, only *primary sources of secondary data* should be used when secondary sources are selected for data collection and use.

When is a source considered to be a primary source of secondary data?

The original person or organization that collected the data is the primary source. For example, the U.S. Census Bureau is the primary source of its data. The Centers for Disease Control and Prevention and the National Center for Health Statistics are key primary sources of secondary data on health care. Using primary sources of secondary data protects against errors that may have been incorporated when data are cited by someone else and then used by the student, researcher, healthcare administrator, public health professional, clinician, policy analyst, or other professional.

▶ Key Sources of Secondary Data on Health Outcomes

A number of primary sources of secondary data exist that can be used to identify health disparities on deaths and death rates as well as in the incidence of disease and illness. Some of these sources are listed in **BOX 4.1.**

- National Vital Statistics System (https:// www.cdc.gov/nchs/nvss/index.htm)
- Compressed Mortality File (https://www .cdc.gov/nchs/data_access/cmf.htm)
- Surveillance Epidemiology and END Results (SEER) (https://seer.cancer .gov/)
- National Longitudinal Mortality Study (NLMS) (https://www.census.gov/did /www/nlms/)
- The World Bank (http://www.worldbank .org/)
- World Health Organization (WHO) Mortality Database (http://www.who.int /healthinfo/mortality_data/en/)
- Henry J. Kaiser Foundation (https://www .kff.org/)
- Human Mortality Database (http://www .mortality.org/)

The process of data analysis is a tedious activity. But, when the highest quality data are used, it becomes revelatory.

What do you mean by "revelatory"?

By "revelatory" we mean that the data reveal new trends, patterns, and information. It is thrilling to form a hypothesis regarding key healthcare variables, to enter the data into a statistical program, and to then examine the findings to determine whether that work has added to the world's understanding of even the smallest of human problems. *Not a single area of health care, education, sociology, and/ or any other field can be advanced without the use of data to serve as both a metaphorical light and roadmap to guide humankind forward!* However, continual quality improvements are needed in the data that are used to create new knowledge in every single field.

What are some areas in which better data are needed to answer current and continuing quality issues in health care?

More and better quality data must be converted into information and knowledge so that healthcare administrators, public health professionals, clinicians, policy makers, and individuals and families can assess health outcomes, systemic contributions by other social systems to those health outcomes, the effectiveness of interventions that are designed to advance health, and to answer other questions.

Where does one obtain these needed data?

There are so very many sources of data. National surveys such as some of those noted have been major sources of data. The electronic medical records that are now used by virtually every medical provider are rich sources of data. Health insurance companies and managed care organizations generate new data every single time an insurance claim is submitted and processed. For several decades, information on certain diseases has been maintained through disease registries, such as those for cancer, organ transplantation, etc.

Virtually every single department and office of the U.S. Department of Health and Human Services has a listing on its website of the data that it collects. For example, the Centers for Medicare and Medicaid Services (CMS) collects and manages a number of datasets. Likewise, the National Institute on Drug Abuse (NIDA), the Agency for Healthcare Research and Quality (AHRQ), and other federal and state-level entities also manage datasets available to the public.

In addition, health organizations collect high-quality healthcare data. For example, the National Association of Health Data Organizations (NAHDO) maintains datasets on insurance. Private organizations that have completed large clinical trials also maintain data.

An additional challenge, and potential frustration, for surveillance, reporting, and therefore responding to, or preventing health disparities has to do with definitions. Readers should pay close attention to how (and whether) data sources define some specific terms that will impact their interpretation, and the ability to compare across data sets or over time. Examples of this include: disability (which will often lump together physical, mental health, intellectual, chronic, acute and aging-related despite the dramatic differences in how these impact individuals), Hispanic versus Latino (people may identify as one but not the other), and binary gender choices (which while not technically have a definitional issue, impacts data collection and therefore our understanding of disparity-related issues).

What should one look for in selecting a large secondary database in the area of health?

Whether in health and/or health care or in housing and energy, data quality is based on the same criteria. **BOX 4.2** summarizes some of the criteria that one would apply when assessing the quality of a secondary dataset.

Can you recommend federal databases that individuals new to health disparities research might wish to use?

BOX 4.2 Assessing the Quality of a Secondary Dataset

Does the dataset include the dependent and independent variables needed to not only describe how change has occurred but to also identify factors that may be associated with or causatively related to that change?

Data can be used from other sources when causal research is being completed as long as it is for the same time period. For example, if a student wished to complete a research paper, thesis, or dissertation on whether subgroup changes in alcohol and other substance use were related to changes in rates of unemployment from 1988–2018, data would be collected from different federal sources. However, many national data sources include information on the hypothesized outcomes and possible correlates of these outcomes. In such cases, the risk of differences in data collection processes that affect data quality are minimized.

Is the dataset sufficiently populated with demographic data, socioeconomic data, health status and behavioral data, and/or data related to all determinants of health so that a more comprehensive health outcome analysis can be done?

Research requires that one first "specify" the model. Model specification refers to the identification of key variables that may be related to the health care outcome. When doing original research, the emphasis is upon independent variables that may be causally related to the dependent variable that other researchers may have overlooked. In the area of health and health care disparities, it is critical to include all key determinants of health outcomes as independent variables. Thus, one may want to assess the dataset to ensure that all key determinants of health are routinely collected in the dataset of interest.

Does the database minimize missing data?

If one wished to compare changes in youth health risk differentials by gender, race/ethnicity, or state, one would consider the Centers for Disease Control and Prevention, Youth Risk Behavior Surveillance Survey (YRBSS). However, as one reviews the data for 2005 and 2015, one would seek to ensure that the same data are available for both years. Thus, it is important to always check the dataset for missing data.

Are data collected for only one point in time or over time?

In some cases, the health or healthcare disparities sought may be **cross-sectional** in nature. **Cross-sectional** data will allow the researcher to identify disparities across various subgroups at one point in time. For example, in completing **cross-sectional** analysis of disparities data for high school students, the Youth Behavioral Risk Behavior Surveillance dataset is oftentimes used. However, this dataset, whether for 2005 or 2015, reveals that youth of "mixed" races/ethnicity have higher risks on most measures than any other group. When this **cross-sectional** data are compared for 2005 and 2015, the portrait is less dismal for it reveals that improvements in health risks have occurred over this ten-year period on most measures collected. It is often important to analyze cross-sectional perspective disparities data over several years. In contrast, some datasets are **longitudinal**. **Longitudinal** datasets collect data for the same individuals over time. The use of such data provides valuable information on cause and effect. Thus, based upon one's research question, one may require a **longitudinal** dataset.

Are new data published for the dataset so that the analysis can be based upon relatively current data?

Some data are published at regular intervals while other data may be released as part of a one-time analysis. It is important to make note of such matters before deciding to use the data for health disparity research.

Is there evidence that the data are accurate?

Data from health disparities interventions, clinical trials, and other original studies can often be licensed for analysis. In doing so, it is important to verify the "cleanliness" of the data. The process begins by studying the data collection protocols used. Inaccurate data are called "dirty data," and their use will permanently tarnish the reputation of the user.

What is the source of the data?

For every dataset used, it is important to ask, "Who collected the primary data used, and what methods did they use? Is there evidence that human error may have occurred at any point in the design and execution of the data collection process?"

Yes. The following subsections describe a sample of databases that contain high-quality data that individuals new to health disparities research may wish to consider.

The Behavioral Risk Factor Surveillance System (BRFSS)

One major factor that impacts health outcomes is human behavior. One federal source of statistical data that can be used to review current and past differences in behavior across subgroups is the Behavioral Risk Factor Surveillance System (BRFSS).

How can we find this dataset, and what types of data are included in it?

The Centers for Disease Control and Prevention (https://www.cdc.gov/brfss/index.html) uses a probability sample that exceeds 400,000 persons age 12 years and older in order to track the changing health behaviors of Americans. The data collected are used to populate the BRFSS.

What is a probability sample?

Numerical data can be collected from individuals in a variety of ways, such as by a census or a probability sample. A **census** is the collection of data from every single individual, household, and/or other entity that is the defined **unit of analysis** for the data collection effort. For example, if we were studying small businesses, then small businesses would be the unit of analysis. Or, if we were studying families, each family would be the unit of analysis. Here, our interest is in the behavior of individuals. Therefore, individuals are our unit of analysis. As of Saturday, January 20, 2018, the population of the United States of America was 327,069,863 persons, according to the U.S. Census Bureau's Population Clock. As you can imagine, it would be far too expensive and time-consuming to collect health data using a census. However, statisticians, through **probability theory**, have found that if appropriate techniques are used to select the units, then the **sample** will have a distribution that approximates that of the universe from which it to drawn.

What are the origins of probability theory?

According to Apostal (1969), probability theory emerged in 1654 from an initial disagreement between the French mathematicians Blaise Pascal and Pierre de Fermat. The concept of probability was the outcome of this dispute. Probability holds that if a "universe" is "sampled" and key laws of probability are followed, the sample's attributes will be extremely close to those of the universe from which it is drawn.

Can we correctly assume that the CDC used a probability sample in selecting the more than 400,000 individuals used to collect data on health behaviors?"

Absolutely! In fact, the BRFSS is one of the most respected surveys in the country.

What are some health behaviors that can be found in the BRFSS?

The BRFSS includes data on alcohol and/or tobacco use, dietary practices, the degree to which physical activities are present in the lives of American residents, risky sexual behaviors, substance use, behaviors associated with injury and/or violence, the presence of chronic health diseases, access and use of prevention-oriented services, perceived overall health status, and other areas. The data are collected on a state-by-state basis and have been collected since 1984.

Can the data be broken down by gender, race/ ethnicity, and other variables?

Yes. In addition, because the data have been collected since 1984, one can also track improvements and/or the worsening of the health status of key groups and subgroups over time.

Is there anything else that is important for a healthcare administrator, public health professional, or clinician to know if they are interested in using the BRFSS to identify disparities?

Current and/or future healthcare administrators, public health professionals, clinicians, and other professionals with an interest in identifying changes in health behaviors within their state and/or within the nation will find that this to one of the easiest databases to use. It is particularly useful in identifying health disparities.

Why would you characterize it as one of the easiest to use?

As you are aware from having had introductory statistics, all observable differences are

not significant. The BRFSS allows those with an interest in how health disparities change over time to calculate a value that describes whether the probability of an observed difference is greater than that which would exist via pure chance. The BRFSS offers the Web-Enabled Analysis Tool (WEAT) for use by researchers to determine whether an observed difference is significant. It also enables you to complete other statistical analyses using cross-tabulations and/or logistics and other forms of regression.

The National Health Interview Survey (NHIS)

The CDC's National Center for Health Statistics is the nation's premier primary source of secondary health data for the purpose of research, including that needed to analyze health disparities. As research on the determinants of health outcomes indicates, socioeconomic factors interact with behavioral variables to ultimately affect health outcomes. The National Center for Health Statistics conducts the National Health Interview Survey (NHIS; https://www.cdc.gov /nchs/nhis/). It includes data that can be used to determine disparities in overall health status, as well as data that can be used to complete a causal analysis in order to determine the role that socioeconomics, cultural differences, individual health behaviors, and other variables may play in contributing to any identified differences in the health conditions of children, adults, and/or families. **BOX 4.3** lists some of the data collected by the NHIS and describes how the dataset can be used to not only identify disparities but also to *explain* them in terms of known determinants of health outcomes.

Is the NHIS data collected using a probability sample?

Yes. The NHIS also uses a probability sample for data collected.

BOX 4.3 National Health Interview
Survey Data

The NHIS can be used to answer research
questions such as:

**To what degree do disparities exist by
subgroup with regard to:**
- Health status?
- Limitations of activity?
- Injury and poisoning?
- Disability?

**To what degree can these observable
differences be explained by differences in:**
- Healthcare access and utilization?
- Health insurance status?
- Family structure?
- Food security?
- Health behaviors?
- Income and assets?
- Other variables?

National Health and Nutrition Examination Survey (NHANES)

A number of datasets are useful in analyzing
the influence of environmental variables on
observed health disparities. One such dataset
is the National Health and Nutrition Examination Survey (NHANES; https://www.cdc.gov
/nchs/nhanes/). NHANES data are collected
using a probability survey. New datasets are
released based on the survey findings every
2 years. This dataset is extremely useful in
questions examining the following:

- Incidence of selected diseases and conditions (including those undiagnosed or
  undetected)
- Children's growth and development
- Incidence of infectious disease
- Overweight and diabetes
- Causes of death
- Mortality by race/ethnicity, income and
  poverty status, education, occupation,
  type of living quarters, language usually
  spoken at home, birthplace, receipt of
  social services

This dataset is an excellent source of information for health disparities research because
it not only includes survey data collected using
a probability sample, but it also includes data
collected through physical examinations. Lab-
oratory tests are administered to those individuals who participate in this survey. DNA
samples are also collected and nutritional status is evaluated.

***This source appears to be very different from
the BRFSS.***

It is quite different, not only in content, but
also because different types of questions can be
asked of the data based upon how and when
it was collected. Specifically, when choosing
large federal datasets to analyze disparities,
we can select between cross-sectional and
longitudinal datasets. As mentioned, **cross-
sectional datasets** include data selected on
a unique set of variables at a particular point
in time. In contrast, **longitudinal datasets**
collect information from the same individuals
and/or families at different points in time.

***How can these types of datasets be used to
identify disparities?***

If, as a learner in the area of health disparities,
you were interested in whether the prevalence
of suicide differed between Asian Americans
versus Caucasians in 2017, a cross-sectional
database would be appropriate.

***Are you saying that we could not compare
data across years for the two groups by using
data from 2000 and 2017?***

Cross-sectional datasets certainly allow such
comparisons to be made. However, the individuals from whom data are collected using
probability-sampling techniques will be different over the two survey years.

How does this make a difference?

If an individual reading this text were interested in the question, "Does tobacco use
differentially impact the development and progression of lung cancer by race/ethnicity over
a period of time?" then a longitudinal dataset

would be needed. In conducting comparative research, it is necessary to minimize change in all variables other than those selected as the independent variables in the study. Maintaining the same set of carefully selected "subjects" in the study lowers the risk that an extraneous factor has had an impact upon the measured relationships between the variables.

Is the National Health and Nutrition Examination Survey a longitudinal survey?

Yes, it is. The NHANES blends interviews and physical exams into research activities in order to collect data from adults and youth regarding their health and eating habits. For over half a century, this survey has informed researchers, physicians, and the general public about the general health activities of the U.S. population.

National Survey of Family Growth (NSFG)

Some researchers argue that differential family structure directly and/or indirectly affects health disparities. In particular, family status appears to be associated with the sexual behavior of youth. For example, Simons et al. (2016) have identified linkages between family structure and the sexual behavior of youth. Kerpelman, McElwain, and Pittman (2016) have also documented various mechanisms through which family structure and interactions can affect the sexual behavior of youth. The National Survey of Family Growth (NSFG; https://www.cdc.gov /nchs/nsfg/index.htm) uses probability sampling to collect data on males and females aged 15 to 44 years by gender, race/ethnicity, family and individual income, sources of income, level of education, and primary language spoken in the home. The database can be used to explore subgroup differences in contraception and sterilization; teenage sexual activity and pregnancy; father involvement; infertility; adoption; breastfeeding; and other variables.

Substantial disparities currently exist by race/ethnicity and gender in terms of prevalence and incidence of HIV/AIDS (CDC, 2018). This database can be used to assess the magnitude of disparities in HIV risk behaviors across various subgroups. But, and this is extremely important, the NSFG can also be used to *conduct a causal study*. As mentioned, **causal research** is conducted in order to identify the extent and nature of cause-and-effect relationships. A causal study can answer questions such as the degree to which HIV risk behaviors differ by degree of fatherhood involvement, family and individual income status, or education across racial/ethnicity and gender groups.

Other National Centers for Health Statistics Datasets

A number of datasets provided by the National Centers for Health Statistics are useful for simply identifying disparities and/or determining whether identified disparities are increasing or decreasing. The National Vital Statistics System (https://www.cdc.gov/nchs/nvss/) dataset can be used to identify patterns of disparities in factors such as:

- Birth and death rates
- Birth weights
- Teen and nonmarital births
- Pregnancy outcomes
- Methods of birth by delivery
- Preterm delivery
- Multiple deaths
- Medical payments
- Breast-feeding only
- Maternal weight
- Infant mortality
- Life expectancy
- Causes of death
- Occupational mortality

But aren't there quite a few studies already out on disparities in these areas?

Many studies have been completed that simply identify the existence of disparities in some of these areas. Nevertheless, some of these areas require additional documentation. For example, a search of health disparities with regard to occupational mortality yields zero citations. The health administration research question, *"Are there disparities in Medicaid payments based upon patients' race/ethnicity?"* appears to have not yet been researched because no studies could be identified that examine this question. This National Vital Statistics System datasets could be used to examine topics such as disparities in breast-feeding between urban and rural women, disparities in breast-feeding between very high-income and very low-income women, and other topics. The types of disparity-related research topics that can be explained using these datasets have not yet been exhausted. But, let's look at a few more data resources.

Health Services Research Information Central (HSRIC)

In some cases, other types of disparity-related information may be needed. For example, the Health Services Research information Central (HSRIC; https://www.nlm.nih.gov/hsrinfo /abouthsr.html) is a site that provides such information on health disparities which has searchable legislation, additional journals, disparity-related meetings that have been held, and other areas.

National Ambulatory Medical Care Survey (NAMCS)

Most of the datasets described thus far are in the area of *health* disparities. A number of other datasets exist that are specific not merely to health outcomes but that also are appropriate to a study of *healthcare* disparities. The National Ambulatory Medical Care Survey (NAMCS; https://www.cdc.gov/nchs/ahcd/index.htm) provides information on persons who receive outpatient medical care. The dataset is populated with data from patients' hardcopy and/or electronic medical records. These records include data on areas such as those listed in **BOX 4.4**.

The NAMCS database is a good one for determining whether differentials exist in initial status and in the outpatient services provided

---

BOX 4.4 National Ambulatory Medical Care Survey Data

- Patient medical record numbers
- Patient descriptive data, including zip code, date of birth, age, sex, ethnicity, etc.
- Source of payment (e.g., private insurance or Medicaid or Medicare)
- Children's Health Insurance Program (CHIP), workers, compensation, self-pay, charity, or other payments made
- Behavioral practices as measured by tobacco use
- Key vital signs as measured by height, weight, temperature, blood pressure, etc.
- Whether the visit is for preventive care, ongoing chronic illness, new problems related to a chronic illness, pre- or postsurgery care, and/or a new health problem
- Whether a visit related to an injury was for an intentional or nonintentional injury
- Degree to which the patient has a primary care physician and a medical "home"
- Type of diagnosis made for each patient
- Medical history
- Types of services received, including health educational counseling, examinations and screenings, lab tests, surgeries, and/or procedures and/or treatment order
- Type of provider who delivered the health care services by training (i.e., physician assistant, nurse practitioner/midwife, licensed vocational nurse, medical health provider, etc.)
- The outcome of any test ordered and the date
- The estimated time spent with the patient and any visit disparities

to different subgroups. Moreover, this database can also be used to assess differences in the need for health care based on age, sex, and/or race/ethnicity. Healthcare administrators can use this database to analyze their own data to determine whether disparities exist by variables such as insurance used, patient zip code, medical condition, and others. Researchers can use this database to assess the type of healthcare administration changes that are needed to reduce remediable differentials in delivery of outpatient services by physician practices.

Outpatient services are not only delivered by various types of physician-owned practices. Hospitals also deliver ambulatory care services to individuals and families who seek primary care through hospital emergency departments. In addition, many hospitals now have outpatient departments and same-day surgery units as a part of the services offered. The National Ambulatory Medical Care Survey dataset can be used in order to identify differences in services provided by these organizations and/or received by various subgroups.

Does this database only include information on hospital ambulatory services?

No, it also includes data from community healthcare centers, which also deliver ambulatory care. Additionally, data on office-based physicians can also be found in this dataset.

The data collected for office-based healthcare professionals and emergency room and outpatient services at the hospitals reflect those collected by the National Ambulatory Medical Care Survey. However, instruments for community health centers also include data that enable analysts to determine whether these unique healthcare delivery organizations provide services to their lower-income patients that are comparable to those delivered by other outpatient providers.

What kinds of data does this survey collect that can be used for such a purpose?"

Data from community health centers and Indian healthcare sites and similar healthcare sites include those listed in **BOX 4.5**.

Can this database can be used to determine whether disparities exist in types of healthcare delivery systems that serve various subgroups?

Yes, it can also be used to assess whether differential health disparities exist among the

---

BOX 4.5   Data Collected by the National Ambulatory Medical Care Survey for Community Health Center Providers

- STD screening and/or treatment policies
- Point-of-service tests offered for STDs
- Documentation of sexual risk behaviors, including substance use, use of condoms, number of sexual partners, types of sexual activities with sex partner, etc.
- HIV infection preventive services
- Degree of cultural competency training
- Familiarity with and adherence to National Standards for Culturally and Linguistically Appropriate Healthcare standards
- Qualifications of the physician, the specific case sites, and/or adherence to other quality measures
- Ratio of full-time and part-time providers per patient;
- Number and ratio of nurse practitioners, physician assistants, nurse/midwives, etc., per patient
- Logging and billing policies for the described personnel time
- Criteria used in reporting client data
- Ownership of the organization
- Characteristics of the electronic health system/electronic medical record system
- Other data

populations of patients served within a primary care organization and/or between different types of primary care organizations.

Are there other highly reliable primary sources of secondary data that can be used to address healthcare disparities?

Numerous other reliable sources of data exist that can be used to analyze whether differential patterns of health care characterize various populations. For example, the National Hospital Care Survey (NHCS; https://www.cdc.gov/nchs/nhcs/index.htm) includes data from other surveys, including the National Hospital Discharge Survey (NHDS; https://www.cdc.gov/nchs/ahcd/index.htm), the National Hospital Ambulatory Medical Care Survey (NHAMCS; https://www.cdc.gov/nchs/ahcd/index.htm), and the Drug-Abuse Warning Network (DAWN; https://www.datafiles.samhsa.gov/study-dataset/drug-abuse-warning-network-2011-dawn-2011-ds0001-nid13747). In addition, data can also be examined from these sources in conjunction with information from the following indexes and databases:

- National Death Index (NDI; https://www.cdc.gov/nchs/ndi/index.htm)
- National Study of Long-Term Care Providers (NSLTCP; https://www.cdc.gov/nchs/nsltcp/index.htm)
- National Nursing Home Survey (NNHS; https://www.cdc.gov/nchs/nnhs/index.htm)
- National Home and Hospital Care Surveys (https://www.cdc.gov/nchs/nhhcs/index.htm)
- National Survey of Resident and Care Facilities (NSRCF; https://www.cdc.gov/nchs/nsrcf/index.htm)
- National Nursing Assistant Survey (NNAS; https://www.cdc.gov/nchs/nnhs/nnas.htm)

Are these the only reliable data sources that can be used to identify health and/or healthcare disparities?

Numerous other reliable sources of data are available for analysis by hospital administrators, public health professionals, clinicians, policy makers, community-based organizations, and/or individuals who wish to understand current patterns.

Are all of the reliable datasets owned by the federal government?

No, a number of reliable datasets exist beyond the federal sector. Datasets that collect healthcare data for each state exist. Data on births, deaths, marriages, divorce, disease prevalence and incidence and other topics are collected. States often have a need for other detailed healthcare information. For example, databases on Certificates of Need applications are maintained at the state level for all 50 states. Analysis of data on the approval or disapproval of these applications for new healthcare facilities could be used to determine if low-income populations are being neglected with regard to availability of care. Similarly, teachers who believe that academic outcomes in their districts are being impacted by lead in the drinking water can test this hypothesis because each state tests water samples for lead in all public schools. States with differential rates of lung cancer can examine the degree to which differences in medical coverage for tobacco use cessation may be associated with differential outcomes. Numerous datasets are available by state. Healthdata.gov can assist readers in identifying data on virtually any health-related topic at the national, state, and community levels.

Does Healthdata.gov assist in finding providers and not merely population data?

Yes, it does. Medicare, Medicaid, hospitals, healthcare quality, patient care, and other topics of interest can be researched using this dataset.

Are there still other databases?

Yes, many other federal and private datasets can be used to identify disparities in health outcomes, disease and illness prevention, screening and diagnosis, and treatment.

The following are additional datasets supported by federal agencies that can be particularly useful in disparities research:

- **Open Payments**: Healthcare manufacturers, group purchasing organizations, and others provide data to the CMS. The Open Payments dataset (https://openpaymentsdata.cms.gov/) can be used to determine whether disparate payments are made to providers and teaching hospitals that are located in zip codes of different socioeconomic status, race/ethnicity, rural/urban location, age group, environmental risk, and other variables.
- **Health Care Common Procedural Coding System (HCPCS)**: The HCPCS dataset (https://www.cms.gov/Medicare/Coding/MedHCPCSGenInfo/index.html) is of particular value to healthcare administrators because it can be used to identify whether miscoding is an administrative problem that is more prevalent in healthcare organizations that disproportionately serve one or more subpopulations.
- **Outcome and Assessment Information Set (OASIS)**: The OASIS dataset (https://www.cms.gov/Medicare/Quality-Initiatives-Patient-Assessment-Instruments/OASIS/index.html) contains data provided by home healthcare providers. It can be analyzed in order to identify differential patterns in overall outcomes. It can also be used to identify baseline and/or continuing differences in the initial patient risk factors.

Chapter Summary

This chapter describes and defines primary versus secondary sources of data. It then identifies a few of the many federal datasets that can be used for health disparities research. As this chapter indicates, an abundance of datasets exist that can be used to identify disparities in health and healthcare outcomes. We urge students of healthcare administration, public health, and clinical care to visit Data.gov. You can search for datasets by organization type, topic category, and other key words at https://catalog.data.gov. By applying the appropriate statistical approaches, virtually any database can be used to identify relevant disparities in health outcomes by subpopulation groups and/or healthcare disparities. Readers are urged to become more familiar with each of the datasets introduced and to begin to identify under-researched areas that can be studied using these datasets.

Review Questions and Problems

1. Choose an area of health disparities that is of interest to you, and identify 3 datasets with information about this area.
2. Review and critique the methods used to collect the information in the datasets collected.
3. Look up every single dataset described in this chapter, and compile a list of research you would like to complete over the course of your career using each dataset.
4. Using PubMed or Google Scholar, compile a list of disparities studies completed from 2010 to the present using one of these datasets and summarize the findings.

Key Terms and Concepts

causal research Research conducted in order to identify the extent and nature of cause-and-effect relationships.

census Collection of data from every single individual, household, and/or other entity that is the defined unit of analysis for the data collection effort.

cross-sectional datasets Datasets that examine a unique set of variables at a particular point in time.

longitudinal datasets Datasets that contain information from the same individuals and/or families at different points in time.

primary data Data collected by a researcher directly from an original source in order to answer one or more research questions. Information that a researcher collects directly from an original source. Healthcare organizations generate primary data that can be used to assess healthcare disparities. For example, The Centers for Disease Control and Prevention (CDC) would be considered a source of primary data whereas the United Way would be considered a secondary source of data.

probability theory The branch of mathematics concerned with the random distribution of quantities.

sample A set of data collected and/or selected from a statistical population.

secondary data Data that were collected by someone other than the user.

unit of analysis The major entity that is being analyzed in a study, such as individuals, groups, social organizations, etc.

References

Apostal, T. M. (1969). *Calculus*, vol. 2. (2nd ed.). New York: John Wiley & Sons.

Centers for Disease Control and Prevention. (2018). The numbers: HIV and AIDS diagnoses. Retrieved from https://www.cdc.gov/hiv/group/racialethnic/africanamericans/index.html

Kerpelman, J. L., McElwain, A. D., Pittman, J. F., & Adler-Baeder, F. M. (2016). Engagement in risky sexual behavior: Adolescents' perceptions of self and the parent–child relationship matter. *Youth & Society*, *48*(1), 101–125.

Simons, L. G., Sutton, T. E., Simons, R. L., Gibbons, F. X., & Murry, V. M., (2016). Mechanisms that link parenting practices to adolescents' risky sexual behavior: A test of six competing theories. *Journal of Youth and Adolescence*, *45*(2), 255–270.

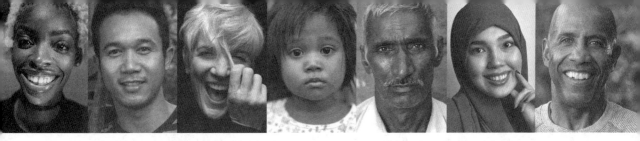

CHAPTER 5

Simple Statistical Tools to Assess Health and Healthcare Disparities

"Whenever we have an opportunity to engage with each other as human beings and to minimize the differences between us based on disparities in resources, then we should do it."

—**William T. Vollmann**, an American novelist, journalist, and war correspondent

LEARNING OBJECTIVES

After completing this chapter, each learner will be able to:

- Identify, compare, and contrast disparities in mortality rates.
- Synthesize information on health outcome disparities and the determinants of health in order to explain the inverted triangle model.
- Converse using the language of basic statistics.
- Calculate disparity ratios using the percentage difference with reference group approach.
- Compare and contrast univariate, bivariate, and multivariate data analysis approaches.
- Explain how nominal, ordinal, interval, and ratio data differ.
- Match tests of significance and other data analysis strategies with the appropriate types of data.
- Use online statistical calculators to identify disparities.

▶ Introduction

Avariety of datasets are available that policy makers and health services researchers can use to identify disparities. Knowledge of statistical techniques is needed in order to analyze the data provided in these datasets so that remediable health and healthcare disparities can be identified and eliminated. This chapter introduces several measures of disease frequency based on the occurrence of disease. Whether you are a current or future healthcare administrator, public health professional, or clinician, an excellent approach to studying health and healthcare disparities is the inverted triangle approach (**FIGURE 5.1**).

According to the inverted triangle approach, one may begin an analysis of subgroup data by identifying disparities in mortality. The researcher should always begin with the most current year for which data are available. The **National Vital Statistics System** (https://www.cdc.gov/nchs/nvss/index.htm), which is part of the Centers for Disease Control and Prevention's National Center for Health Statistics, is the most reliable primary source of secondary data on deaths, death rates, life expectancy, and infant mortality by race/ethnicity, gender, age, geographic area, and cause of deaths.

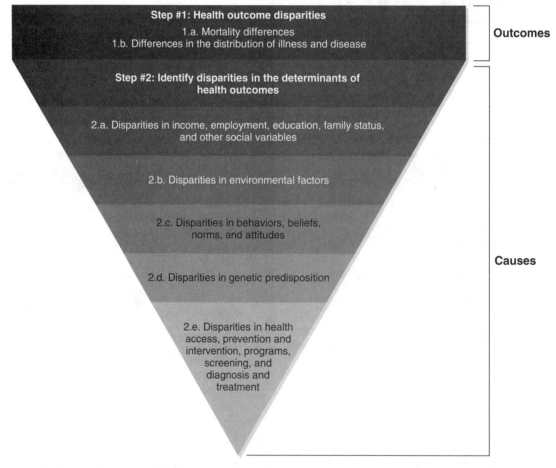

Step #1: Health outcome disparities

1.a. Mortality differences
1.b. Differences in the distribution of illness and disease

Outcomes

Step #2: Identify disparities in the determinants of health outcomes

2.a. Disparities in income, employment, education, family status, and other social variables

2.b. Disparities in environmental factors

2.c. Disparities in behaviors, beliefs, norms, and attitudes

2.d. Disparities in genetic predisposition

2.e. Disparities in health access, prevention and intervention, programs, screening, and diagnosis and treatment

Causes

FIGURE 5.1 Inverted triangle approach.

The importance of this resource cannot be overemphasized.

How does the National Vital Statistics System obtain data on mortality?

Collecting data on mortality levels and rates is an arduous task. The National Vital Statistics System's staff rely on records submitted to state registration offices by funeral directors and/or their staff. Physicians, medical examiners, and coroners are also key elements in the data collection process. The National Center for Health Statistics works closely with these state registration offices. The data are received, reviewed for errors and omissions, and then entered into a centralized database that exists as part of the Vital Statistics Cooperative Program.

The magnitude of the data involved in this process is such that a lag occurs between the most current data available for analysis at any given point in time. Accordingly, data published in 2018 report mortality data for 2016 and data published in 2017 report data for 2015. For the remainder of this chapter, we will examine final data for 2015, which were published in 2017 by the National Vital Statistics System (Murphy, Xu, Kochanek, Curtin, & Arias, 2017).

As you can imagine, it is difficult to simply look at data on morbidity and mortality and identify health disparities. However, a variety of statistical tools can be used to analyze data to determine whether health and healthcare disparities exist so that the first stage in the inverted triangle model can be completed.

▶ Measures of Disease Frequency

When reviewing data on health disparities, a variety of measures are used. It becomes virtually impossible to assess the presence of health and/or healthcare disparities without familiarity with these measures. For example, approximately 2,712,630 persons or .844%, of the overall population who were alive as of January 1, 2015, died during the year (Murphy et al., 2017). However, deaths are not measured for reporting based on absolute numbers or upon percentage rates. Rather, incidence rates are used. Other measures are applied in the quantification of other health measures. In the following sections, we will introduce you to some of the commonly used measures that are applied in discussions of health disparities.

Count

The **count** is the simplest way to measure disease frequency in epidemiology.

What is epidemiology?

Epidemiology is an area in the field of health that focuses upon the frequency, prevalence, distribution, and causes of illness and disease in various populations and subpopulations.

So how do we measure disease or illness frequency using a count?

The measure, which we call a count, provides an aggregate portrait of the number of cases (individuals) that meet a particular definition of having a specific disease or health issue. However, the use of this measure will provide false information if the size of the designated population is unknown. For example, **TABLE 5.1** provides the "counts" of heart disease deaths in five states.

So, based on this data, can one say that Iowa is better off than any of the other four states because it has the lowest number of deaths due to heart disease?

That is, indeed, the problem with simple counts. One cannot draw such a conclusion unless the total population of Iowa is known. Specifically, in order to transform a "count" into information that is of value, additional operations must be completed. In Table 5.1 the column "Annual Crude Death Rate" in combination with the total population is used to calculate the death rate due to heart disease per 100,000 population.

Location	Count Number of Deaths Due to Heart Disease (A)	Total Population of Persons Alive (Estimated) (B)	Annual Crude Death Rate = Count (A)/Total Population (B) × 100,000
Iowa	6,813	3,123,899	218.10 per 100,000
Florida	45,441	20,271,272	224.2 per 100,000
Nevada	6,114	2,890,845	211.5 per 100,000
Pennsylvania	32,042	12,802,503	250.3 per 100,000
Washington	11,025	7,170,351	153.8 per 100,000

TABLE 5.1 Deaths Due to Heart Disease in 2015 in Five U.S. States

Murphy, S. L., Xu, J. Q., Kochanek, K. D., Curtin, S. C., & Arias, E. (2017). Deaths: Final data for 2015. Table 12. Number of deaths, death rates, and age-adjusted death rates for major causes of death: United States, each state, Puerto Rico, Virgin Islands, Guam, American Samoa, and Northern Marianas, 2015. *National Vital Statistics Reports, 66*(6). Hyattsville, MD: National Center for Health Statistics. Retrieved from https://www.cdc.gov/nchs/data/nvsr/nvsr66/nvsr66_06.pdf

I've often heard the term "proportion" used in health care. What is a proportion?

A proportion in health is used to answer the question, "What percent of a total population in an area experienced a certain health condition?" Now remember, the total population in an area will consist of those who did not have the illness plus those who did. Accordingly, the denominator of a proportion will always consist of the whole of the population.

Proportion

Thus, a **proportion** is a measure that requires that the denominator is always a sum of the total population. It can be calculated by dividing the number of identified "cases" by the "total population." The formula for a proportion is:

$$\text{Proportion} = \frac{x}{x+y}$$

x = e.g., Number of persons with influenza on your campus
y = e.g., Number of persons without influenza on your campus
$x + y$ = e.g., Total population on your campus

Could you give us an example?

Imagine that you live in a small community of 1,105 residents, and 140 persons have hypertension and 965 persons do not. Thus, the proportion of persons with hypertension in the community is 140/1,105, or 12.7%. The proportion of persons without hypertension is 965/1,105, or 87.3%. But, the total population is 1,105 or 100% of residents. As you can see, in both cases, the numerator (x) is part of the denominator ($x + y$: the total population). In epidemiology, the term proportion is used to describe the fraction of the total population that is affected by illness or disease.

Oh, I see...the total population is always the number with, plus the number without!

Ratio

The ratio is another key measurement concept for persons interested in health disparity. A **ratio**, like a proportion, is a fractional relationship between the numerator and denominator. However, when one divides one quantity by another but, and this is important, the two quantities may not "belong to each other."

In this case, they should not be added. The formula for a ratio is:

$$\text{Ratio} = \frac{x}{y}$$

Some research in health disparities use relative comparisons which is usually referred to as ratio. For example, the measure of persons without shots to persons with flu shots is a ratio. Similarly speaking, the ratio of the females to males in the population is also a ratio. But, in this case, the numerator and denominator are independent of one another.

What do you mean by independent?

By independent, we mean mutually exclusive. That is, they do not belong to each other. Assume for a moment that you wish to conduct research to determine whether there is a relationship between the ratio of females to males and the incidence of sexually transmitted diseases in a county. Because the biological definition of males and females is mutually exclusive, one can easily calculate a ratio.

I think I understand ratio. So, what other measures are used in health disparity research?

Rate

The rate is still another important term. The epidemiological definition of **rate** is a type of ratio – one number divided by another number. Two of the most common rates calculated in health care are the prevalence and the incidence. While both of these measures are rates, they are calculated differently.

How so?

Prevalence and Incidence

Let's begin with the prevalence. The **prevalence rate** is the proportion of the total population or subpopulation affected by a condition over a specified time period (e.g., one month, one year) or single point in time. For example, Skinner, Ravanbakht, Skelton et al. (2018) report that the prevalence of overweight was higher among non-Hispanic African American (37.8%), and Hispanic (45.9%) children, while Asian American (23.2%) children had much lowest prevalence.

The **incidence rate** is a rate which can be defined as the number of new cases of diseases, or deaths, per defined time period. The incidence rate differs from the prevalence in that it measures the total number of cases or disease, the incidence, on the other hand, measures only *new cases*. Consider the formula for the incidence:

$$\text{Incidence} = \frac{\text{Number of new cases of disease}}{\text{Person-time of population "at-risk"}} \times 1{,}000$$

There are three important key elements in the calculation of an incidence: (1) the numerator only refers to new diseases/events; (2) a denominator refers to the population "at-risk", and (3) the specific amount of time (person-time) within which the population is at-risk. The incidence also incorporates a multiplier; hence, the unit may be 1,000 persons, 10,000 persons, or 100,000 persons a year. For disease occurrence, we would refer to the "annual" incidence of disease x as 33/100,000 or 33 cases per 100,000.

The concept of prevalence and incidence has been grossly simplified here in order to better support the process of using these measures to identify disparities. Both prevalence and incidence are used to summarize disparities in rates of illness and disease.

Can you give us more detail on the applications of rates?

Crude rates, specific rates, and adjusted rates are also important measures. **Crude rates**, mean that they are not "refined" rates. Thus, crude rates are simply calculated by the number of affected cases divided by the total study population. Sometimes the crude rate can be misleading, because it does not consider possible systematic differences in a population, such as differences by demographic group (e.g., age, gender, race, education, etc.). Thus, one should be cautious when comparing populations using crude rates. Nevertheless, the crude rate is still an important measure that is simple and easy to compute. Consider the formula for the crude death rate:

$$\text{Crude death rate (CDR)} = \frac{\text{Annual death count}}{\text{Reference population (at midpoint of year)}} \times 1{,}000$$

Can you show me an example?

Okay, let's say that in 2015 the death count in the United States was 2,712,360. In contrast, the U.S. population on June 30, 2015, was 321,032,786. The crude death rate is thus:

$$CDR = \frac{2{,}712{,}360}{321{,}032{,}786} \times 1{,}000$$
$$= 8.44 \text{ per } 1{,}000 \text{ people}$$

In contrast, **specific rates** and **adjusted rates** are "refined" rates. They can be used to make comparisons more accurately. A *specific rate* is a type of rate considering only a unique group such as gender, age groups, race, etc. Example of gender-specific rates is defined as a rate for females or males only. An *adjusted rate* is a statistically adjusted summary rate that removes the effects of selected variables (such as race/ethnicity or gender) on the data analysis. The procedure of removal of the effects of the variable results in a comparison without prejudice between groups where differentials may be present with respect to these variables.

But why do we multiply by 1,000?

By definition, a rate is calculated using a numerator, a denominator, and a number that we call a multiplier. In health care, the multiplier is normally 1,000, 10,000, or 100,000. The purpose of a multiplier is to make it simple when presenting a rate. That is, to avoid presenting a number with too many decimal places (ideally up to 2 decimal places e.g., 8.44 per 1,000 people).

Note that when describing rates, one should always include "per 1,000" or the unit of analyses selected for expressing the rate (e.g., per 100,000, per 10,000, per 1,000, or per 100). No one form for the description of rates is standard. For example, statistics regarding teen pregnancy rates are usually reported in "per 1,000 population", and death rates and causes of death (heart disease, cancer, stroke, diabetes, etc.) are usually reported in per "100,000 population" unit format.

How to maximize "truth" when using numbers

When rates, ratios and/or other measures are calculated, they must be presented and interpreted in a way that does not distort the message. Although some people find comfort in the objectivity of numbers, numbers can actually present a distorted view of reality. First, it is critical to note that all numbers presented are not statistics. For example, let's say that 1,000,000 current or future healthcare administrators read this book and 100% of these 1,000,000 readers are surveyed. The survey then reveals that 800,000 readers felt that the information supports their understanding of health disparities. Thus, 80% of the readers have provided favorable responses. From a research perspective, this number, 80%, although a number, is not a statistic. Rather, it comprises a parameter.

What is a parameter vs. a statistic?

A **parameter** is a number based upon the entirety of the target population. A **statistic** is a number that is derived from a sample taken from a total of the target population. As a result, a statistic is *less reliable*. Accordingly, steps must be taken to ensure the accuracy of a statistic. These steps include ensuring that the sample is selected based upon probabilistic approaches. Health disparity analysis at the population level is based on statistics. For a particular healthcare institution, such as a specific hospital or nursing home, data are available for the entire universe of consumers. Thus, the data are parameters and not statistics. Therefore, the data used in disparity analysis at the national level is statistical, or based upon a sample. As a result, it is important to read the methodologies section when using federal, state, or local datasets so that the validity and reliability of the numbers used can be assessed.

What are validity and reliability?

Data that measure that which it purports to measure is considered to be **valid**. That is, the measurement instrument measures that which it purports to measure. Data measurements that produce the same value independently of user, time, or place are said to be **reliable**. That is, the measurements are consistent over time.

Can you provide an example?

The exams that healthcare administration students take in their university classes are supposed to measure students' grasp of the readings, assignments, and other learning activities to which the students have been exposed over the period covered by the exam. If the exam covers content that was not assigned, then the test is *invalid*. Similarly, if the instructor administers the same test to the same student two, three, or four times within a 24-hour period and the student obtains approximately the same results (if the student has not completed additional studying and/or checked answers from prior tests), this means that the test is *reliable*.

▶ Using Statistics to Identify Health Disparities

As discussed, the concept of health disparities is a statistical concept. Statistical data serve as the informational pool that is used to identify whether a health disparity exists between selected groups and/or subgroups. Similarly, statistical approaches are used to assess the size of an identified disparity. All sources of statistics include a methodology that describes how the data were collected, cleansed, analyzed, and presented. But when primary sources of secondary data are used to identify disparities, the data must be further manipulated in order to calculate a health disparity measure.

But exactly what kinds of questions can healthcare administrators answer through the use of parameters?

Datasets generated within healthcare organizations enable healthcare administrators to answer questions on healthcare disparities, such as those listed in **BOX 5.1**. The questions in Box 5.1 are just a few examples. Numerous other healthcare disparity questions can be answered using data internal to the organization. Oftentimes, the data are used to calculate *health disparity measures* at the institutional level.

What is a health disparity measure?

A **health disparity measure** is a figure that summarizes the width of differentials in health outcomes between populations and/or subpopulations relative to each other. It is extremely critical that health disparity measures be accurately and fairly calculated. Statistical methods can sometimes distort the data. It is imperative that this be avoided because health disparity indices or ratios can be used to further inflame group and subgroup tensions. Accordingly, some key guidelines are presented in **BOX 5.2** that can be followed to ensure that health disparity measures are not presented in a way that supports abuse and/or misuse during this period of contemporary tribalism and subtribalism.

How do we calculate a health disparity?

Harper (2011) identified 20 statistical techniques for calculating health disparities. However, because a number of these methods assume a detailed knowledge of statistics, their inclusion would contradict the purposes of a multi-purpose, cross-disciplinary text that current and future health managers and other groups and individuals can immediately use to identify health disparities. Indeed, most health disparities measures that are reported

---

BOX 5.1 Questions on Healthcare Disparities That Can Be Answered with Data Internal to the Healthcare Organization

- Do quality measurement surveys such as the Health Care Effectiveness Data and Information Set (HEDIS) and others reveal differences in measured outcomes between subgroups?
- Are there differences in queues by subgroup?
- In applying location analysis for new facilities, are low-income and/or other neighborhoods differentially "weighted" in the location model used to complete the analysis?
- To what degree do initial differences in patients' conditions "explain" differential health outcomes for the same illness/disease?
- Do missed appointments differ by subgroup and, if so, to what degree do such variables explain differences in patient outcomes?
- Do average days of service, per week day, or month, differ between patient subgroups with the same diagnosis and same disease stage?
- Are there differences in early patient admission data for a hospital's different intensive care units over a given year by patient subgroups with the same illness treatment?
- Do total expenditures for an accountable care organization differ per assigned beneficiary for different subgroups?

BOX 5.2 Preventing Misuse of Health Disparity Data

- While it is often stated that "a picture is worth a thousand words," do not use images of objects to describe disparity measures. The visuals used can imply that the differences are much greater than they actually are.
- Use no more than two decimal points when reporting disparity ratios or indices. Note that health disparity measures are approximations. Multiple digits after the decimal may convey the sense that the disparity measure is more precise and accurate than it actually is.
- Be sure to cite the reference group used as the measure of comparison and the rationale for the use of the selected reference group. The use of only one subpopulation as a reference group without the provision of a rationale can imply superiority.
- Determine whether the disparity is to be measured from a favorable or nonfavorable perspective. For example, it is reported that less than 10% of the U.S. population has no health insurance. Thus, this statistic is reported from an unfavorable perspective. It would be more impactful to say that more than 90% of the U.S. population now has health insurance.
- Make note of how the groups are ordered when the disparity is reported. This is because research from psychology reveals that negative information has more impact than positive information. For example, Thompson (2007) reports on some of the scholarly research that reveals a human tendency to remember "bad" things more often than "good" things. In addition, the serial position effect in psychology indicates that humans are more likely to remember the first and last items (Frensch, 1994).

---

at the public level bypass these more complex statistical approaches. For example, the U.S. Department of Health and Human Services often utilizes the maximal rate difference approach, which is the simplest method of calculating a disparity.

The **maximal rate difference** is calculated by simply subtracting the lower from the higher value for a particular healthcare variable. This absolute difference is then tracked over time to determine whether the disparity is increasing or decreasing.

Could you provide an example?

Males in the United States had a life expectancy at birth of 76.3 years in 2015. Life expectancy for females was 81.2 years (Xu, Murphy, Kochanek, & Arias, 2016). The maximal rate difference approach involves simply subtracting these two values; that is, subtracting 76.3 from 81.2 to find the difference, which is 4.9 years. This value is the male/female disparity rate. This figure is then compared against the difference found in subsequent or past periods to determine whether disparities are improving and/or worsening.

Is this a good approach for healthcare administration students and/or healthcare professionals to use?

No, with tremendous respect for the work of the Department of Health and Human Services, this is not the approach that would be the most useful to a healthcare administrator, a clinician, a public health worker, and/or the general public. An absolute disparity such as this does not allow for relative comparisons in the present period. A *relative measure* provides more information, allowing the healthcare administrator to answer the question, "How much longer do women live than men percentage wise?" *Absolute differences* cannot serve as a basis for such a comparison. Accordingly, the subsections that follow introduce a simple method of calculating disparities that is extremely useful to both public health students and personnel, healthcare administration students, and clinicians. This health disparity measurement process can also be quickly and accurately used by policy makers, consumers, and other stakeholders.

How do we determine whether there are disparities in death rates between different groups?

Percentage Difference

To determine whether a disparity in death rates exists between different groups and subgroups, the simplest technique is to calculate the **percentage difference** with a reference group. **TABLE 5.2** uses non-Hispanic White Americans as a reference group for calculating percentage differences. White Americans are usually used as the reference group because of their position as the majority population in the United States. However, in doing so, analysts oftentimes fail to

TABLE 5.2 The Use of a Percentage Difference with Reference Point to Identify 2015 Death Rate Disparities by Race/Ethnicity

Race/Ethnicity	Death Rate per 100,000	% Difference	Higher or Lower Than Reference Group?
White, non-Hispanic Americans	753.2	—	—
African Americans, non-Hispanic	876.1	+16.32	Higher
Latino/Hispanic Americans	525.3	−30.26	Lower
American Indians/Alaskan Natives	805.7	+6.9	Higher
Asian/Pacific Islander Americans	396.2	−47.4	Lower

Murphy, S. L., Xu, J. Q., Kochanek, K. D., Curtin, S. C., & Arias, E. (2017). Deaths: Final data for 2015. Table 1: Number of deaths, death rates, and age-adjusted death rates, by race and Hispanic origin, and sex: United States, 1940, 1950, 1960, 1970, 1980, 1990, 2000, and 2010-2015. Pg. 22. *National Vital Statistics Reports, 66*(6). Hyattsville, MD: National Center for Health Statistics. Retrieved from https://www.cdc.gov/nchs/data/nvsr/nvsr66/nvsr66_06.pdf

mention that *even White Americans experience unfavorable health disparities.*

As Table 5.2 indicates, the death rate per 100,000 was 16.32% higher for non-Hispanic African Americans than for non-Hispanic White Americans. However, despite the active assumptions made by many that health disparities always favor the majority group via the highly divisive concept of "white privilege," these data, assuming that the public sector's data are reasonably correct, demonstrate that disparities in health outcomes as measured by death rates favor White Americans only with regards to African Americans and Native Americans. As Table 5.2 indicates, in 2015 African Americans had the highest death rate per 100,000; American Indians/Alaskan Natives had the second highest death rate, and White Americans the third highest. However, Latinos/Hispanics had a death rate that was 30.26% lower than White Americans, and Asian/Pacific Islanders had a death rate that was 47.4% lower than that of White Americans.

What simple analytical tool was applied in order to "cause" these basic data to "give up" this information?

The basic mathematical procedure of calculating the percentage difference with reference group yields this finding.

How do we calculate percentage difference?

BOX 5.3 describes how to calculate the percentage difference *without* a reference group to determine whether a disparity exists. **BOX 5.4** describes how to calculate the percentage difference *with* a reference group. Note that a percentage difference with no reference group is calculated differently than a percentage difference with a reference group. The percentage difference without a reference group is the difference that exists between two of the same health measures at the same point in time as a percentage of the average of both values. A percentage difference without a reference point assumes that the two values are of equal significance.

A percentage difference *without* a reference point provides a completely different disparity rate than when a reference point is used. As can be seen, the difference in the death rates of whites and Latinos is 35.6% when no reference point is used (not adjusted), but 30.26% when a reference point is used (adjusted). That is, when White Americans are used as the reference group, it reveals that Latinos have a death rate that is 30.26% lower than the rate that exists for this reference group. Thus, the choice of mathematical technique affects the magnitude of the disparity. Note that you could also calculate rates with any specific

---

BOX 5.3 How to Calculate Percentage Difference *Without* a Reference Group

Step 1: Calculate the difference by subtracting the smaller value from the larger value.

Death rate for White Americans = 753.2 (per 100,000)
Death rate for Latino Americans = 525.3 (per 100,000)
753.2 − 525.3 = 227.9 (per 100,000)

Step 2: Average the two totals.

(753.2 + 525.3)/2 = 639.25

Step 3: Divide the difference by the average.

227.9/639.25 = 0.356

Step 4: Convert the decimal to a percentage by multiplying by 100.

0.356 × 100 = 35.6%

This tells us that Latino Americans had a death rate per 100,000 that was 35.6% lower than that of White Americans in 2015.

BOX 5.4 How to Calculate Percentage Difference *with* a Reference Group

Step 1: Identify the two groups, and choose one as the reference group.

Death rates per 100,000 with White Americans as the reference point.

Death rate = 753.2 (per 100,000)

Step 2: Choose the comparison group.

Death rates per 100,000 with Latino Americans as the comparison group = 525.3

Step 3: Calculate the difference.

753.2 − 525.3 = 227.9

This number tells us that Latino Americans have a death rate per 100,000 that is 227.9 points lower than that of the reference group.

Step 4: Divide this difference by the value of the reference group (as is done in calculating a percentage change rather than a percentage difference).

227.9/753.2 = 0.303

Step 5: Convert the decimal to a percentage by multiplying by 100.

0.303 × 100 = 30.3%

This tells us that Latino Americans had a death rate per 100,000 that was 30.26% lower than that of White Americans in 2015.

group of the population used as a reference. The specific groups can be calculated based on gender, age, race (see Table 5.6), cancer site, cause of death, etc.

Throughout this text, racial/ethnic and other subgroup disparities will be calculated using percentage differences with White Americans as a reference point. The reason for this choice is to begin to shift the discussion away from the conflict paradigm that assumes that White Americans are the only beneficiaries of the current American healthcare system while all minorities are the "losers." However, the choice to use the term "Americans of European descent" or "White Americans" as the reference group at some points was made because the terms subordinate race as a biological concept to a term that reflects continent of origin. Again, the primary question that this text addresses is, "What are some remediable health disparities that affect various subgroups of humans who live in American society and how can these be addressed?"

The conflict model suggests that males are more favored by the healthcare system.

However, close examination of these supposedly "dominant groups" reveals that every group and/or subgroup in American society experiences positive and negative disparities. Provided with such a framework, it becomes possible for policy makers, healthcare administrators, and others who influence change to seek to apply strategies that benefit the collective of groups and subgroups that live in the United States.

As noted earlier, Box 5.4 describes the steps used in calculating a disparity rate *with* a reference group. The methodology is even simpler than when no reference group is used. Mathematically, one applies the procedure used to calculate a percentage change. This is because the objective of disparity analysis as currently framed is to answer the hidden question, "How much worse are various subgroups than those populations who are viewed as being the dominant group?" In this regard, persons without disabilities would be used as the reference group in seeking to uncover health disparities between the disabled and the non-disabled. Likewise, a majority of

Americans live in urban areas relative to rural areas. Thus, urban dwellers would be used as the reference group in measuring rural/urban health disparities.

As mentioned, this latter set of procedures was used in the computations in Table 5.2 and will be used throughout this text as the topic of health and healthcare disparities is pursued. Additional instructions regarding the measure of health disparities can be found in Keppel et al.'s (2005) classic article.

Identifying Health Disparities: Other Approaches

The percentage differences methods are excellent and simple starting points for identifying health disparities. However, as one analyzes the data in Table 5.2, which reveal that Latino Americans and Asian Americans have rates of mortality per 100,000 that are below those of both White, Native, and African Americans, it becomes clear that this simple analysis does not lend insight into the *causes* of the observed disparities. One statistical technique that can be used to begin to identify patterns that might explain such differences is to stratify the data by other variables. This process of stratification is referred to as *bivariate analysis*. The type of analysis that we just completed is referred to as *univariate analysis*.

What do you mean by univariate and bivariate analysis?

Univariate analysis involves the process of organizing, describing, and summarizing data along one dimension. For example, with regards to the data on death rates per 100,000, we described the data by one variable only—race/ethnicity.

Bivariate analysis can be described as the process of analyzing data across two or more variables in order to determine whether there appears to be a relationship between those factors. For example, could there be a relationship between death rates for African,

Native and White Americans and the age distribution of the population? Bivariate analysis can be used to gain insights into such a question. In order to maximize knowledge from bivariate analysis as a source of measurement for disparities, the analysis must address two questions:

1. Are there *observable* differences between the death rates per 100,000 for persons age 65 and older and persons younger than age 65?
2. If so, are there differences by race/ethnicity in the representation of persons age 65 or older?
3. Do these differentials intermediate the differences in mean life expectancy by race/ethnicity?
4. If so, are these observable differences sufficiently large as to not occur through chance alone?

The first question can easily be answered by constructing a distribution table and examining the death rates per 100,000 by age and race/ethnicity, as in the example in **TABLE 5.3**.

TABLE 5.4, assuming that the data for each subgroup are not characterized by severe unreliability associated with underreporting, displays observable inequalities at each of the older age groups by race/ethnicity even without applying difference analysis with a reference group. These differences signal the need to answer the second question: Are the observable differences significant?

The concept of significance in the area of health can be answered from two perspectives: clinical and statistical. Differences can be clinically significant but not statistically significant. *Clinical significance*, also referred to as *practical significance*, is of greater concern to healthcare providers and public health personnel. This is because their interest is to answer the question of whether a certain intervention or treatment they provided has been effective. However, healthcare administrators seeking to uncover disparities are more interested in whether observable differences in health outcomes are

TABLE 5.3 Death Rates by Age 65+ and Race/Ethnicity for Both Sexes (per 100,000), 2015

Age Range	Non-Hispanic White Americans	Non-Hispanic African Americans	American Indian/ Alaska Native	Asian/Pacific Islander Americans	Latino/ Hispanic Americans
65–69	1,464.5	2,069.7	1,627.1	712.2	1,099.0
70–74	2,286.1	2,964.9	2,578.8	1,166.9	1,678.8
75–79	3,655.3	4,311.4	3,794.0	2,000.1	2,670.2
80–84	6,176.9	6,427.4	5,770.0	3,592.7	4,556.7
85 and over	14,324.3	12,364.4	9,792.4	8,653.4	9,585.2

Murphy S.L., Xu, J., Kochanek K.D., Curtin, S.C., & Arias, E. (2017) Deaths: Final data for 2015. Table 2. Number of death and death rates, by age, race and Hispanic origin, and sex: United States. 1. National Vital Statistics Reports 66(6) pg. 24, Hyattsville, MD: National Center for Health Statistics.

statistically significant. As is known, some numbers may be different from each other but the breadth of the difference is so small as to be meaningless. Statistical significance is a measure of whether the magnitude of the differences in values between two groups is too large to have occurred by chance. A *p*-value helps to identify if a difference between groups is due to chance or not. Chance can be indicated by a larger *p*-value whereas a smaller *p*-value may indicate that the difference between the groups may be due to another factor and not chance alone.

Assessing Statistical Significance

Current and future healthcare administrators will be held accountable if data reveal the presence of observable patterns of disparities in health or healthcare outcomes. Accordingly, the healthcare administrator may be required to select an in-house and/or contractual statistician to complete tests of significance to determine whether observed differences are statistically significant. Multiple types of tests of significance can be used based upon the type of data and the size of the dataset. Chi-square

tests and *t*-tests are oftentimes used in disparities analysis. In this case, the statistician would apply a *t*-test to the data as the test of significance.

What is a t-test and how does it differ from a chi-square test?

A chi-square test is used to determine whether two or more sets of values have frequencies that are significantly different. Chi-square tests are therefore used when values are expressed as frequency and percentages. A *t-test* is a statistical tool that is used to assess whether the means of two or more populations are equal or not sufficiently different as to be considered unequal. For example, we will state two hypotheses with regard to our question about death rates and age and race/ethnicity:

H_0:There are no differences in death rates per 100,000 by race/ethnicity for persons in the United States age 65 and older.

H_1:H_0 is false.

We can see that H_0 can be false in two ways. It can be false because there are differences in

TABLE 5.4 Frequency of Weapons Carrying Status by Race/Ethnicity Among Youth, 2015

Race/Ethnicity	Carried Weapons		Did Not Carry Weapons		Total	
	n	%	n	%	n	%
White Americans	6,530	18.1	29,547	81.9	36,077	100
American Indian/ Alaskan Natives	152	22.4	526	77.6	678	100
Hispanic	4,823	13.7	30,381	86.3	35,204	100
Black	1,272	12.4	8,986	87.6	10,258	100
Asian	600	7.1	7,850	92.9	8,450	100
Multiple Race Americans	669	20.8	2,547	79.2	3,216	100
Native Hawaiian/Pacific Islander	87	–	–	–	87	–
Missing Data on Weapons	290	–	–	–	290	–
Total	14,423	16.2%	79,837	83.8%	94,260	100%

Centers for Disease Control and Prevention. High School Youth Risk Behavioral Surveillance System. 2015 Results. https://nccd.cdc.gov/youthonline /App/Default.aspx

death rates per 100,000 between the racial/ethnic groups that are greater than those of White Americans as the reference group. H_0 can also be false because there are differences between the two groups that are less than the rate for White Americans. Because two options are available, the statistician will apply what is called a *two-tailed t*-test. If you only want to know whether other ethnic/racial groups had unfavorable disparities relative to the reference group, the statistician will apply a *one-tailed t*-test.

Because the data are from a national database and the findings have been isolated so that there is no relationship between the subgroups,

the statistician will use a *t*-test for independent samples. If the disparity analysis is for one particular healthcare organization, the statistician will decide whether the data are independent.

If I can hire a statistician, why do I need to know all of this?

Knowledge of statistics is necessary for anyone involved in healthcare administration, public health, or clinical health. Evaluation of health and healthcare involves data. Healthcare administration involves data. Public health involves data. Medical care by physicians and/ or nurses involves data. While healthcare professionals in leadership positions may not be required to perform the test of significance directly, *they cannot speak with the statistician nor interpret the findings in the absence of a familiarity with the language of statistics.* In the current many-cultural world of American society, all health institutions deliver services to numerous groups and subgroups. Assessing the existence of observable differentials by group and subgroup will inevitably be required.

What if I work for a nonprofit that has no funding for a statistician?

Current and future healthcare leaders, like the rest of the world, live within an environment in which knowledge is at one's fingertips within less than a second if the right search terms are used. Therefore, it should be less than surprising that any current or future healthcare leader can actually conduct a two-tailed *t*-test for independent samples within minutes using an online *t*-test calculator that can be accessed on your computer, laptop, tablet, or cell phone. While currently underused in the field of health care, these online statistical calculators should become a standard part of a healthcare professional's tools much like the arithmetical calculator. But, to accurately use and interpret findings from these simple tools, some of the conceptual language of statistics must be known. In addition, statistical calculators and smartphone apps can be purchased that can perform these statistical tests.

Despite their broad application and utility, *t*-tests can only be used if the data are interval or ratio. They cannot be used with nominal or ordinal data.

What do you mean by interval, ratio, ordinal, and nominal data, and how does this relate to health disparities measures?

Data can be interval, ratio, ordinal, or nominal:

- **Interval data** are quantitative data that do not have a true "zero" but that are, nevertheless, numerical. Temperature is measured on an interval scale. Interval data can be used with *t*-tests.

- **Ratio data** are measured using numbers that have a true zero. Ratio data can also be expressed as fractions.

- **Ordinal data** are based upon order. When data such as that from the Behavioral Risk Factor Surveillance Survey asks respondents to rank their own health status as excellent, good, fair, or poor, the data are ordinal.

- **Nominal data** are not quantitative but can be distinguished by name or category. In health disparity research, data collected by sex, race/ethnicity, rural/urban status, and sexual preference involve nominal variables.

It is important to determine whether it is meaningful to measure the distance between two possible data points. Interval or ratio scales provide greater statistical flexibility compared to nominal and ordinal scales because interval and ratio data are continuous scales that can easily be converted into categorical scales (i.e., ordinal and nominal).

Could you provide another example?

Say that you are interested in whether sex disparities exist in a pool of healthcare providers who are active physicians. Sex is a categorical variable; thus, it is nominal. You can do research that provides "frequencies" or "counts" of the total number of physicians and the total number of physicians who assigned themselves to the category of male or female. You can then calculate a percentage. That percentage tells you whether a difference exists in the proportion of males and females who are active physicians ("active" being physicians who are currently practicing medicine).

Let's say the proportions are different and that the differences do not reflect the proportion of males and females in the population. Can we say that disparity exists and apply a t-test to see if it is significant?

We can say a disparity exists, but we cannot use a *t*-test with nominal data. Rather, we can use a chi-square test. As mentioned, a **chi-square test** is a statistical tool that is used to determine whether differences between two categories of variables are statistically significant. Chi-square tests can be used with nominal or ordinal data but not with interval or ratio data. For example, you could use a chi-square to analyze whether there is a statistically significant difference in the percentage of males and females who rate their health as "excellent" or "good" versus "fair" or "poor."

How can we use a chi-square test to determine whether a significant difference exists?

As is true with any test of significance, certain guidelines must be met regarding sample size and other variables. If these guidelines are met, the online calculators that were discussed earlier can be used to calculate a *p*-value (**BOX 5.5**). (As mentioned earlier, the *p*-value is critical in disparity analysis for this value tells us whether observed differences by subgroups are of such a magnitude as to be considered as a major disparity.)

Does this mean that as healthcare professionals, we can ignore differentials between subgroups that are not significant?

Absolutely not! By addressing even small differentials, health care professionals can contain them so that they do not grow larger.

Can you provide an example of when to use a chi-square test?

As an example, you could use a chi-square test to determine if the genotype in a certain community differs from that of the nation as a whole. For example, your research question could be, "Do White Americans who live in Appalachia have a genotypic distribution that is significantly different from those who live in Massachusetts?" Again, because the variable *genotype* is nominal, a chi-square could be used to determine whether any identified differences are significant. Similarly, if you wanted to explore the relationship between the prevalence of cancer between Mormons and Protestants in Utah, you could also use a chi-square test. Table 5.4 is an example of data that you, the reader, could use to calculate a chi-square test. However, because this table is constructed from data found on the Centers for Disease Control and Prevention, Youth Risk Behavioral Surveillance Survey data website, statistical significance can be calculated directly on the website.

The data in the table reveal interesting information regarding health disparities by race/ethnicity regarding high school students who decided to carry a weapon in 2015. Specifically, the contingency table reveals that the group with the highest percent of high school youth who carried weapons in 2015 were American Indian/Alaskan Natives youth (22.4%), Multiple Race youth (20.8%), and White or Caucasian youth (18.1%). The key

---

BOX 5.5 Examples of Online Calculators for Performing Chi-Square Tests

Social Science Statistics Chi-Square Calculator for 5 × 5 (or less) Contingency Table:
   http://www.socscistatistics.com/tests/chisquare2/Default2.aspx
Social Science Statistics Easy Chi-Square Calculator:
   http://www.socscistatistics.com/tests/chisquare/Default2.aspx
iCalcu.com Chi-Square Calculator (unlimited size contingency table):
   https://www.icalcu.com/stat/chisqtest.html
Stat Trek Chi-Square Calculator:
   stattrek.com/online-calculator/chi-square.aspx
Math Cracker Chi-Square Test of Independence:
   https://mathcracker.com/chi-square-test-of-independence.php

question becomes, "Are these differences statistically significant?"

Rather than focusing upon all youth who carried a weapon in 2015, let's assume that we only wish to know whether there are statistically significant differences between the three youth groups who were most at risk of carrying a weapon. As mentioned, when we review the data in the table, we notice that the three groups of youths who had the highest rate of weapon-carrying were White American youth, Native American youth, and Multiple Race youth. When the data are entered into a chi-square calculator, the results in **TABLE 5.5** below are revealed. Whether a Pearson's chi-square, a likelihood ratio chi-square or Fisher's exact chi-square is used, we see that the *p*-value is less than zero. Thus, there are statistically significant differences in weapon carrying among these groups.

Had the data in these contingency data been analyzed by race and gender, it would have indicated that male high school youth of European descent were significantly more likely to carry a weapon in 2015. Researchers Kann, McManus, Harris, et al. (2016) state, "Nationwide, 16.2% of students had

carried a weapon (e.g., gun, knife, or club) on at least 1 day during the 30 days before the survey (Table 9). The prevalence of having carried a weapon was higher among male (24.3%) than female (7.5%) students; higher among white male (28.0%), black male (17.6%) and Hispanic male (20.2%) than white female (8.1%), black female (6.2%) and Hispanic female (7.1%) students, respectively. . . ." Thus, adding gender provides even more insight to those students most at risk of carrying weapons in 2015. Yet, because of the disciplinary nature of the field of health disparities, health care administrators, public health professionals, clinicians, educators, parents, community groups, policy makers, nor researchers have yet partnered in an effort to identify the causes of this high risk behavior across these critical subgroups. Moreover, even if these differences were not statistically significant, it is extremely clinically significant that youth in high school in 2015 felt a need to carry weaponry. Many of these youth are now in college. Causal research is needed to understand and remediate the circumstances generating large numbers of males across races/ethnicities to carry weapons. This

TABLE 5.5 Summary of Chi-square Test Analysis Between Race/Ethnicity and Weapons Carrying Status

Race/Ethnicity	Carried Weapons	Did Not Carry Weapons	Total
White Americans	6,530	29,547	36,077
American Indian/ Alaskan Natives	152	526	678
Multiple Race Americans	669	2,547	3,216
Total	7,351	32,620	39,971

Pearson chi2(2) = 21.8203, Pr <=0.000
Note: Pearson chi square calculations did not include Native Hawaiian/Pacific Islander data and/or any missing data.
Likelihood ratio chi2(2) = 21.0625, Pr < 0.000
Fisher's exact test = <0.000
Source: Calculated by authors with data found at the CDC High School Youth Risk Behavioral Surveillance System. Youth Who Carried Weapons, 2015.

example of a contingency table clearly demonstrates the criticality of linking statistical findings to transdisciplinary actions.

Are there any online calculators that can be used to duplicate the results just discussed?

Examples of Data on Ordinal Scales

The previous example demonstrated the use of chi-square tests to analyze data on a nominal scale. However, class rankings based on grade point average in nursing or medical school is an example of ordinal scale. Some data regarding health disparities can be on ordinal scale. Say that your hypothesis is that your 10th class reunion from medical school will include more students who were in the top half of the class rankings rather than those in the bottom half. Now, if you think about class rankings, simply because you were first in your class does not allow you to say that you, as a medical student, were 99% "better" than your classmates. It simply says that if you line everyone up by grade point average, you would hold the position of first place. Similarly, if you consider socioeconomic status, your classmates can be assessed as poor, middle class, and/or wealthy. These are rankings, but they are not mathematically meaningful terms. Accordingly, rank order characterizes *ordinal* scale. As you can see, these are *discrete* and *noncontinuous* variables.

Examples of Data on Interval Scales

An interval scale is the most useful for the purposes of analyzing health and/or healthcare disparities. The reason is that such data are measured on a continuous and numerical scale with equal intervals. However, interval scale does *not* have a fixed zero point (i.e., zero is arbitrary, not fixed). Age is an interval variable because it is on a continuous and numerical scale and is based on equal intervals. Also, age 0 can be culturally determined. In the United States, for example, a child's first year is defined as birth to 12 months. However, society could have just as easily decided that birth to 24 months comprises 1 year. Other examples of interval scale include temperature (Celsius or Fahrenheit), intelligence quotient, etc. A *t*-test and other statistical approaches can be applied to such data as long as the intervals are equal in length. Note, however, that such data cannot be multiplied or divided. For example, a summer temperature of 90°F does not mean that it is twice as hot as a winter temperature of 45°F. In health care, the difference between a temperature of 101°F is not statistically significantly different from a temperature of 98.6°F, although the difference is extremely significant from a clinical perspective.

Examples of Data on Ratio Scales

Ratio scales are the same as the interval scales except that the measurements are based on true numbers (i.e., they have a fixed zero). All mathematical operations can be applied to such measurements, and the results can be meaningfully interpreted. Weight is a ratio variable. Thus, an individual who weighs 300 pounds is twice as heavy as an individual who weighs 150 pounds. Other examples of ratio scales include healthcare costs, number of people in a household, height, annual income, etc. Zero in the natural number scale means that nothing exists. As a student, if you have zero income, you have nothing, but a temperature of zero does not mean that there is no temperature.

▸ Matching the Type of Data with the Analytical Approach

Different tests of significance are used based on the type of data. **TABLE 5.6** provides information on how to match data with the correct data analysis strategy. It is critical that

	TABLE 5.6 Matching Tests of Significance with the Appropriate Scale and Other Data Analysis Strategies	
Data Type	**Data Summary Strategy**	**Examples of Tests of Significance and Goodness-of-Fit Tools**
Nominal data	Frequency Percentages Means and standard deviations cannot be performed Display using bar charts or circle graphs rather than line graphs	Chi-square test Fisher's exact test Repeated measures analysis (to assess causation) Logistical regression (to assess causation) Contingency tables (to assess association) Simple logistic regression (to assess causation) Multiple logistic regression (to assess causation) Discriminant analysis (to assess causation) Other
Ordinal data	Frequency, median, mode In some cases a mean with the variance and standard deviation can be used Display data using a bar chart (because the data are not continuous)	Wilcoxon-Mann-Whitney test (to assess significance) Kruskal-Wallis (to assess significance) Wilcoxon signed ranks (to assess significance) Friedman test of logistic regression (to assess causation) Nonparametric correlation (to assess association) Other
Interval data	Mean, median, and mode with variance and standard deviation Line graphs	Kruskal-Wallis test of significance Paired *t*-tests of significance One-way repeated measures and other forms of ANOVA Friedman test (for nonparametric data) Correlation coefficient for association Multiple line regression and other forms of regression (for causal analysis) Factor analysis
Ratio data	Mean, median, and mode with variance and standard deviation as measures of dispersion Line graphs	Paired *t*-tests Independent *t*-tests Analysis of variance to compare mean or if the data do not fit the assumption for the above tests of significance All types of regression analysis for causal analysis

you know the information in this table. As a healthcare administrator and/or public health personnel, resources may be misused if they are directed toward the remediation of observed differences that are not statistically significant (the exception is in the area of clinical care). The table that follows includes examples of tests of significance and goodness of fit tools. Goodness of fit refers to the degree to which one's sample data complies with that expected from a normal distribution.

Table 5.6 describes how to summarize data by type. It also lists techniques for analyzing the significance and observable differences.

Can you explain these tests in greater detail?

A basic statistics course is normally a prerequisite for courses that use this text. The purpose of this chapter is that of describing how these tools that you have previously encountered can be used to identify the potential presence of health and/or healthcare disparities Table 5.5 includes statistical tests to assess causality. Please refer to an introductory statistics text for further information. The next section describes basic language healthcare administrators, public health leaders, or clinicians need to know to contract with a statistician.

Multivariate Analysis

In your discussions with a statistician, a number of multivariate analytical techniques will be outlined. Again, while you, as a healthcare administrator, public health worker, or clinician, will not be required to apply these analytical approaches, you will need to have the level of statistical literacy necessary (1) to understand the approaches proposed and discussed by the statistician and (2) to understand the interpretation of the findings after the data have been analyzed.

But what is "multivariate analysis"?

As discussed earlier, health outcomes are primarily the result of the following: (1) personal and behavioral characteristics, (2) socioeconomic factors, (3) environmental forces, (4) clinical care, and (5) genetics. Within each of these categories, a number of subcategories exist. For example, personal behaviors surrounding many substance use disorders that may affect retention in treatment programs include the type of substances used, the length of usage, the number of previous treatment attempts, the number of substances used, and other factors. The degree to which each of these variables are present may differ based on the group or subgroup. **Multivariate analysis** is a statistical approach that allows the statistician to simultaneously assess the impact of variables such as these upon a dependent variable. In this case, the dependent variable could be retention in the treatment program at a facility that you manage.

Correlation Analysis

Before engaging in multivariate analysis, a theoretical or conceptual model is needed that identifies independent variables that may be causally linked with the observed health disparities. **Correlation analysis** is a first step toward the identification of a possible association between key variables. For example, you could select an independent variable and a dependent variable that are disparately distributed by race/ethnicity and/or other identified subgroup to create a graph called a **scatterplot** (**FIGURE 5.2**). In this example, the scatterplot uses the independent variable of Global Assessment of Functioning (GAF) scores as a factor that may be associated with the length of time that a substance user remains in treatment (the dependent variable). Although correlation analysis is bivariate in nature rather than multivariate, it generally is used to signal the need for a multivariate analysis.

What is a Global Assessment of Functioning Score?

In mental health, various assessment tools are used to measure the degree of mental health need. Persons scoring 91–100 are assumed to have excellent mental health status, while individuals scoring 71–90 are considered as having mild mental health concerns.

Assessing Whether a Relationship Exists Between Variables

How can this information be used to determine whether a relationship exists between retention in a substance abuse program and mental health?

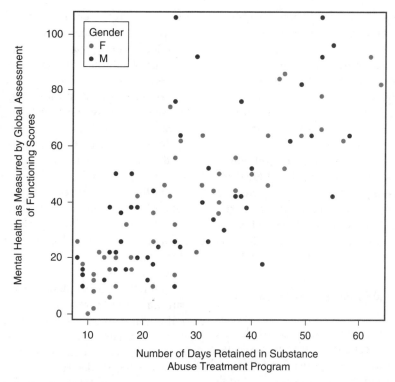

FIGURE 5.2 Example of a scatterplot.

- The statistician will calculate a *correlation coefficient* that identifies the strength of the identified relationship between the number of days retained in a substance abuse treatment program and GAF score for all participants in a 6-month non-residential treatment program or a 3-month residential treatment program.
- Correlation coefficients fall between 0 and 1. A coefficient of zero indicates that no change in the dependent variable takes place when there is a change in the independent variable.
- A correlation coefficient of 1 reveals that every unit change in the independent variable leads to a unit change in the dependent variable.

In the scatterplot in Figure 5.2, the correlation analysis may reveal that every person who did not complete the substance abuse treatment program had a mental health score

between 40 and 70 (independent of race/ethnicity). However, if a greater percentage of those with mental illness was not disproportionably clustered within one of the subgroups, but was normally distributed across subgroups, the disparity in program completion rates can be shown to be related only to the intervening variable, mental illness, rather than to lower-quality substance use disorder treatment by subgroup. It is important to note that this bivariate analytical strategy, correlation analysis, *reveals association and not causation*. Multivariate analysis must be applied in order to assume causation. However, correlation analysis is useful in building the causal model.

Factor Analysis

Factor analysis is a multivariate approach that can be used to reveal which of a large number of variables should be used in a causal analysis. Similar to correlation analysis, it is used to assist in constructing the conceptual model. By "specifying the model," we are referring to the process of identifying those independent variables that, collectively, may explain a significant proportion of the change in the dependent variable, which, in our example, is retention or dropout in a substance use disorder treatment program.

Factor analysis is the "parent" of what is now called *data mining*, a field of study that is not hypothesis driven, like multivariate analysis, but which is instead *hypothesis seeking*. Data mining falls into the category of *exploratory research*, whereas most multivariate analytical approaches are considered *conclusive research*.

How would a factor analysis be used in our example?

The healthcare administrator may ask the statistician who is conducting the disparity study to complete factor analysis in order to "search" for a list of subcategories of personal, lifestyle, socioeconomic, clinical, genetic, and environmental variables that may be causally related to mental health and, as a result, to retention in a substance use disorder treatment program.

Multiple Regression

Multiple regression is a primary tool that a statistician hired by a healthcare manager will use in a health disparities study. **Multiple regression** can be defined as a statistical methodology that allows causation to be *identified and measured*. Thus, the statistician will use this approach to not only confirm the existence of disparities but also to identify how much each variable in the specified model contributes to the identified disparity. A variety of types of multiple regression analysis are available.

Logistic regression is oftentimes used in the analysis of health disparities. This is because there are only two possible disparity outcomes. Either there is the odds that a disparity is present or there is no odds of a disparity. In terms of this approach, the outcome is defined as being categorical. Logistic regression is probably one of the approaches that the selected statistician will recommend.

Hierarchical linear modeling is, in many respects, a superior approach that a healthcare manager may wish to request the statistician to consider. It is a particularly useful approach in disparities research because if comprehensive data are available, it will allow the statistician to simultaneously assess the impact of the patient-level variables, institutional variables, provider/clinician-related factors, social determinants, environmental factors, genetic variables, and other clusters of the determinants of health outcomes.

Other multilevel models that the healthcare administrator may wish the statistician to address in terms of their appropriateness to the disparities study in question are *random effects multilevel models*, *mixed models*, *nested models*, and other models. Other types of regression include traditional linear regression, ridge regression, and the relatively new jackknife regression. Again, a healthcare administrator is not required to have a detailed knowledge of the differences in these analytical techniques but will benefit from having a familiarity with the analytical language used to conduct disparity studies. Every current and/or prospective healthcare administrator, public health professional, or clinician should ask their statistician, "What analytical approach do you propose to use given our datasets and research needs, and why do you think that approach is most appropriate?"

Other Types of Multivariate Analysis

One particularly important form of multivariate analysis is **analysis of variance (ANOVA)**, a multivariate approach that is most often used with categorical data such as gender, types of mental illness, and/or other nominal data.

Please remind me once more of the definition of nominal data?

Recall that *nominal data* refers to qualitative data such as names, categories, etc. For example, male and female are nominal variables. The term *health care administrator* is a nominal variable. Data that use categories such as true or false comprise nominal data. However, because disparities research most often uses continuous variables, such as death rates, prevalence, and/or incidence of illness and diseases and other numerical values as the unit of analysis, neither analysis of variance (ANOVA) nor multiple analysis of variance (MANOVA) is an approach that the healthcare administrator's statistician will usually consider.

Path analysis is an analytical approach that identifies correlations across and between different hypothesized independent variables. As such, it can be applied to an analysis of health disparities. Specifically, path analysis can be used by the healthcare manager's statistician to determine how strong the relationships are among the multitude of variables that are causally related to health disparities. Indeed, for the most part, the conversation between the healthcare administrator and the statistician will be based upon a discussion of which type of regression analysis will best uncover the "causes" of the confirmed disparities in outcomes. Again, whereas the statistician will be the "expert," the healthcare manager must be prepared to serve as an active participant in the conversation.

Chapter Summary

This chapter addressed the question, "How do we identify the presence of health disparities from a statistical viewpoint?" It began with a discussion of the simplest basic processes for analyzing health care data such as counts, ratios, etc. Toward that goal, data on health disparities in health outcomes as measured by death rates were described and used as sample data. This chapter also reviewed the different types of data and emphasized the importance of properly matching the analytical process

with the type of data. An example was also used to demonstrate the use of chi-square analysis as a tool for assessing significance when nominal variables are being analyzed. These data were then analyzed to demonstrate difference analysis and difference analysis with a reference point. The differential roles of univariate, bivariate, and multivariate analysis were described. Finally, key statistical information that a health care professional needs in order to converse with a statistician was introduced.

Review Questions and Problems

1. In Table 5.2, data were introduced that reveal that not all health disparities in death rates "favor" White, non-Hispanic Americans. Using this data, write an essay (250 to 350 words) explaining whether you believe that the data for the minority populations cited may be incorrect because of data underreporting. Be sure to cite the sources used.

2. Review the data in the following table on death rates among children by race/ethnicity using difference analysis with a reference group. Then answer the questions that follow. Be sure to show all calculations.

Disparities in Death Rates for Children Younger Than 1 Year (both sexes) By Race/Ethnicity			
White (including Hispanics)	Black/African American (including Hispanics)	American Indian/ Alaska Native	Asian/ Pacific Islander
499.5	1,062.1	459.2	399.0

Murphy S.L., Xu, J., Kochanek K.D., Curtin, S.C. & Arias, E. Deaths: Final data for 2015. Table 1-15. Number of deaths and death rates, by age, race, and sex: United States, 2015. National Vital Statistics Reports 66(6), Hyattsville, MD: National Center for Health Statistics. 2017.10

A. Based on the data, how much higher was the death rate per 100,000 for African American children younger than 1 year of age than was the case with white children?

B. Assuming that the data above are correct, how much higher was the death rate for white children younger than 1 year of age than for Native American children?

C. Assuming that the data above are correct, how much higher was the death rate per 100,000 for white children younger than 1 year of age than for Asian/Pacific Islander children?

D. How are you affected by the above disparities from a subjective perspective?

3. Using the research on early childhood deaths in question 2, if you were the administrator of a maternal and child health clinic, describe (in 250 or more words) some of the strategies you would use to improve the healthcare outcomes for children younger than 1 year of age across the described racial/ethnic groups. What precautions would you advise the parents to take to support the efforts of your clinic?

4. You are the administrator of a community center that provides services to patients who are HIV positive. Your clinic has been cited as having one of the highest racial/ethnic death disparity rates in the state. Write a brief screenplay of 250 to 350 or more words that describes a meeting between you, a statistician, and any other staff you wish to include. Then create a video of the scene with your phone and critique your performance based on whether you seemed knowledgeable and confident as a health administrator conversing with a statistician.

5. Differentiate between primary and secondary sources of data.

6. Compare and contrast the terms *prevalence* and *incidence*.

7. The authors interchange names for some of the ethnic groups. For example, the authors have chosen to use the terms "White", "Caucasian," or "Americans of European Descent" to describe the same population. Do these terms reduce or increase the intergroup tensions that are implicit to discussions of social/ethnic disparities?

8. Compare and contrast the terms *difference analysis* and *difference analysis with reference group*.

9. What is a *t*-test, and when and why is it used?

10. What are the differences between univariate, bivariate, and multivariate analysis? When is each used?

11. Why do the authors recommend linear hierarchical analysis over logistic regression?

Key Terms and Concepts

adjusted rate A type of "refined" rate that can be used to make comparisons more accurately. It is also a statistically adjusted summary rate.

analysis of variance (ANOVA) A statistical method that tests general differences among two or more means.

bivariate analysis The process of analyzing data across two or more variables in order to determine whether there is a relationship among those factors.

chi-square test A statistical tool that is used to determine whether differences between two categories of variables are significantly associated.

correlation analysis Statistical evaluation of the association and strength of the connection that exists between two variables.

count The simplest way to measure disease frequency in epidemiology. It is the number of how many cases (individuals) meet a particular definition (have a disease or health issue).

crude rates A summary rate that expresses how many cases existed in a population during a given time period.

factor analysis A statistical method by which a larger set of variables are reduced in order to reveal the cause and effect relationship between variables and/or to support a hypothesis.

health disparity measure A measure that summarizes the width of differentials in health outcomes between populations and/or subpopulations relative to one another.

hierarchical linear modeling or multilevel modeling is used to analyze hierarchical data.

incidence rate The number of new cases of diseases or deaths per defined unit. The unit may be 1,000 persons, 10,000 persons, or 100,000 persons a year.

interval data Quantitative data that do not have a true "zero" but are numerical.

logistic regression A statistical method that is used to identify an outcome from the analysis of one or more independent variables.

maximal rate difference Maximal rate difference is the method that is used by the federal government for calculating disparities. This method is simply based upon subtracting the lower value from the higher value.

multiple regression Statistical tool that allows causation to be identified and measured.

multivariate analysis A statistical approach that allows the statistician to simultaneously assess the impact of multiple variables upon a dependent variable.

National Vital Statistics System Part of the Centers for Disease Control and Prevention's National Center for Health Statistics, this agency is the most reliable primary source of secondary data on deaths, death rates, life expectancy, and infant mortality by race/ethnicity, gender, age, geographic area, and cause of deaths.

nominal data Data that are distinguished by name or category, such as sex, race/ethnicity, rural/urban status, or sexual preference.

ordinal data Data that are based upon order.

parameter A number based upon the entirety of the target population.

path analysis A statistical analysis tool used to assess relationships that exist between variables.

percentage difference The difference, categorized in percent format, between two variables. The calculation of the percentage difference can be accomplished by taking the difference between the two values and dividing it by the average of the two values.

prevalence rate The percentage of the total population or subpopulation affected by a condition in a specified time period.

proportion A measure in a form of ratio in which the numerator is also included as part of denominator. It can be calculated by dividing the number of interested cases [A] by the total cases [B].

rate A type of proportion that incorporates a given time period into the denominator. The numerator represents the cases that met the definition, and the denominator includes all cases that may or may not meet the definition.

ratio A fractional relationship between the numerator and denominator. You divide one quantity by another but the two quantities do not belong to each other.

ratio data Numbers that have a true zero and can be expressed as fractions.

reliable Data measurements that produce the same values independently of user, time, or place.

scatterplot A scatter graph or scatterplot consists of a series of plots that outline the connection between two sets of variables (or data).

specific rates A type of "refined" rate that can be used to make comparisons more accurately.

statistic A number that is derived from a sample taken from a total of the target population.

t-test A statistical tool that is used to assess whether the means of two or more populations are equal or not sufficiently different as to be considered unequal.

univariate analysis The process of organizing, describing, and summarizing data along one dimension.

valid Data that measure that which it purports to measure.

References

Centers for Disease Control and Prevention. High School Youth Risk Behavioral Surveillance System. 2015 Results. https://nccd.cdc.gov/youthonline/App/Default.aspx

Frensch, P. A. (1994). Composition during serial learning: A serial positive effect. *Journal of Experimental Psychology, Learners, Memory and Cognition. 20*(2), 422–442.

Harper, S. (2011). Methods and tools for measuring health inequalities across nominal social groups. Academy Health Workshop on Measuring Health Inequalities, Seattle, Washington, June 12.

Kann, L., McManus, T., Harris, W. A., Shanklin, S. L., Flint, K. H., Hawkins, J., . . . Zaza, S. (2016). Youth Risk Behavior Surveillance--United States, 2015. Morbidity and Mortality Weekly Report. Surveillance Summaries. Volume 65, Number 6. Centers for Disease Control and Prevention.

Keppel, K., Pamuk, E., Lynch, J., Carter-Pokras, O., Insun, K., Mays, V., . . . Pearcy, J. (2005). Methodological issues in measuring health disparities. *Vital Health Statistics.* National Center for Health Statistics. Series 2(141), 1–16.

Murphy, S. L., Xu, J. Q., Kochanek, K. D., Curtin, S. C., & Arias, E. (2017). Deaths: Final data for 2015. *National Vital Statistics Reports, 66*(6). Hyattsville, MD: National Center for Health Statistics. Retrieved from https://www.cdc.gov/nchs/data/nvsr/nvsr66/nvsr66_06.pdf

Skinner, A. C., Ravanbakht, S. N., Skelton, J. A., Perrin, E. M., & Armstrong, S. C. (2018). Prevalence of obesity and severe obesity in US children, 1999–2016. Pediatrics, e20173459.

Thompson, A. (2007). Bad memories stick better than good. Live Science, https://www.livescience.com/1827-bad-memories-stick-good.html

Xu, J. Q., Murphy, S. L., Kochanek, K. D., & Arias, E. (2016). Mortality in the United States, 2015. NCHS Data Brief, no 267. Hyattsville, MD: National Center for Health Statistics.

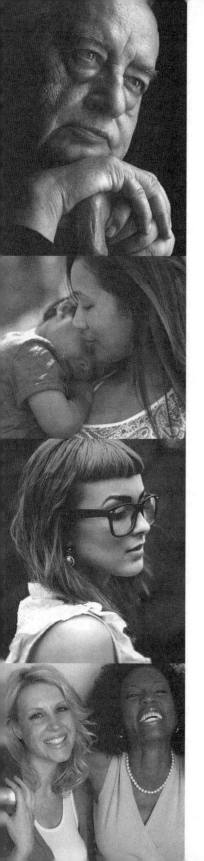

PART III

Disparities in Health Care

"Humanity's greatest advances are not in its discoveries, but in how those discoveries are applied to reduce inequity. Whether through democracy, strong public education, quality health care, or broad economic opportunity, reducing inequity is the highest human achievement."

—**Bill Gates**, June 2007, Howard University Commencement

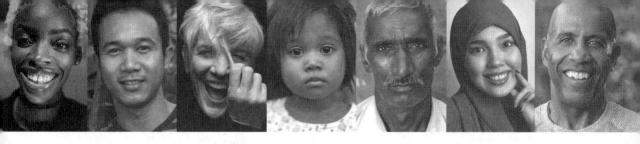

CHAPTER 6

Physicians, Healthcare Quality, and Health Disparities

"The secret of quality is love. You have to love your patients, you have to love your profession, you have to love your God."

—**Azedis Donabedian**

LEARNING OBJECTIVES

After completing this chapter, each learner will be able to:

- Define the term *panel size*.
- Identify trackable measures in the National Healthcare Quality and Disparity Report.
- Assess the accuracy of statements in this chapter by using data from the 2016 *National Healthcare Quality and Disparity Report* (2017) to recalculate cited findings regarding healthcare quality and disparities.
- Use data from the 2016 *National Healthcare Quality and Disparity Report* to identify new findings regarding physicians, race/ethnicity, and poverty with regard to healthcare quality disparities.
- Summarize research findings regarding physicians and health care disparities.

▶ Introduction

In some respects, physicians and other healthcare providers can be viewed as foundational to the American healthcare system. Accordingly, it becomes appropriate to ask the following question: "Despite the oath taken by physicians to do no harm to their patients, do physicians support disparities in the distribution of illness and disease across subpopulations in their delivery and management of the healthcare services provided?" Before further exploring this question, it is important to provide key background information regarding this highly

critical component of the American healthcare system.

▶ Physicians as a Component of the American Healthcare System

The United States has a population of more than
300 million men, women, and children. This
patient pool embodies persons of various races/
ethnicities, income levels, gender choices, educational and income backgrounds, behavioral
choices, varying health risks, and healthcare
needs. Young et al. (2017) indicate that, as of
2016, approximately 953,695 actively licensed
physicians provided health care to the American population. This represented an increase
of 12.9% from 2010, when the physician count
was 850,085. Based upon the most recent data
available at the time of this research, the ratio
of physicians to the total U.S. population was a
mere 2.55 physicians per 1,000 persons in 2015
(World Bank, 2016). This number ranked below
the following countries who had more physicians per 1,000 persons: Ireland (2.8), United
Kingdom (2.8), Luxembourg (2.9), Ukraine
(3.0), France (3.2), the Netherlands (3.35),
Australia (3.37), Andorra (3.69), Argentina
(3.76), Iceland (3.8), Spain (3.87), Malta (3.9),
Uruguay (3.94), Bulgaria (4.0), Belarus (4.07),
Sweden (4.11), Switzerland (4.11), Germany
(4.13), Norway (4.42), Portugal (4.43), Georgia
(4.78), Austria (5.15), Greece (6.26), Monaco
(6.65), Cuba (7.52), and a number of other
countries. Such data suggest that in the United
States, a country in which the provider infrastructure delivers health care based on market
conditions, patients may have to engage in a
greater competition for services given that the
United States has fewer physicians per 1,000
persons in the population. Such circumstances
alone could support the emergence of health
disparities within the American healthcare

system. Moreover, the physician pool is disparately distributed by state. For example, Massachusetts and other northeastern states have
higher physician-to-population ratios.

Why is this important?

When the ratio of physicians to the overall
population is low, two outcomes normally
occur. First, access to medical care becomes
limited based on the percentage of the residents of that state who have public and/or
private health insurance. Second, in order to
accommodate the insured populations, physicians have larger panel sizes.

What do you mean by "panel size"?

Panel size is the total number of patients that
a physician sees on a regular basis. The term is
most frequently applied to primary care physicians. This is because specialist care is not
designed to occur on a continuous basis.

So panel size is the physician's workload?

Not quite. The physician's **workload** is the total
sum of time associated with all activities completed as part of the delivery of health care. It
includes time spent with patients, as well as time
spent reviewing patient files, writing prescriptions, communicating with labs, completing
referrals, managing the clinical and administrative team, and completing other tasks.

Why is panel size important?

A number of studies have found that larger
panel sizes are sometimes related to lower quality of care. For example, Dahrouge et al. (2016),
in a study of 4,195 physicians with panel sizes
ranging from 1,200 to 3,900 patients, found
that while the medical management of chronic
diseases appeared unaffected by panel size,
some areas showed decreases in quality. Specifically, as panel size increased, the probability
was greater that patients would be hospitalized
for conditions that could have been treated on
an outpatient basis. The study also revealed a
slight drop in the comprehensiveness of medical care that occurred with larger panel sizes.
Murray, Davies, and Boushon (2007) found

an optimal-size patient panel improves patient outcomes. Accordingly, one can hypothesize that disparate geographic outcomes may occur between states with lower and higher physician-to-population ratios. Moreover, to the degree that those states include diverse subpopulations, this variable itself may reflect differential subgroup outcomes in the quality of medical care.

In addition, panel size may differentially affect healthcare outcomes by disease status. For example, Angstman et al. (2016), in a study of data from 36 family practitioners, found an inverse relationship between panel sizes greater than 2,959 patients and poorer quality of care for patients with diabetes. Thus, panel size may also generate documented disparities in healthcare outcomes among subgroups such as Latino Americans, African Americans, Native Americans, and Asian Americans, because these groups have higher prevalence rates of diabetes.

What is the point you are trying to make here?

The critical point is that there is an urgent need to not only identify the presence of statistically and clinically significant differences in physician health care, but that it is equally important to explore causation that extends beyond the hypothesis that direct and/or systemic discrimination is the operative variable "causing" such confirmed differences. This chapter examines physicians as merely one component of overall quality outcomes in the American healthcare system.

▶ Characterizing Disparities in Healthcare Quality in the United States

Healthcare outcomes based on physician practices do not occur in isolation. Rather, they take place within the context of the broader economy. Accordingly, it becomes useful to review healthcare outcomes across hospitals, physician practices, and other components of the American healthcare system as a context for examining its individual components. Moreover, this is one approach that warrants adoption by healthcare administrators, public health professionals, and clinicians.

Are you saying that before healthcare providers and professionals examine their specific subsystem, they should have an understanding of how the healthcare system as a whole is performing?

Yes, a noncontextualized assessment and evaluation of performance can be extremely distorting given that environmental forces serve as the context in which the healthcare system's subsystems operate. One useful data source for quickly summarizing the performance of the overall healthcare system is the U.S. Department of Health and Human Services' Agency for Healthcare Research and Quality, 2016 **National Healthcare Quality and Disparities Report**. The report, published in 2017, is available at www.ahrq.gov/research /findings/nhqrdr/index.html. Data used in this report are compiled from the Administration for Children and Families, Centers for Disease Control and Prevention, Health Resources and Services Administration, Centers for Medicare and Medicaid Services, Indian Health Services, National Institutes of Health, and other federal sources.

The initial online report is released in July of each year, and a hardcopy of the report is published each September. The edition of this document published in July 2017 revealed a number of interesting patterns that have implications for health disparities in physician practices. This edition reports data for 2000 to 2014. **BOX 6.1** presents some of these trends with regards to quality of access.

What do these data reveal?

The data in Box 6.1 reveal an urgent need to improve healthcare access for all Americans while seeking to identify and address causes of differences in improvement to access for selected subgroups.

BOX 6.1 Quality Changes in the Delivery of American Healthcare

Access to health care is necessary in order for healthcare providers and healthcare institutions to deliver services. The 2016 *National Healthcare Quality and Disparities Report,* published in 2017, uses 20 measures to assess *quality of access.*

- From 2000 to 2014, 35% of the access measures revealed significant quality improvement.
- One access variable that improved significantly was the decrease in the percentage of Americans who were uninsured from 2000 to 2014. This trend also continued into 2016 according to the report.
- However, subgroup differences occurred in terms of improvements in access from 2000–2014. (2016 National Healthcare Quality and Disparities Report, Appendix B)
  - Access improved on 0% of the measures for impoverished versus high-income Americans.
  - Access improved on 0% of the measures for Americans of African descent relative to Americans of European descent.
  - Access improved on 0% of the measures for Native Hawaiians or other Pacific Islanders relative to White Americans.
  - Access improved on 0% of the measures for Native Americans/American Indians and Alaska Natives relative to White Americans.

Data from: U.S. Department of Health and Human Services, Annual National Healthcare Quality and Disparities Report AHRQ Publications No. 17-0001, July 2017 (www.ahrq.gov/research/findings/nhqrdr/index.html).

Is access a primary measure of healthcare quality?

An abundance of research reveals that access alone is insufficient. Once care has been accessed, the maximization of health outcomes requires the inclusion of other quality standards. First, the care should be customized and delivered in a way that is responsive to the needs of each individual patient. Thus, clinical care must be provided, but patients must also be comfortable with their providers and the providers must assist patients in navigating the complex American healthcare system. This area of quality is referred to as *person-centered care,* and it is measured by 12 variables in the *2016 National Healthcare Quality and Disparities Report.*

Have quality improvements occurred based on this measure?

Yes, Americans in general experienced a 75.0% improvement in the receipt of **patient-centered care** from 2000 to 2014.

What other measures are used to gauge changes in quality of care?

Other quality measures include determining the incidence of medical errors. Those persons who receive health care should not be injured or made worse off by the experience. This is critical, because some researchers have found that medical errors are the third leading cause of death in the United States (Makary & Daniels, 2016).

Note that medical care contributes only 10% to 20% to overall health outcomes. Individual behaviors contribute much more. Thus, assessment of healthcare quality also includes a number of measures that assess whether the healthcare provider and/or provider institution supported primary and/or secondary prevention by asking questions on *healthy living.* Excellent quality in health care also requires that providers deliver treatments that reflect the highest standards of evidence and that patients remain adherent to recommended treatments and health practices. Thus, a number of measures assess *effective treatment.*

Patients receive care from many components of the American healthcare system. For example, prescriptions must be called into pharmacies. Similarly, patients will go to the medical lab for blood tests or other diagnostic procedures. These tests must be conducted to ensure reliable results. Referrals are made by primary care physicians to specialists. Family members must be informed of the health status of a patient if he or she is incompetent. As a result, case management services are needed. The quality measure that assesses the coordination of all of these services is called *care coordination*. Finally, despite the presence of insurance, individuals and families are responsible for co-pays, deductibles, and other forms of cost sharing. Thus, *care affordability* is required.

Just based on this short discussion, one can see that a comprehensive assessment of healthcare quality requires an examination of a wide range of measures. The 2016 *National Healthcare Quality and Disparities Report* presented 172 quality measures for the 2014–2015 reporting period. On a positive note, improvements occurred on 99, or 57%, of these measures. **BOX 6.2** presents information on documented improvements over the period of 2000 to 2014.

To what degree did these improvements in quality reach various subgroups?

When these quality measures are analyzed by race/ethnicity, income group, insurance status, and urban/rural living status, among other divisions, the data reveal that there is an urgency to promptly and effectively address ongoing healthcare disparities within the U.S. healthcare system. **BOX 6.3** summarizes some of the healthcare disparities by race/ethnicity

that can be identified in the 2016 *National Healthcare Quality and Disparity Report*.

What do you mean by "net quality loss or gain"?

In Box 6.3 we present the concept of *net quality loss or gain*. Note that the authors created this disparity construct. Because the cited subgroups received both better and worse quality outcomes on various measures, it was necessary to introduce one single measure that took both quality losses and gains into consideration. The net quality loss or gain is computed by simply adding together the percent loss and percent gain.

Differences in Healthcare Quality by Income Group

Some analysts have suggested that differential income subgroups experience greater disparities in health outcomes and healthcare services than those disparities that are operative by race/ethnicity (Myers, 2009). As the data in **BOX 6.4** indicate, the net impact of disparities in healthcare quality by income status for 2014–2015 did, in fact, exceed those differences observed by race/ethnicity. Note that *poor* refers to individuals whose annual incomes place them at or below the federally defined poverty line. *Low income* refers to families that spend a greater proportion of overall income on food, shelter, clothing, etc., than is true for families on average. *Middle income*

BOX 6.2 Improvements in Healthcare Quality as Documented in the 2016 National Healthcare Quality and Disparities Report from 2000 to 2014

- Overall, improvements were seen in 57.56% of healthcare measures.
- Person-centered care measures improved by 83.33%.
- Patient safety measures improved by 65.63%.
- Healthy living measures improved by 61.11%.
- Effective medical treatment measures improved by 52.78%.
- Care coordination measures improved by 48.39%.
- Availability of affordable health care improved by 14.28%.

Data from: U.S. Department of Health and Human Services, Annual National Healthcare Quality and Disparities Report AHRQ Publications No. 17-0001, July 2017 (www.ahrq.gov/research/findings/nhqrdr/index.html).

BOX 6.3 Observable Disparities in Healthcare Quality by Race/Ethnicity, 2014–2015

- For 12.64% of the quality measures, African Americans experienced better quality of care than their white counterparts. African Americans received worse quality of care than whites for 42.3% of the measures. This resulted in a *net negative quality gap* of 29.66%.
- Asian Americans received better quality of care on 33.74% of the measures relative to White Americans and worse care on 19.3%. Thus, Asian Americans experienced a *net positive quality gap* of 14.44%.
- American Indians/Alaska Natives received better scores on 12.9% of the quality measures compared to White Americans but worse scores on 33.33%. This resulted in a net negative quality disparity of 20.43%.
- For Americans who were Native Hawaiians and Pacific Islanders, scores were higher on 24% of the quality measures compared to White Americans and worse on 28%, for a net quality loss of 4%.
- Hispanic/Latino Americans received a better score than their non-Hispanic White American counterparts on 22% of the quality measures. They received worse scores on 38.69% of the measures, for a net quality gap of 16.69%.

Data from: 2016 National Healthcare Quality and Disparities Report. Rockville, MD: Agency for Health Care Research and Quality; July, 2017. AHRQ Pub. No. 17-0001; http://www.ahrq.gov/research/findings/nhgrdr/nhgrdr16/index.html9

BOX 6.4 Disparities in Healthcare Quality Outcomes by Income, 2000–2014

- Based on 123 quality measures, poor populations rated higher than higher-income groups on only 8 (6.5%) healthcare quality measures. Poor subgroups did worse that higher-income groups on 69 (56%) of the measures. Thus, their net quality loss was 49.5%.
- Low-income groups ranked better than higher-income groups on only 4 (3.25%) healthcare quality measures. Low-income groups did worse than higher-income groups on 69 (56.0%) of healthcare quality measures, for a net disparity loss of 52.72%.
- Middle-income groups received better health care on only 3 (2.4%) healthcare quality measures relative to high-income groups. Middle-income groups scored worse on 52 (42.28%) of quality measures. Thus, the net quality disparity loss was 39.88%.

Data from: U.S. Department of Health and Human Services, Annual National Healthcare Quality and Disparities Report AHRQ Publications No. 17-0001, July 2017 (www.ahrq.gov/research/findings/nhqrdr/index.html).

is defined as having an income that ranges from 67% to 200% of the U.S. median income (Pew Research Center, 2015). High income is defined as median incomes that exceed 200% of the U.S. median income for their family size.

What could account for the fact that net quality disparity loss scores are so high for middle-income groups relative to higher-income groups?

The overall healthcare quality scores support the continuing theme of this chapter of the urgency of using the simple tools of disparity analysis to broaden knowledge of differences in

healthcare outcomes wherever they exist. The data demonstrate that there is an urgent need to address differentials in healthcare quality between middle-income and higher-income Americans. Many healthcare administrators, public health personnel, and clinicians have failed to pose the question, "Do healthcare disparities differ between middle-income and higher-income Americans, and, if so, what are the causes and solutions?"

Many policy makers, community healthcare administrators, public health professionals, and clinicians do not normally classify middle-income persons as experiencing healthcare disparities. However, was this group disadvantaged in terms of improvements in healthcare quality for the period from 2000 to 2014?

The *2016 National Healthcare Quality and Disparity Report* can be used to answer the question, "For groups who experienced disparities in the year 2000, did any improvements in these disparities occur over the 14-year period?" Data from the 2016 *National Healthcare Quality and Disparity Report* reveal the patterns listed in **BOX 6.5**.

But didn't we just look at healthcare disparities?

We did. In Boxes 6.3 and 6.4 the research question was, "Given that healthcare quality became better, stayed the same, or became worse overall for the American population, how were all changes distributed across these three categories by race/ethnicity and income over this time period?" Now the question is, "Given that disparities in the various healthcare quality measures existed in the years up to 2000, the baseline year, did improvements occur in these baseline disparities by race/ethnicity and income when the 2014 data are examined?"

Could you give us an example?

If the difference between these research questions is not clear consider the following example. Let's say that from 1990 to 1999, Asian Americans had less access to care than whites on 50% of the criteria used to measure access to care. Then, over the period of 2000 to 2014, Asians still had less access to care on 50% of the variables used to measure access to care. These data will reveal that disparity levels neither worsened nor improved between the two periods for this measure. Rather, the change is 0%. Thus, no change in disparities occurred. This example may help clarify the data that are summarized in Box 6.5. To reiterate, in Boxes 6.3 and 6.4 healthcare quality changes between 2000–2014 were compared with the previous time interval in order to learn whether healthcare quality differences had improved in that time period.

What about other subgroups?

As is often discussed, persons with private insurance are advantaged in receiving healthcare relative to persons without insurance. Over the 2000–2014 time period, persons with public insurance and/or with no insurance experienced

---

BOX 6.5　Healthcare Quality Disparities by Race/Ethnicity and Income

- African Americans improved on 12 quality measures compared to White Americans over the last time period.
- Asian Americans, a group whose adverse disparities have oftentimes been overlooked because of a failure to view each Asian group separately, experienced *no improvements* in baseline disparities on any single measure and actually experienced a worsening of healthcare quality disparities on two measures when the two time periods are compared.
- Americans who are classified as Native Hawaiians and Pacific Islanders, another group considered as "doing well," experienced *zero improvements* in disparities in healthcare quality between the two time periods.
- American Indians/Native Americans and Alaskan Natives and Hispanic/Latino Americans, both groups with well-identified healthcare disparities, experienced improvements in disparities on 3 and 11 quality measures, respectively.
- Poor individuals experienced improvements in baseline disparities on 13 measures. Low-income persons had quality improvements on only seven quality measures.
- With regards to middle-income versus higher-income households, no improvements occurred on any healthcare quality measures when two time intervals are compared.

better outcomes on at least some quality measures compared with the previous time period. Likewise, persons across the entire continuum of rural to large central metro areas experienced better outcomes in some quality of care areas for the 2000–2014 measurement period. Yet, the data show that middle-income persons/households experienced no change in the quality of their health care over the entirety of the 2000–2014 period when compared with a previous period.

▶ Differences in Health Quality Outcomes Based on Differences in the Physician-to-Population Ratio

Let's find out if the physician-to-population ratio has an impact on healthcare quality. If you have not already done so, please download the U.S. Department of Health and Human Services' *2016 National Healthcare Quality and Disparities Report* which was published in 2017 www.ahrq.gov/research/findings/nhqrdr/index.html. You will use the data in the report to walk through the example presented in this section, which uses the sample data shown in **TABLE 6.1**. Note that the data are considered secondary data. Consider the following situation. Imagine that you and your family are listening to a newscast. The newscaster presents the data that we just described and, on the basis of the data, concludes that the American healthcare system is rife with net disparities in the quality of health care provided based on differential race/ethnicity and income status as a result of class and racial/ethnic discrimination. As the head of a large hospital, you are asked to comment. The question becomes, "How can you determine whether it is actually differences in the physician-to-population ratio that are associated with the observed

outcome?" The following is one way you can proceed in answering this question.

Step 1: Identify the best possible sources of data on physician-to-population ratios and on healthcare quality, key demographics, and socioeconomic variables by state.

Step 2: Create a table like that shown in Table 6.1. Populate the table with data, ensuring that all data are for the same year. The dependent variable is the one you wish to explain. The independent variables are the ones that you believe helped to "cause" the dependent variable to change. In this case, the quality of health care by state is the dependent variable. The total number of active physicians per 100,000 population is one of the independent variables. The percent of population in poverty and the percent of the population in each state who are minority are the other two independent variables (these data were taken from the Bureau of the Census). Healthcare quality data were taken from the *2016 National Healthcare Quality and Disparities Report*.

Step 3: Summarize the data by finding a mean for each set of states:

1. The 12 states with the highest overall quality of care
2. The 9 states with the lowest overall quality of care
3. The 9 states with the fewest racial and ethnic disparities in quality of care
4. The 12 states with the most racial/ethnic disparities in quality of care

Step 4: Now compare the outcomes by asking, "How did states with the highest and lowest quality of health care differ in terms of the mean number of active physicians per 100,000 population, the percentage of the population that was minority, and the percentage of the population that was impoverished?"

TABLE 6.1 Sample Data for Case Study

State Quality of Care[a]	Total Active Physicians per 100,000 Population[b]	% of Total Population Who Are Minority[c]	% of Total Population in Poverty[d]
States with the Highest Overall Quality of Care (2016)			
Midwest 1. Iowa	211.0	12.10	12.2
2. Minnesota	282.9	17.49	11.5
3. Nebraska	226.0	18.63	12.4
4. North Dakota	237.9	17.38	11.5
5. Wisconsin	254.9	17.00	13.2
Northeast 6. Delaware	266.8	35.33	12.5
7. Maine	313.8	5.21	14.1
8. Massachusetts	432.4	24.80	11.6
9. New Hampshire	300.3	7.78	9.2
10. New Jersey	290.1	42.48	11.1
11. Pennsylvania	306.4	21.35	13.6
12. Rhode Island	346.5	24.51	14.3
	$N = 12$ $\Sigma = 3,469.0$ Mean = 289.08	$N = 12$ $\Sigma = 244.06$ Mean = 20.33	$N = 12$ $\Sigma = 147.2$ Mean = 12.26
States with the Lowest Overall Quality			
South and Southwest 1. Arkansas	198.1	25.53	18.9
2. Kentucky	225.1	13.67	19.1

(continues)

TABLE 6.1 Sample Data for Case Study *(continued)*

State Quality of Care[a]	Total Active Physicians per 100,000 Population[b]	Percentage of Total Population Who Are Minority[c]	Percentage of Total Population in Poverty[d]
States with the Lowest Overall Quality			
3. Louisiana	240.9	40.01	19.8
4. Mississippi	184.7	42.23	21.5
5. New Mexico	235.3	60.36	21.3
6. Oklahoma	201.8	29.98	16.6
7. Texas	213.3	55.70	17.2
8. West Virginia	246.7	6.54	18.3
Midwest 9. Indiana	222.6	18.87	15.2
	$N=9$ $\Sigma=1,968.5$ Mean = 218.72	$N=9$ $\Sigma=292.9$ Mean = 32.54	$N=9$ $\Sigma=167.9$ Mean = 18.6
States with the Fewest Racial and Ethnic Disparities			
West and Midwest 1. Idaho	189.6	16.16	14.8
2. Kansas	214.2	22.00	13.6
3. North Dakota	237.9	12.38	11.5
4. South Dakota	231.4	15.95	14.2
5. Utah	207.5	19.52	11.7
6. Wyoming	196.7	14.89	11.2
South 7. Kentucky	225.1	13.67	19.1

8. Tennessee	247.1	24.46	18.3
9. Virginia	255.9	35.68	11.8
	$N = 9$ $\Sigma = 2{,}005.4$ Mean $= 222.82$	$N = 9$ $\Sigma = 174.71$ Mean $= 19.41$	$N = 9$ $\Sigma = 126.2$ Mean $= 14.02$

States with the Most Racial and Ethnic Disparities

Northeast 1. Massachusetts	432.4	24.80	11.6
2. New York	353.8	42.75	15.9
3. Pennsylvania	306.4	21.35	13.6
Midwest 4. Illinois	271.5	36.99	14.4
5. Indiana	222.6	18.87	15.2
6. Iowa	211.0	12.10	12.2
7. Minnesota	282.9	17.49	11.5
8. Ohio	279.8	18.98	15.8
9. Wisconsin	254.9	17.00	13.2
South 10. North Carolina	244.0	35.04	17.2
Southwest 11. Texas	213.3	55.70	17.2
West 12. Arizona	234.0	42.81	18.2
	$N = 12$ $\Sigma = 3{,}306.60$ Mean % $= 275.55$	$N = 12$ $\Sigma = 343.88$ Mean % $= 28.66$	$N = 12$ $\Sigma = 176.0$ Mean % $= 14.66$

[a] Based on U.S. Department of Health and Human Services. (2017). *2016 National Healthcare Quality and Disparities Report*. AHRQ Publications No. 17-0001. Retrieved from www.ahrq.gov/research/findings/nhqrdr16/index.html

[b] Based on Center for Workforce Studies. (2015). *State physician workforce data book*. Association of American Medical Colleges for Table 1.1, Active Physicians per 100,000 Population by Degree Type, 2014. July 1, 2014, population estimates are from the U.S. Census Bureau. Physician data are from the 2015 AMA Physician Masterfile (December 31, 2014).

[c] Based on National Center for Health Statistics, Bridged-Race Population Estimates, 1990–2014 Results. Available on CDC WONDER Online Database. Retrieved from http://wonder.cdc.gov/bridged-race-v2014.html

[d] Based on 2014 data from Glass, B. (2016). Selected economic characteristics by state: 2014 and 2015. U.S. Census Bureau. Retrieved from https://www.census.gov/data/tables/2016/demo/income-poverty/glassman-acs.html

Why do we ask this question? Our hypothesis is that the states with the higher quality health care will have a greater physician-to-population ratio and a lower percentage of minorities and impoverished persons. This hypothesis appears logical given that (1) physician care correlates with better health based upon numerous studies and (2) the data presented in the chapter revealed that healthcare quality measures differed by race/ethnicity.

Step 5: Next, compare the data by asking, "Did the states with the fewest overall racial and ethnic disparities in healthcare quality and the states with the most overall racial/ethnic disparities in healthcare quality differ in terms of the number of active physicians per 100,000, the mean percentage of the states' population that was minority, and the mean percentage of the states' population who were impoverished?"

Here, your hypothesis is that states with a higher physician-to-population ratio, a lower percentage of minorities, and a lower percentage of impoverished persons will be represented among the states with the fewest disparities.

Should we calculate tests of the significance?

Perhaps, but first let's use the raw data in our fully populated table to calculate central tendencies so that we can answer the questions. Please remember to check your calculations several times so that we have no errors.

Now that we've completed the analysis by walking through the steps, how can we interpret these findings?

The data provide some very interesting information. We identified the 12 states with the highest overall quality scores based on data in the *2016 National Healthcare Quality and Disparities Report* (which reports on 2014 data). These states included five states in the Midwest and seven states in the Northeast. These high-quality states were then compared with those with the lowest overall healthcare quality.

You can see that geographic region is associated with the quality of overall health care in the United States. These geographic disparities in quality are such that of the nine states with the lowest quality, all except one were located in the South or Southwest. Indiana, which is a Midwestern state, was the only state outside of the South included among those with poor healthcare quality. These findings suggest that healthcare administrators, public health personnel, and clinicians in these states have cause for concern, particularly given that healthcare quality disparities can contribute to higher death rates (Baciu, Negussie, Geller et al., 2017).

Why are those states with the best healthcare quality located in the Midwest and the Northeast?

Recall that five Midwestern and seven Northeastern states are those with the best healthcare quality. Why might this be the case? A causal study using multivariate analysis would be required to answer such a question. However, before completing a study of causation, it is necessary to generate a hypothesis. Earlier we discussed variables at the state level that may be related to quality of care: the number of physicians per 100,000 population, race/ethnicity, and poverty rates. Accordingly, the mean number of doctors per 100,000 population for the low-quality and the high-quality states was calculated. In addition, the mean percentage of the population who were minorities was estimated for the high- and low-quality state groupings. Finally, the mean percent of the population in each state with individual and/or family incomes at or below the federally defined poverty level was calculated for the low- and high-quality states. Unsurprisingly, the mean number of active physicians per 100,000 population was higher in the high-quality states compared with the low-quality states.

What were the numbers, and were the differences statistically significant?

The mean number of physicians in the high-healthcare quality states was 289.08 versus

218.72 in the lowest-quality states. Thus, the mean number of physicians was 32.16% higher in those states with the highest healthcare quality than the mean for the states with the worst overall healthcare quality. Although no tests of significance were completed, the preliminary data suggest that there is a need for additional inquiry into the role that physicians play in the quality of healthcare outcomes both within and between states.

However, the data also reveal that healthcare quality is associated with both the percentage of minorities and with the proportion of low-income persons in a state. States with the lowest overall healthcare quality had a 32.54% mean proportion of minorities relative to 20.33% for states with the best healthcare quality. Thus, states with the lowest overall quality also had a 60% greater proportion of minorities than states with the highest quality. No tests of significance were completed. However, these preliminary data demonstrate a basis for the inclusion of racial/ethnic minorities in a causal model of these healthcare quality disparities.

One may hypothesize that the proportion of impoverished persons also affected whether a state was included among those with the best or worst healthcare quality. On average, 12.26% of the population were poor in the states with the best healthcare quality. The percentage was 18.6% in the states with the worst healthcare quality. Thus, mean poverty rates were 51.71% higher in the states with the absolute worst health quality.

What do these data suggest?

They suggest a need for a more sophisticated causal model to identify the relationship between the health care outcomes of states and the physician-to-population ratio, the percentage of the population who are low income, and the percentage that belong to minority groups.

Should we examine other variables?

Possibly, but because we have so few states, we would not want to be guilty of what is called *overfitting* or *underfitting* the model if we were to conduct a causal analysis. Underfitting or overfitting a regression refers to having too few (underfitting) or too many (overfitting) independent variables for the dataset used in a regression analysis.

So, is that a problem in this exercise?

No, it is not a problem with the exercise we performed here because we are simply engaging in exploratory research to demonstrate the importance of always asking new questions of datasets when one is in search of disparities.

How were these variables—the number of physicians per 100,000, the percentage of minorities, and the percentage of a state's population who are impoverished—associated with the states with the fewest and the most disparities in healthcare quality?

The patterns identified were quite interesting and, in one instance, somewhat surprising. The states with the most racial disparities had a higher number of physicians per 100,000 population than the states with the least disparities! Specifically, states with the *fewest* disparities had a mean of 222.82 physicians per 100,000 relative to 275.55 per 100,000 for the states with the most racial/ ethnic disparities. Thus, the states with the most disparities had 23.66% more active physicians than those states with the fewest disparities.

The reason behind this finding is not clear. However, the data suggest that there is a need to review research on physicians and disparities in order to identify those variables that may be operative.

But what about the question of whether race/ ethnicity and poverty interfere with healthcare quality?

The data also revealed that, whether via discrimination, cultural factors, the environment, or other variables, race/ethnicity is associated with quality disparities in health care. Those states with the fewest disparities in healthcare quality had, on average, populations that were 19.41% minority. Those states with the most racial/ethnic disparities were 28.66% minority. Thus, states with the worst disparities were 47.66% more heavily populated by racial/ethnic minorities.

What about poverty rates?

In this case, the differences in poverty rates appeared to be relatively minor. The states with the least disparities had a mean poverty rate of 14.02%. The states with the most disparities had a mean poverty rate of 14.66%. Thus, the states with the most disparities had a poverty rate that was only 4.56% higher.

Based on this simple analysis, the data indicate that poverty has no relationship to healthcare quality disparities. In fact, the mean poverty rate was actually the same when accounting for a margin of error in the states with the least healthcare quality disparities and the states with the worst disparities (14.02% vs. 14.66%). This is only a 4.5% difference.

But these findings seem to contradict what we believe about disparities?

You might be surprised by these findings. Most racial and ethnicity disparities among the states are *not* disproportionately in the Southern and Southwestern states, except for North Carolina, Texas, and Arizona but rather in the Northwest and Midwest. Even more surprising, the states with the worst healthcare quality disparities had the highest physician-to-population ratios. The data also show that there is a higher percentage of minorities in the population of the states with the worst healthcare quality disparities but with very little differences in poverty rates.

What could account for these findings?

We can't say exactly. However, this exercise revealed that states that had the worst healthcare quality outcomes also had a higher number of physicians per 100,000 population and larger minority populations. This could indicate a need for the physicians to deliver culturally competent medical services to their patients in those states. But, this was solely a descriptive exercise. Perhaps one of our readers will conduct a conclusive research study on some of the issues raised by this exercise.

Chapter Summary

This chapter shifted the focus of discussion from health disparities to health care disparities. Toward this goal, it began with an overview of physicians per population in the United States versus other countries. It then explored changes in health care quality. The chapter then introduced the question, "What role do physicians play in healthcare quality disparities?" The data introduced demonstrate that physicians are particularly positioned to address disparities in healthcare quality. An exercise was then completed that sought to extract new knowledge regarding the relationship between the physician population ratio in the United States and measured quality in health care. The discussion was further extended to an analysis of the relationship between the physician/population ratio by state and disparities in health care quality. The analysis revealed the surprising finding that the physician/population ratio was actually higher in states with the "worst" health disparities. This finding suggested a need for further research.

Review Questions and Problems

1. Complete research on the physician/population ratios and maternal death rates by state. Use an online statistical calculator to calculate the correlation coefficient. Is the correlation strong, moderate, or weak? Is the correlation positive or negative? Is it significant at the $p < .01$, $p < .05$, or $p < .10$ level?

2. Now complete research on maternal deaths in the most impoverished states versus the states with the lowest poverty rates as a function of the number of doctors per population. Does it appear that there may be a relationship?

3. Write a well-researched 1,000-word essay on physicians and health disparities. Does this literature review suggest that physicians are major contributors to health disparities?

Key Terms and Concepts

National Healthcare Quality and Disparities Report Annual report produced by the U.S. Department of Health and Human Services that documents health and healthcare measures for the U.S. population.

panel size The total number of patients who see a physician on a regular basis.

patient-centered care A collaborative form of health care and decision-making that involves healthcare providers, patients, and their families wherein the main goal is to strategize a customized and comprehensive healthcare plan.

workload The total sum of time associated with all activities completed as part of the delivery of health care. Includes time spent with patients, as well as time spent reviewing patient files, writing prescriptions, communicating with labs, completing referrals, managing the clinical and administrative team, and completing other tasks.

References

Angstman, K. B., Horn, J. L., Bernard, M. E., Kresin, M. M., Klavetter, E. W., Maxson, J., . . . Thacher, T. D. (2016). Family medicine panel size with care teams: Impact on quality. *Journal of the American Board of Family Medicine, 29*(4), 444–451.

Baciu, A. National Academies of Sciences, Engineering, and Medicine (2017). Communities in Action: Pathways to Health Equity. Washington, D.C.: The National Academies Press. https://doi.org/10.17226/24624

Dahrouge, S., Hogg, W., Younger, J., Muggah, E., Russell, G., & Glazier, R. H. (2016). Primary care physician panel size and quality of care: a population-based study in Ontario, Canada. *Annals of Family Medicine, 14*(1), 26–33.

Mackary, M. A., & Daniel, M. (2016). Medical error—the third leading cause of death in the U.S. *BMJ, 353*, i2139. doi.org10.136/bmj.i2139

Murray, M., Davies, M., & Boushon, B. (2007). Panel size: how many patients can one doctor manage? *Family Practice Management, 14*(4), 44–51.

Myers, H. F. (2009). Ethnicity and socio-economic status-related stresses in context: An integrative review and conceptual model. *Journal of Behavioral Medicine, 32*(1), 9–19.

National Academies of Sciences, Engineering, and Medicine (2017). Communities in Action: Pathways to Health Equity. Washington, D.C.: The National Academies Press. https://doi.org/10.17226/24624.

Pew Research Center. (2015). The American middle class is losing ground: No longer the majority and falling behind financially. Washington, D.C. Retrieved from http://www.pewsocialtrends.org/2015/12/09/the-american-middle-class-is-losing-ground/

U.S. Department of Health and Human Services, Agency for Healthcare Research and Quality. (2017). *National Healthcare Quality and Disparities Report*, AHRQ Publications No.17-0001. Retrieved from https://nhqrnet.ahrq.gov/inhqrdr/reports/qdr

U.S. Department of Health and Human Services, Agency for Healthcare Research and Quality. (2017). *National Healthcare Quality and Disparities Report*, Appendix B: Trends in Access, Quality and Disparities for Measures in 2016 Report. Content last reviewed July 2017. Agency for Healthcare Research and Quality, Rockville, MD. http://www.ahrq.gov/research/findings/nhqrdr/nhqdr16/appendixb3_qualitytrends.html

World Bank. (2017). Physicians (per 1,000 people). Retrieved from https://data.worldbank.org

Young, A., Chaudry, H. J., Pei, X., Arnhart, K., Dugan, M., & Snyder, G. B. (2017). A census of actively licensed physicians in the United States, 2016. *Journal of Medical Regulation, 103*(2), 7–21.

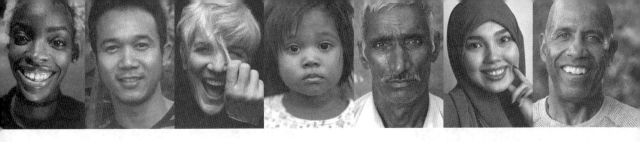

CHAPTER 7

Healthcare Disparities in Physician Practices

"The good physician treats the disease; the great physician treats the patient who has the disease."

—**William Osler** (1849–1919), a Canadian physician and one of the four
founding professors of Johns Hopkins Hospital

▶ Introduction

When secondary data on disparities in healthcare quality are examined, an interesting pattern emerges—the states with the greatest healthcare quality disparities also have the highest mean number of physicians per 100,000 persons. That is, states with the "worst" health disparities have a higher number of physicians relative to their population than states with better measures of healthcare quality. This empirically verifiable trend suggests that it may be useful to review literature on healthcare disparities in physician practices in order to identify factors that may be associated with these unusual findings.

What does empirical mean?

Empirical refers to information and knowledge that transcends theory. Empirical data are generated by statistical observation of real-life experiences and/or via experiment or data analysis.

▶ Physician Practices and Patient Communication

Physicians are assigned the duties of diagnosing and treating illness and disease and, more recently, of engaging in activities that involve the prevention of illness and disease. This aspect of medicine is called **primary prevention**. Physicians also assist in secondary prevention. **Secondary prevention** involves the provision of treatment that reduces the odds of the recurrence of illness and disease. Physicians also support the patients in the self-management of chronic diseases. **Patient self-management** refers to patients engaging in activities that can reduce the progress of their disease and decrease or prevent the appearance of symptoms associated with their disease. For all of these tasks, physicians and patients communicate with one another. Accordingly, the question arises, "Do problems in physician–patient communication occur in some physician practices?"

Evidence exists that some patients do perceive themselves as encountering problems in the area of physician–patient communication. For example, Hawkins and Mitchell (2018), in an analysis of the views of a group of African American males, confirmed that the participants felt that communication barriers existed between themselves and their providers.

Such a finding is not new. Earlier studies have identified differences in physician–patient communication as a source of differences in the quality of the healthcare experience. Siminoff, Graham, and Gordon (2006) applied communication analysis to audiotapes of physician–patient encounters. They observed a bilateral form of communication inadequacies. Specifically, patient and physician communications were more active among majority (White) group patients with higher income

and education. Additionally, younger patients asked more questions than older ones. These findings indicate that there may be a need to not merely educate clinicians regarding the improvement communications across all patients but to also educate patients to formulate and ask more questions related to their condition.

In other instances, research has indicated that while some physicians do make an effort to communicate with patients across educational, racial/ethnic, and income differences, communication failures are magnified because physicians do not adequately translate clinical terminology into easy-to-understand language. Kelly and Haidet (2007), using the Rapid Estimate of Adult Literacy in Medicine (REALM) to measure the literacy level of patients by race/ethnicity and gender, found that contrary to the use of racial/ethnic stereotypes, physicians disproportionately assumed that the literacy levels of African American and Latino patients were significantly higher than they actually were. Thus, rather than "talking down" to them, they "talked up" to them and, as a result, created a communication failure. Street et al. (2009) suggest that such issues transcend mere politeness and patient comfort. Rather, physician–patient communications literally affect patient outcomes by impacting patient compliance with treatment and access to service.

In still other instances, physician–patient miscommunications were related to the fact that the two groups literally spoke different languages (Cooper & Powe, 2004). The researchers recommended increases in physician–patient language concordance as a needed strategy.

Are these issues still a problem today? These studies are rather dated.

Yes, the studies listed thus far are rather dated. However, these studies are specifically cited before discussing more recent research in order to determine whether some of these matters have continued into the present.

Have issues of physician–patient communication been resolved?

More recent research suggests that although the importance of physician–patient communications has been more widely recognized and addressed through the **cultural competency model**, barriers to high-quality health care remain. Cultural anthropologists define culture as the total way of life of a people. It references language and language use, food consumed, clothing worn, housing, art, dance, norms regarding social behavior, religion, and intrapersonal thought. Values, beliefs, and attitudes are each components of the culture of a people (Schultz and Lavenda, 2009). However, Spencer-Oatey (2012) demonstrates that culture is far more definitionally complex than that which has been standardized via the influence of cultural anthropologists. Accordingly, the entire groups and subgroups of humans are judged based upon the crispness and fluidity of their speech; the nature, type, and cost of the clothing that they wear; the loudness or softness of their speech as they enter into a room; the complexity of the musical constructions that they prefer; and other differentials in their ways of life. As Spencer-Oatey's (2012) article confirms, each of the various definitions of culture explicitly and/or implicitly generates feelings, emotions, and/or behaviors which support the ranking of other humans as superior and/or inferior.

For example, the field of consumer behavior in marketing is replete with stories of the difficulties experienced by American and European businesspersons in seeking to establish trade relations with business owners from Japan, China, and other Asian businesses (Jiang and Wei, 2012). Dictionary.com, Collins Dictionary, *Merriam-Webster*, and others have now institutionalized the term "Ugly Americans" as one which characterizes tourists whose cultural behaviors abroad relegate the United States to the ranks of the "culturally inferior." Accordingly, it is less than surprising

that workshops and seminars were developed and offered to increase the skills of American businesspersons in interfacing with their counterparts in other countries. Knight (1999) provides a review of some of these efforts. The concept of cultural intelligence (CQ) has now been integrated into the field of international business (Ott & Michailova, 2018). Moreover, Alon et al. (2016) confirm that the cultural intelligence quotient of business professionals is associated with improved outcomes.

Accordingly, the notion that, like business professionals, healthcare professionals can also be trained to improve their interactions with persons who are culturally diverse has been activated. Whether the nature of the behavioral differences is a result of nationality, language, and/or differences in language use, dress, speech, beliefs, and/or differential ways of life that result from religion, socioeconomic class, gender orientation, or any other stratifier, the concept of cultural competence has emerged in health care as one approach to a reduction in health disparities. Cultural competency as defined by Cross et al. (1989) implies that this term references a set of compatible actions and policies that are adopted by professionals and their organizations that will enhance outcomes when services are provided across cultures. While the exact words used have been modified by other writers over time, the concept of being trained to better understand the way of life of those with whom one "does business" began with marketers and has remained the essence of the cultural competency model that exists in health care.

However, more refined knowledge relative to the causes of the problem is now known. Additionally, the mechanisms through which health outcomes are affected by physician–patient communications have been better specified.

Indeed, cultural competency training has been introduced as a key tool for the improvement of differences in physician–patient communication. Research by Betancourt, one of the pioneers in the field of health disparities, and colleagues (2003) used a literature review to summarize and categorize the use of various "cultural competence interventions" to address provider–patient miscommunication issues. Strategies included (1) increased representation of traditionally defined health disparity populations in the fields of healthcare administration, public health, and clinical health care; (2) education of providers on issues related to the treatment of patients across racial/ethnic, socioeconomic, and other subgroups; (3) the use of cultural interpreters when needed; and, (4) other strategies. These methods continue to be used today. Jongen et al. (2017) state that, "Improving the cultural competence of the health workforce is the original and still the most common cultural competence intervention strategy" (pg. 49).

Nevertheless, recent research demonstrates the continuation of patient-based, physician–patient communication problems. Moreover, it appears that these communication problems involve patients as well as providers. For example, Ricker et al. (2018) found that when genetic test results indicating a genetic predisposition to cancer are communicated to patients, Latino patients are less likely to communicate this information to their providers and Asian patients are less likely to urge family members to also be tested. Such communication challenges reduce cancer prevention opportunities.

Duberstein et al. (2017), in a study of 977 patients with incurable cancer, discovered that barriers existed preventing the linkage of patients with education about end-of-life care because of a refusal of some patients to confront the incurable nature of their disease. These researchers also found that African Americans and Americans of Asian/Pacific Islander descent were less likely to embrace end-of-life care because of a refusal to accept their status than was the case with their Caucasian counterparts. Thus, even if professional interpreters are used, problems are encountered as these interpreters seek to have a conversation in which the patient does not wish to participate (Rhodes et al., 2018).

A variety of quality differentials may exist in physician care other than in physician–patient interactions. Foo et al. (2017) conducted research on physicians in Detroit, Michigan, by making audiotapes of physician–patient conversations. Analysis of the conversations revealed that the degree of relevant physician empathy differed based on the race/ethnicity of the patient and the physician. In other words, the dehumanizing component of subgroup loyalties can be so strong that some physicians feel no emotional response to the health problems of patients with discordant race/ethnicity. Nagarajan, Rahman, and Boss (2016), in a study of parental satisfaction with pediatrics care, found that parents of minority children had a level of satisfaction that was 30% to 50% less than their nonminority counterparts in the areas of care that involved cultural responsiveness and communication. This suggests that some physicians fail to respond with caring and/or sympathy even when the patients are children.

Such patterns, however, are interactive. Perceptions of bias may cause some people to even avoid contact with physicians. For example, Saadi, Himmelstein, and Woolhandler (2017), using data from the Medical Expenditure Panel Survey (MEPS), found that, when holding other variables constant, race/ethnicity impacted whether those with neurological disorders selected to visit emergency departments for health care rather than seek care from a neurologist. Stated differently, patients who perceive their physicians to be biased against them will avoid direct contact *even when their conditions are serious.*

▶ Implicit Bias

Some recent studies have discovered that implicit racial/ethnic bias continues in the realm of health care. For example, Maina (2018) documented the existence of implicit racial bias in pediatric care. **Implicit bias** occurs when beliefs, attitudes, and values regarding various subgroups are operative at a subconscious level.

If healthcare providers and professionals are not conscious of their bias, how can they be held responsible for it?

Selmi (2017) makes an interesting argument. This legal scholar suggests that individuals can easily recognize and uncover the biases, prejudices, and other attitudes that can adversely impact the lives of others. Accordingly, he suggests that persons who analyze differences in outcomes among subgroups cease and desist from the use of implicit bias as a framework for explaining actions based upon biased beliefs and behaviors.

How strong is the evidence that implicit bias creates healthcare disparities?

Implicit bias is widespread in healthcare and can be identified in numerous areas of health care (The Joint Commission, 2016). In their publication, *Quick Safety*, The Joint Commission, an accreditation and certification health care non-profit, lists some areas where implicit bias among health care providers of European descent have led to disparities. For example, they cite the decreased likelihood that a physician will recommend the use of chemotherapy for African American men with prostate cancer as opposed to their Caucasian counterparts, the lower rates of pain medication prescriptions given to people of color, the greater number of prescribed heart disease interventions given to Caucasians, and others. Blair, Steiner, and Havranek (2011) provide multiple hypothetical examples of how physician responses to patients can occur as a function of implicit bias by race/ethnicity. For example, these researchers found that implicit bias played a role in certain treatment recommendations given to a patient of African descent. Green, Carney,

Pallin et al. (2007) found that implicit bias was active in physicians who were responsible for the medical treatment of patients with thrombolysis and myocardial infarction. Specifically, even though the physicians did not show a preference for any one particular type of patient, they harbored implicit bias regarding the anticipated cooperation levels of African American patients. These beliefs affected their prescribed medical procedures. Barr (2014), an MD/PhD who is an acknowledged authority on health care disparities, cites the discovery that cancer specialists in the State of California less often provided bone marrow transplantation to Americans of African descent as the trigger for the writing and publication of his text, Health Disparities in the United States: Social Class, Race, Ethnicity & Health (2014).

Such examples demonstrate how implicit bias can transcend direct physician–patient communications and literally affect the screening, diagnosis, and treatment of patients. Shiela Tolentino (2018), a University of Nevada, Las Vegas student who conducted research on diabetes and Asian Americans, discovered that implicit bias is of such strength that of the 26 medical practice guidelines on diabetes analyzed, only 7 of them direct providers to screen Asian Americans for diabetes at a lower body weight than other ethnic groups. Similarly, a group of researchers (O'Brien et al. 2016) discovered that the 2015 clinical screening guidelines for abnormal blood glucose levels (dysglycemia) and type 2 diabetes written by the United States Preventive Services Task Force (USPSTF) contained insufficient cutoff criteria regarding age and body weight which could lead to a large number of undiagnosed patients. Specifically, when creating the screening guidelines for dysglycemia and type 2 diabetes, the USPSTF did not take into account the increase in the number of younger and lighter-weight minorities who may have these conditions. Rather, the screening guidelines were written for adults who were between 40 and 70 years old and overweight or obese. Thus, physicians, following the parameters of the screening criteria, were not screening younger non-Caucasian persons and those with lower body weights. Due to the findings of these researchers, the USPSTF has since recommended that physicians expand the screenings to include phraseology such as "racial/ethnic groups… that may be at increased risk for diabetes at a younger age or at a lower body mass index" (USPSTF, 2018). Thus, clinical screening guidelines that bypass directions for physicians regarding certain groups of people may inadvertently cause health disparities. Additionally, Suneja et al. (2016) reviewed data from the National Cancer Database for the period 2002–2011. Their analysis revealed that even with insurance, persons infected with HIV were significantly ($p < .05$) less likely to receive cancer treatment than were patients without HIV. The assumption by the authors is that this outcome occurred as a result of implicit and not explicit bias.

Woodhead et al. (2016), in a study of 4,056 Great Britain primary care patients with several mental health disorders and 270,669 patients without mental health disorders, discovered that the mental health patients were less likely to receive state-of-the-art treatment for heart failure and coronary heart disease. Similarly, Virani et al. (2014) conducted a study from 2010–2011 with 972,532 persons with coronary heart disease, peripheral artery disease, and ischemic stroke. Care for these illnesses was received from 130 Veterans Health Administration facilities. The study revealed that females were significantly ($p < .0001$) less likely to receive the statins and/or high-intensity statins that medical practice guidelines recommend as the state-of-the-art treatment. Again, the assumption of the authors is that no intentionality was present in these physician actions and that implicit bias was operative.

Is there evidence that implicit bias may be associated with disparities in screening and diagnosis also?

Lamontague-Godwin et al. (2018) conducted an analysis of 1,448 research studies from the United States, Australia, Hong Kong, and Canada to determine whether disparities exist in physical health screenings between patients with severe mental illness and those without this condition. This study indicated that persons with severe mental illness were less likely to be screened for metabolic syndrome, breast cancer, and other conditions. Brown and Jones (2016) documented mental and medical health disparities in screening and diagnosis for transgender veterans.

Murphy et al. (2018) provide one option that can reduce such disparities by providers. These researchers advance the argument that physicians can literally use the medical interview to identify social and other health risk factors. In addition, the medical interview provides an opportunity for physician–patient communication to be broadened so that a relationship is established. The establishment of a relationship with the patient will reflect itself in all aspects of care from screening and diagnosis to treatment according to these authors.

As the cited studies reveal, research indicates that implicit bias is also operative based upon socioeconomic status, sexual orientation, age, gender, mental illness, substance use status, and other variables. They even found evidence that some providers exhibit implicit bias against persons who are obese.

But don't patients also embody implicit bias?

Yes, patients do bring their own implicit and explicit biases into the healthcare setting based upon their past experiences. Researchers have reported numerous cases of majority patients who have refused to be served by minority physicians. Evidence also exists of minority patients who distrust their majority providers. For example, Abigail Sewell (2015) found that in the areas of technical judgment and interpersonal competence, patients of African descent were less likely to trust their physicians. Other researchers have had similar findings. Armstrong et al. (2007), by analyzing data from the Community Tracking Study, found that both Latinos/Hispanic and

African American patients reported greater distrust than did Caucasian patients. However, one factor that has increased both internal and external bias has been the use of a zero-sum game model for the analysis of bias and the framing of solutions to its reduction and elimination.

What do you mean by zero-sum game?

A **zero-sum game** refers to situations in which resources are fixed and gains or losses experienced by one group are at the expense of the gains or losses of another group. As a result, in order for lower-status groups to "win," higher-status groups must "lose." Research by Wilkins et al. (2015) that examined traditional disparities based on race/ethnicity and gender found that White Americans and males, as the historically high-status groups in U.S. society, have disproportionately embraced the belief that win-win solutions do not exist in terms of disparity outcomes in American society.

Win-win solutions will benefit everyone. A better educated, healthier population will make all persons in the United States better off. However, change may be slow. Ashraf, Lester, and Weil (2009) emphasize that investments into better health outcomes, when introduced into the **disparities chain**, may take as many as 30 years to positively impact the country's gross domestic product (GDP). Thus, they suggest that investments into improving health outcomes should be based simply on the argument that everyone benefits if the U.S. population is healthier as a whole.

How is health related to economic growth?

A healthier population is far more productive than one burdened by chronic health issues. Increased productivity means that more goods and services will be generated at a lower cost. People will be able to save more and their salaries will go further. Similarly, a better educated workforce will also lead to an increase in new businesses and higher productivity in existing businesses. Additionally, education generates higher levels of reported happiness, less

crime, and other social benefits (Trostel, 2015; Oreopoulos & Salvanes, 2011; Justice Policy Institute, 2007). As you can see, attitudes, beliefs, and behaviors that are supportive of all subgroups are a win-win strategy for humanity.

When did health disparities as an area of health and health care emerge?

▶ # History of Efforts to Track and Improve Health Disparities

Until the publication of the now historic Institute of Medicine's report, *Unequal Treatment* (2002), disparities in health care were an institutionalized component of the American healthcare system. Whether the folkways that were implicit to the American healthcare system involved unspoken norms with regard to race/ethnicity that supported patient self-assignment to culturally concordant providers, and/or the acceptance of variability in wait times, unpleasant patient–physician interactions, differential prescriptions for common illnesses and diseases, cultural norms among selected subgroups that supported greater reliance on alternative medical remedies, and/or other factors, differentials in healthcare treatment were interwoven into the fabric of virtually all aspects of the U.S. healthcare system.

Once such practices were empirically confirmed and made visible, the first wave of "humankind advocates" began to protest and advocate for change. In response, Congress mandated a shift in norms by mandating that the Agency for Healthcare Resource and Quality (AHRQ) track progress in improvements in health care for different subgroups through the collection and analysis of healthcare disparities data on an annual basis. This drive toward change was also accelerated by increased funding for the analysis of health disparities data in conjunction with recommended strategies to advance the rates of change.

Previous research revealed a need for the expansion of key preventative measures to all subgroups. Accordingly, interventions were funded to support increases in **preventive screenings**. Many diseases, if identified in the early stages, can be cured. Thus, empirically verified differences in breast cancer and/or colorectal cancer screenings were addressed through various health educational promotion messages to the targeted groups. Resources also were directed toward providers to motivate them to remind their diverse patient panels to follow recommended screening guidelines.

Can you provide some examples of preventive care services that were found to have been characterized by disparities?

Many, many areas of disparities were identified. Disparities were identified in flu and pneumonia vaccinations among Medicare beneficiaries (Winston et al., 2006). More recently, disparities have been identified in preventive services among nursing home residents (Travers, 2017). Patient-based differences even existed in testing to track changes in eye pressure that suggested the presence of glaucoma (Murakami et al., 2011). Once disparities were identified, efforts were made to reduce them. For example, when disparities in screening for osteoporosis were identified (Miller et al., 2005), improvements were made in the use of x-rays to identify signs of osteoporosis among all older females (Gillespie & Marin, 2017). Numerous other changes were implemented.

Moreover, quality measurements were expanded for use throughout the healthcare system. Providers were made accountable if the data revealed subgroup differences. In addition, data were reviewed to determine whether medical practice guidelines for diseases such as diabetes mellitus, hypertension, rheumatoid arthritis, chronic kidney disease, and other diseases were differentially applied across subgroups without a clinical basis for disparate care. And, returning to our earlier discussion of physician–patient communications and the overall provider–patient relationship, customer service and other measures of the physician–patient relationship were also included as part of the annual measure of disparities in healthcare.

Have disparities continued in many of these areas?

To a large degree, yes, disparities have continued. However, note that the more important question is not whether they have continued but whether they are improving! Fiscella and Sanders (2016) found that while progress has been slow, progress has been made in many, but not all, areas.

Why aren't physicians doing more to eliminate disparities?

Physicians alone cannot fully remediate these matters. Healthcare administrators, public health professionals, researchers, and policy makers, as well as individuals who are a part of subgroups with disparate healthcare experiences all have a role to play in eliminating disparities.

Wait, are you "blaming the victim" for subgroup disparities?

Absolutely not. However, it is a mathematical fact that any time two or more "values" encounter each other, both "values" determine the magnitude of the outcome. Accordingly, although individuals can be viewed as having unequal power, all individuals have some degree of power.

What do you mean by "power"?

Consider some of the following definitions of **power**:

- Possession of control, authority, or influence over others (*Merriam-Webster*, n.d.)
- In physics, the amount of energy put out or used in a given amount of time (Dictionary.com, n.d.)
- In mathematics, how many times to use the number in a multiplication, written as a small number to the right and above the base number (Dictionary.com, n.d.)

Why are you using definitions of power from physics and math?

We use such definitions because humans are made of matter and thus behave like all other matter in the universe. Humans have energy and when that energy is expended, it generates a reaction.

Are you saying that individuals can apply their energy toward creating large or small changes in their circumstances?

Yes, even the simplest experiments in a physics lab confirm such a statement.

What about the definition of power as a number multiplied times itself, with the number of times indicated by an exponent?

This very important definition of power suggests that every single individual has, at a minimum, the power to affect his or her own life and, based upon the exponent, the power to multiplicatively affect the lives of others.

History is replete with examples of individuals who used their internal power to initiate change in various aspects of the human condition. Moreover, these were individuals who were very similar to those persons who are now reading this chapter.

Chapter Summary

This chapter examined physician-based healthcare disparities. Physicians are a core component in health care. Accordingly, this chapter explored some of the mechanisms that may be operative between physicians and their patients that can result in health disparities. Physician–patient communication, implicit bias, patient bias, and the mistaken belief that health, education, socioeconomic, and other gains by one subgroup reduces outcomes for another subgroup are factors that are cited as causal elements in the equation that generates healthcare disparities. The need for systemic changes in public policy and across the health care spectrum were also discussed. The chapter concludes by asserting

that both physicians and patients require behavioral change in order to reduce disparities in health outcomes.

Review Questions and Problems

1. As a current and/or future healthcare administrator, public health professional, and/or clinician, please carefully answer each question below.
    A. When you search deeply within, identify aspects of the "culture" of various racial/ethnic groups, gender minorities, urban populations, religious subgroups, or other subgroups listed below that "disturb" you when encountered.
        a. Ways of dress
        b. Use of speech
        c. Music
        d. Other
    B. What are some of your explicit biases toward any subgroup?
    C. What are some of your implicit biases?
2. Create a fictional dialogue that describes how you would respond to a patient and his/her family who insulted you as you sought to deliver services.
3. Use your telephone to do a self-video on how to improve physician/patient communications.
4. List some types of communication techniques that could be used to strengthen the understanding between physicians and patients, i.e., using teletype or a sign language interpreter for patients who are deaf.
5. List and explain another example where empirical data have been used.

Key Terms and Concepts

cultural competency model Based upon the belief that educating individuals and groups regarding quality of life of different subgroups will allow them to reduce bias and discrimination.

disparities chain Refers to the historic and contemporary factors that interactively affect current and future outcomes.

empirical Information and knowledge that transcends theory. Data generated by statistical observation of real-life experiences and/or via experiment or data analysis.

implicit bias Beliefs, attitudes, and values regarding various subgroups that are operative at a subconscious level.

patient self-management Provision of services and/or support so that a patient can manage a chronic disease.

power The ability to exercise control over human and/or non-human resources within a physical and/or human environment.

preventive screenings Examinations and tests designed to detect certain diseases in their early stages when a cure is more likely.

primary prevention Activities that involve the prevention of illness and disease.

secondary prevention Activities that prevent the recurrence of illness and disease.

zero-sum game Situations in which resources are fixed and gains or losses experienced by one group are exactly balanced by the gains or losses of the other group.

References

Alon, I., Boulanger, M., Elston, J. A., Galanaki, E. Martinez de Ibarreta, C., Meyers, J., Muñiz-Ferrer, M., & Vélez-Calle, A. (2016). Business Cultural Intelligence Quotient: A Five-Country Study. *Thunderbird International Business Review, 60*(3), 237–250. https://doi.org/10.1002/tie/21826

Armstrong, K., Ravenell, K. L., McMurphy, S., & Putt, M. 2007. Racial/ethnic differences in physician distrust in the United States. *American Journal of Public Health, 97*(7), 1283–1289.

Ashraf, Q. H., Lester, A., & Weil, D. N. (2009). When does improving health raise GDP? *NBER Macroeconomics Annual, 23*, 157–204.

Barr, D. A. (2014). Health Disparities in the United States, 2nd Edition, Johns Hopkins University Press, Baltimore, preface, xii.

Betancourt, J. R., Green, A. R., Carrillo, J. E., & Ananeh-Firempong, O. (2003). Defining cultural competence: A practical framework for addressing racial/ethnic disparities in health and health care. *Public Health Reports, 118*(4), 293–302.

Blair, I. V., Steiner, J. F., & Havranek, E. P. (2011). Unconscious (implicit) bias and health disparities: Where do we go from here? *The Permanente Journal, 15*(2), 71–78.

Brown, G. K., & Jones, K. T. (2016). Mental health and medical health disparities in 5135 transgender veterans receiving healthcare in the veterans health administration: A cast control study. *LGBT Health, 3*(2), 122–131.

Cooper, L. A., & Powe, N. R. (2004). Disparities in patient experiences, health care processes and outcomes: The role of patient-provider racial, ethnic, and language concordance. Commonwealth Fund, New York. Retrieved from http://www.commonwealthfund.org /publications/fund-reports/2004/jul/disparities-in -patient-experiences–health-care-processes–and -outcomes–the-role-of-patient-provide

Cross, T., Bazron, B., Dennis, K., & Issacs, M. (1989). Towards a Culturally Competent System of Care, Volume 1. Washington, D.C.: Georgetown University Child Development Center, CASSP Technical Assistance Center.

Dictionary.com. (n.d.). Power. Retrieved from http://www.dictionary.com/browse/power?s=t

Duberstein, P. R., Chen, M., Chapman, B. P., Hoerger, M., Saeed, F., Guacial, E., & Mack, J. W. (2018). Fatalism and educational disparities in beliefs about the curability of advanced cancer. *Patient Education and Counseling, 101*(1), 113–118.

Fiscella, K., & Sanders, M. R. (2016). Racial and ethnic disparities in the quality of health care. *Annual Review of Public Health, 37*, 375–394.

Foo, P. K., Frankel, R. M., McGuire, T. G., Zaslavsky, A. M., Lafata, J. E., & Tai-Seale, M. (2017). Patient and physician race and the allocation of time and patient engagement efforts to mental health discussions in primary care: An observational study of audio recorded periodic health examinations. *Journal of Ambulatory Care Management, 40*(3), 246–256.

Gillespie, C. W., & Morin, P. E. (2017). Trends and disparities in osteoporosis screening among women in the United States, 2008-2014. *The American Journal of Medicine, 130*(3), 306–316.

Green, A. R., Carney, D. R., Pallin, D. J., Ngo, L. H., Raymond, K. L. Iezzoni, L., & Banaji, M. R. (2007). Implicit bias among physicians and its prediction of thrombolysis decision for black and white patients. *Journal of General Internal Medicine, 22*(9), 1231–1238.

Hawkins, J. M., & Mitchell, J. (2018). The doctor never listens: Older African American men's perceptions of patient–provider communication. *Social Work Research, 42*(1), 57–63.

Institute of Medicine. (2002). *Unequal treatment: Confronting racial and ethnic disparities in health care.* Washington, D.C.: National Academies Press.

Jiang, J., & Wei, R. (2012). Influences of culture and market convergence on the international advertising strategies of multinational corporations in North America, Europe and Asia. *International Marketing Review, 29*(6), 597–622. http:// doi:10.1108 /02651331211277964

Joint Commission (The) (2016). Implicit bias in health care. Quick Safety. 23, pgs. 1-4.https://www .jointcommission.org/

Jongen, C., McCalman, J., Bainbridge, R., & Clifford, A. (2017). Health workforce development interventions to improve cultural competence: cultural competence in health 49-64, Springer Briefs in Public Health book series.

Kelly, P. A., & Haidet, P. (2007). Physician overestimation of patient literacy: A potential source of health care disparities. *Patient Education and Counseling, 66*(1), 119–122.

Knight, G. (1999). International services marketing: review of research, 1980-1998, *Journal of Services Marketing, 13*:4/5, 347–360, https://doi.org/10.1108/088760499102 82619

Lamontagne-Godwin, F., Burgess, C., Clement, S., Gasston-Hales, M., Greene, C., Maryande, A., … Barley, E. Interventions to increase access to or uptake of physical health screening in people with severe mental illness: a realist review. *BMJ Open*, 2018 8(2):e019412 doi:10.1136/bmjopen-2017-019412

Maina, I. (2018). A systematic review of implicit racial bias on healthcare. *Pediatrics, 141*(1). Retrieved from http://pediatrics.aappublications.org/content/141/1 _MeetingAbstract/337

Merriam-Webster. (n.d.). Power. Retrieved from https:// www.merriam-webster.com/dictionary/power

Miller, R. G., Ashar, B. H., Cohen, J., Camp, M., & Coombs, C. (2005). Disparities in osteoporosis screening between at-risk African-American and white women. *Journal of General Internal Medicine, 20*(9), 841–851.

Murakami, Y., Lee, B.W., Duncan, M., Kao, A., Huang, J. Y., Singh, K., & Lin, S. C. (2011). Racial and ethnic disparities in adherence to glaucoma follow-up visits in a county hospital population. *Arch Ophthalmol,* Jul;*129*(7), 872–878. doi: 10.1001 /archophthalmol.2011.163.

Murphy, K. A., Ellison-Barnes, A., Johnson, E. N., & Cooper, L. A. (2018). The clinical examination and socially at-risk population: The examination matters for health disparities. *Med Clin N AM 102*(3), 521–537.

Nagarajan, N., Rahman, S., & Boss, E. F. (2016). Are there racial disparities in family-reported experiences of care in inpatient pediatrics? *Clinical Pediatrics, 56*(7), 619–626.

O'Brien, M.VJ., Lee, J.VY., Carnethon, M.VR., Ackermann, R.VT., Vargas, M.VC., Hamilton, A., . . . Feinglass, J. (2016) Detecting Dysglycemia Using the 2015 United States Preventive Services Task Force Screening Criteria: A Cohort Analysis of Community Health Center Patients. *PLOS Medicine.* July 12, 2016. https://doi .org/10.1371/journal.pmed.1002074.

Oreopoulos, P., & Kjell G. Salvanes. (2011). Priceless: the nonpecuniary benefits of schooling. *Journal of Economic Perspectives, 25*(1), 159–184. doi: 10.1257 /jep.25.1.159

Ott, D. L., & Michailova, S. (2016). Cultural intelligence: a review and new research avenues. *International Journal of Management Reviews, 20*(1), 99–119.

Page, A., Petteruit, A., Walsh, N., & Ziedenberg, J. Justice Policy Institute (2007). Education and Public Safety. http://www.justicepolicy.org/images/upload/07-08 _rep_educationandpublicsafety_ps-ac.pdf

Rhodes, M., Fletcher, M. D., Blumen-Field, F., & Jacobs, E. (2018). Challenges faced by professional interpreters during discussions of end-of-life. *Journal of Pain and Symptom Management, 55*(2), 658–659.

Ricker, C. N., Koff, R. B., Qu, C., Culver, J., Sturgeon, D., Kingham, K. E., Lowstuter, K., . . . Idos, G. E. (2018). Patient communication of cancer genetic test results in a diverse population. *Translational Behavioral Medicine, 8*(1), 85–94.

Saadi, A., Himmelstein, D. U., Woolhandler, S., & Mejia, N. I. (2017). Racial disparities in neurologic health care access and utilization in the United States. *Neurology, 88*(24), 2268–2275.

Schultz, E.A., & Lavenda, R.H. (2009). Cultural anthropology: A perspective on the human condition. New York: Oxford University Press, Incorporated, 2009.

Selmi, M. (2017). Paradox of implicit bias and a plea for a new narrative. George Washington University Law School, Public Law Research Paper No. 2017-63, Available at: http://www.ssrn.com/abstract=3026381

Sewell A. (2015). Disaggregating ethnoracial disparities in physician trust. *Social Science Research, 54*(1) 1–20.

Siminoff, L. A., Graham, G. C., & Gordon, N. H. (2006). Cancer communication patterns and the influence of patient characteristics: Disparities in information-giving and affective behaviors. *Patient Education and Counseling, 62*(3), 355–360.

Spencer-Oatey, H. (2012). What is culture? A compilation of quotations. GlobalPAD/University of Warwick. http:///www.warwick.ac.uk/globalpadintercultural.

Street, R. L., Jr., Makoul, G., Arora, N. K., & Epstein, R. M. (2009). How does communication heal? Pathways linking clinician–patient communication to health outcomes. *Patient Education and Counseling, 74*(3), 295–301.

Suneja, G., Lin, C. C., Semard, E. A., Han, X., Engels, E. A., & Jemal, A. (2016). Disparities on cancer treatment among patients infected with the human immunodeficiency virus. *Cancer, 122*(15), 2399–2407.

Tolentino, S. M. (2018). Disparity notes for primary care physicians who treat Asians with diabetes. Unpublished paper, UNLV, Dept. of Health Care Administration and Policy.

Travers, J. L., Schroeder, K. L., Blaylock, T. E., & Stone, P. W. (2017). Racial/ethnic disparities in influenza and pneumococcal vaccinations among nursing home residents: a systematic review. *The Gerontologist*, https://doi.org/10.1093/geront/gnw193.

Trostel, P. It's not just the money: The benefits of college education to individuals and to society. VOCEDplus. http://hdi.voced.edu.au/10707/38472

Virani, S. S., Woodard, L. D., Ramsey, D. T., Urech, T. H., Akervel, J.M., . . . Petersen, L. A. (2014). Gender disparities in evidence-based statin therapy in patients with cardiovascular disease. *The American Journal of Cardiology, 115*(1), 21–26. doi: http://doi.org/10.1016/j.amjcard.2014.09.041

Wilkins, C. L., Wellman, J. D., Babbit, N. G., Toosi, N. R., & Schad, K. D. (2015). You can win, but I can't lose: Bias against high-status groups increases their zero-sum beliefs about discrimination. *Journal of Experimental Social Psychology, 57*(1), 1–14.

Winston, C. A., Worthy, P. M., & Lees, C. K. (2006). Factors associated with vaccination of Medicare beneficiaries in five US communities: results from the racial and ethnic disparities immunizations initiative survey 2003/. *Journal of the American Geriatrics Society, 54*(2), 303–310.

Woodhead, C., Ashworth, M., Broadbent, M., & Matthew, A. C. (2016). Cardiovascular disease treatment among patients with severe mental illness: A data linkage study between primary and secondary care. *British Journal of General Practice, 66*(647), e374-381. doi: 10.3399/bjgp16X685189. Epub 2016 Apr 25.

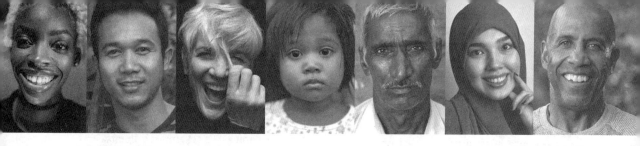

CHAPTER 8

Reducing Healthcare Disparities Through Physician–Patient Partnerships

"…instead of empowering users for a preset goal, we should let them determine a role for themselves…"

—**Kamal Jethwani**, MD, MPH, & **Jodi Sperber**, PhD (2017), authors of an article - Who Gives Us the Right to "Empower" Patients? on NEJM Catalyst

LEARNING OBJECTIVES

After completing this chapter, each learner will be able to:

- Discuss current issues in physician–patient relationships that can lead to healthcare disparities.
- List key elements of self-management.
- Describe the goal of a behavioral change contract.
- Summarize, analyze, and assess the value of websites and smartphone apps as self-management tools.
- Summarize and extend guidelines that healthcare professionals can offer to patients on using websites and smartphone apps to support their partnerships with their physicians.
- Describe the potential role that telemedicine can play in strengthening physician/patient partnerships.

▶ Introduction

In the United States, life expectancy varies by subgroup. In addition, various subgroups also experience differences in the need for medical treatment due to variations in the prevalence and incidence of major illnesses and diseases. Indeed, when changes in the causes of death are analyzed by racial/ethnic subgroup, differential healthcare needs are revealed. For example, diseases of the heart have remained the number one cause of death for Americans of European and African descent since 1950 (National Center for Health Statistics, 2015). Moreover, although data are not available for Native Americans and Americans of Spanish descent over the same time interval, diseases of the heart are now the number one cause of death for these populations as well and the second leading cause of death for Asian Americans and Pacific Islanders. However, significant differences exist in the death rates from these two diseases for various subgroups. Moreover, as one explores the top ten causes of death by subgroup, differences not only exist in the ranking of the causes of death, but differences also exist in the physician and patient's "partnerships" that develop in the management of specific illnesses or diseases. Stated differently, patients and physicians must partner together in ensuring that the patient's healthcare needs are met. Such a statement is applicable whether the disease is malignant neoplasm, unintentional injury, diabetes mellitus, chronic liver disease/cirrhosis, and/or other areas for which healthcare interventions are available. This chapter describes some ways in which these partnerships can be facilitated.

▶ Partnering with Healthcare Providers in Reducing Healthcare Disparities

Considerable attention has been directed toward increasing the adoption of preventive behaviors as a tool for reducing healthcare disparities. And, indeed, the public health sector has provided leadership in this area. As a result of such efforts, disparities have been improving in many arenas. For example, influenza and pneumonia were identified as areas with disparities in death rates by race/ethnicity, as well as other factors. Cordoba and Aiello (2016) identified race/ethnicity, income/wealth, education, and stress levels as factors associated with influenza and pneumonia morbidity and mortality. As of 2000, influenza vaccination was a preventive measure characterized by severe disparities. However, these disparities had narrowed by 2015 as a direct result of patients and providers working in tandem (**TABLE 8.1**).

As demonstrated in Table 8.1, the disparity rates for influenza vaccinations were reduced between 2000 and 2015. In 2000, 52.1% more White Americans than African Americans selected to receive vaccinations. For Latino/Hispanic Americans, the disparity rate was 70.1%—the highest of all groups. However, 3.22% more American Indians/Alaskan Natives received influenza vaccinations than their White American counterparts. By 2015, White American influenza vaccine rates had increased, and 12.47% more White Americans than American Indian/Alaskan Natives had received the vaccination. This trend was also observable in the rates for Asians, who experienced a 27.0% vaccination rate in 2000, compared to the rate for White Americans, which was 11.5% higher (30.1%). However, in 2015 the vaccination rate among White Americans (44.2%) was lower compared to Asians, who received the influenza vaccination at a rate of 47.0%. Thus, a reverse disparity had occurred. That is, White Americans had a disparity rate that was 6.33% lower than that for Asians. Thus, each subgroup significantly increased the number of influenza vaccinations over the 15-year time period.

What prompted these changes?

These improvements occurred because physicians encouraged their patients to receive these immunizations and because more patients were

TABLE 8.1 Personal Behaviors: The Receipt of Influenza Vaccinations

Disparity question: How much higher were influenza vaccination percentages for White Americans in 2000 and 2015 compared with other racial/ethnic groups?

	% Receiving Influenza Vaccine, 2000	% Difference	% Receiving Influenza Vaccine, 2015	% Difference	Assessment of Change
White (non-Hispanic) Americans[a]	30.1	Reference	44.2	Reference	—
African American (non-Hispanic)	19.8	White Americans' vaccine rates were 52.1% higher	35.7	White Americans' vaccine rates were 23.8% higher	Major decrease in disparity rate
Latino/Hispanic	17.7	White Americans' vaccine rates were 70.1% higher	31.2	White Americans' vaccine rate were 41.67% higher	Major decrease in disparity rate
American Indian/ Alaskan Native Only	31.1	White Americans' vaccine rates were 3.22% lower	39.3	White Americans' vaccine rates were 12.47% higher	Major increase in disparity rate
Asian Only	27.0	White Americans' vaccine rates were 11.5% higher	47.0	White Americans' vaccine rates were 6.33% lower than those for Asians	Major decrease in the disparity rate. However, a reverse disparity occurred.

[a] This table uses non-Hispanic White Americans as the reference group.

Based on National Center for Health Statistics. (2017). Health, United States, 2016: With Chartbook on Long-term Trends in Health. Table 68. Hyattsville, MD.

willing to be vaccinated! Accordingly, these data reveal the power of patient–physician partnerships. As the data reveal, by 2015, the percentage of all racial/ethnic groups who chose to receive an influenza vaccination had increased. Accordingly, the disparity rates narrowed. Unfortunately, in some cases, the rate for White Americans fell behind those for some other subgroups. This suggests a need to direct more outreach to *all* racial/ethnic groups. These changes in disparities reflect the success of health promotion campaigns by public health professionals, healthcare providers more aggressively offering vaccinations to all populations, and an increase in patients' willingness to receive this important preventive measure.

What about changes in disparities for other subgroups?

Much attention has been directed toward disparities by race/ethnicity, sex, and age. But what about disparities by income? When the data for vaccination rates and income are examined, disparities in accessing influenza vaccinations actually worsened between 2000 and 2015 (**TABLE 8.2**). We hypothesize that this occurred because neither health administrators, public health professionals, nor clinicians sufficiently targeted health disparity reduction strategies toward different income groups. Or, stated differently, strong patient–physician partnerships around the issue of immunizations did not occur across income groups.

As Table 8.2 indicates, disparities in the receipt of influenza vaccinations were not as severe by income in 2000 as in 2015. For example, higher-income persons, as defined by those with annual incomes 400% or greater than the federally defined poverty level, had influenza vaccination rates that were only 26.4% higher than those below poverty level, 3.9% higher than those with incomes that were

TABLE 8.2 Narrowing of Disparities in Personal Behavior Disparities in the Receipt of Influenza Vaccinations Between Lower- and Higher-Income Groups Using the Highest Income Group as the Reference Group: 2000 vs. 2015

Income Group[a]	% Receiving Influenza Vaccine, 2000	% by Which the 400% (% of poverty level) or More Income Group Compare to This Income Group	% Receiving Influenza Vaccine, 2015	% by Which the 400% (% of poverty level) or More Income Group Compare to This Income Group
Below 100%	23.1	+ 26.4	33.6	+ 50.0
100% to 199%	28.1	+ 3.9	37.0	+ 36.2
200% to 399%	29.6	− 1.35	41.2	+ 22.3
400% or more	29.2	-	50.4	-

[a] The percent of poverty level is based on U.S. Bureau of the Census poverty thresholds.
Constructed by the authors from data found in National Center for Health Statistics. Health, United States, 2016: With Chartbook on Long-term Trends in Health. Hyattsville, MD. 2017. Table 68.3.

100% to 199% greater than poverty level, and 1.35% lower than those with incomes that were 200% to 399% above the poverty line in 2000. By 2015, these disparities had worsened. Persons with the highest levels of income were 50% more likely to have been vaccinated for influenza than those in the poorest group, 36.2% more likely to have been vaccinated than those with incomes 100% to 199% above poverty level, and 22.3% higher than those with incomes 200% to 299% above poverty level.

What happens to these data when income is held constant? That is, can racial/ethnic differences be observed at each income level?

When income is held constant between various racial/ethnic groups, it reveals that other variables within the disparity chain are operative that generate different behavioral choices. However, it also illustrates the criticality of income in the disparity chain because the differential vaccination rates were "worse" between lower- and higher-income White Americans than between higher- and lower-income African Americans. Public health interventions appear to have bypassed campaigns to close this gap (**TABLE 8.3**).

Table 8.3 demonstrates that income subgroup had a greater impact than race/ethnicity on whether a patient received an influenza vaccination by 2015. The differentials were relatively small by income group for both races/ethnicities in 2000 but, by 2015, differential patterns of behavior had emerged.

TABLE 8.3 Differences in Influenza Vaccination Rates by Race/Ethnicity and Income Group[a]

	% Receiving Influenza Vaccine, 2000	% Receiving Influenza Vaccine, 2015
White Americans		
Below 100%	27.8	34.9
100% to 199%	33.1	41.7
200% to 399%	32.5	44.4
400% or more	30.5	52.2
African Americans		
Below 100%	20.0	30.2
100% to 199%	21.3	33.9
200% to 399%	19.5	36.1
400% or more	19.2	43.3

[a] The income groups (percentages) in this table above depict the percent of poverty level based on U.S. Bureau of the Census poverty thresholds.
Constructed by the authors from data found in National Center for Health Statistics. Health, United States, 2016: With Chartbook on Long-term Trends in Health. Hyattsville, MD. 2016. Table 68.

With a vaccination rate of 52.2%, the highest-income White Americans were 20.55% more likely to obtain an influenza vaccination than African Americans (43.3%) in the same income bracket. In the 200% to 399% income bracket, White Americans (44.4%) were 22.99% more likely to have an influenza vaccination than African Americans in the same income group (36.1%). In the 100% to 199% bracket, White Americans (41.7%) were 23.00% more likely to be vaccinated against influenza than their African American counterparts (33.9%). For the below 100% poverty groups, the disparities were far less severe. The lowest-income White Americans (34.9%) were 15.56% more likely to obtain an influenza vaccination than the lowest-income African Americans (30.2%). *In other words, behavioral disparities that affect health outcomes were less severe in the lower-income brackets than at the higher-income brackets.* Thus, physician–patient partnerships are needed to address these disparities by income and race/ethnicity.

Are you saying that disparities by income for this preventive measure subordinate disparities by race/ethnicity?

Yes, that is the case. Thus, the question becomes how physician–patient partnerships can support reductions in these healthcare disparities. In addition, current and future healthcare administrators, public health personnel, and clinicians can ask, "What can we do to support behavioral change in all subgroups characterized by health disparities?" Specifically, healthcare personnel will need to support the adoption of preventive and personal behaviors around self-management while simultaneously ensuring that clinicians remind patients of the importance of vaccinations and other preventive measures. Likewise, public health campaigns to educate all subgroups regarding the importance of vaccinations and other preventive measures must continue.

▶ Supporting Behavioral Change as a Strategy to Reduce Health and Healthcare Disparities

Despite the critical roles played by healthcare administrators, public health professionals, and clinicians in healthcare delivery, most programs of study do not offer interdisciplinary courses on behavioral change. Yet, a growing body of research now suggests that healthcare administrators, in seeking to reduce costs and elevate efficiency, may wish to consider introducing programs on behavioral change into the patient services offered by their healthcare institutions. Likewise, healthcare administrators can work in partnership with public health personnel to ensure that population-level, evidence-based measures are introduced into communities. Similarly, as part of the shift from curative to preventive medicine, physicians and other providers can directly support behavioral change with individuals and families.

What are some of the findings from this growing body of research on behavioral change?

In an analysis of habits, which are behavioral responses that have become automated when confronted by certain stimuli, Gardner (2018) emphasizes the strength of the nature of *behavioral continuity* rather than *behavioral change*. Specifically, Gardner (2018) argues that replacement behaviors, once initiated, must be "shielded" from exposure to the old cues until they, too, become automated. This research suggests that programs to promote "healthy" behaviors may require interventions across the various health disciplines. For example, public health professionals can identify the growing number of clinical trials and outcomes that test habit-based interventions. These findings and materials can then be made available to clinicians for dissemination to patients and their families. Health insurance companies can also disseminate materials to their enrollees. Healthcare administrators can schedule training for the providers and other staff at their institutions.

Gardner, Lally, and Wardle (2012) assert that to significantly affect change, physicians and other clinical personnel may wish to disseminate a behavioral change toolkit. These toolkits must be developed to support the patient in the continuous repetition of behaviors at the same time each day until the new behavior becomes automated.

Pomey et al. (2015) emphasize the importance of patient-centered care to any process of change. While our recommendation has not yet been tested, we hypothesize that patient-centered care be expanded to include the use of a behavioral change contract. The **behavioral change contract** would include (1) the patient's diagnosis; (2) the physician's treatment plan; (3) a detailed list of the behaviors that the patient must make to support maximum quality of healthcare and health outcomes; and (4) a detailed discussion of the potential impacts of a failure to choose to adopt the "prescribed" treatment upon the projected quality and length of the patient's life. Finally, and perhaps most important, is the patient's signature next to the checkbox that denotes his or her agreement with the contents of the contract, selecting from one of the following:

- "I will make the prescribed behavioral changes because I wish to maximize the length and quality of my life."
- "I will not comply with the proposed behavioral change recommendations and confirm that I am willing to reduce the length and quality of my life in order to gain the pleasures I receive from sustaining my current behavioral patterns."
- "I want to change my behaviors but I realize that altering existing habits will be difficult and, at this time, I do not wish to invest the time or energy. Accordingly, I do not choose to accept and implement the Behavioral Change Toolkit."

The signed behavioral change contract would become a part of the healthcare record of each patient served.

Stewart (1995), as well as others, has confirmed a relationship between health outcomes and physician–patient communications. However, some studies have revealed that in many cases, physicians "soften" their warnings regarding the patient's present and future health status (Monden et al., 2016; Girgis, 2017). However, when patients have choices that will affect their outcome, perhaps the message needs to be hardened. We hypothesize that the use of a contract that "spells out" the impact of a continued lifestyle pattern in clear and "hard" terms will motivate behavioral change.

▶ Self-Management: The Foundation of Physician–Patient Partnerships

Physicians, public health professionals, and healthcare administrators must aggressively market self-management to patients as an element in any patient-based behavior change campaign. Even insurance companies may wish to consider the inclusion of self-management in the language of their policies. **Self-management** is defined as the adoption of behaviors that maximize treatment outcomes and minimize the progression of a disease. Self-management may include actions such as those listed in **BOX 8.1**.

Healthcare administrators, public health professionals, and clinicians can make a business

> **BOX 8.1** Examples of Disease/Illness Self-Management Practices That Can Reduce Health Disparities
>
> - Medication adherence—taking medications prescribed, in the amount prescribed, and at the recommended intervals—is a form of self-management.
> - Disease and/or illness monitoring is a form of self-management that requires individuals to use various tools and/or procedures to check for and track signs that the conditions associated with their disease/illness are improving or worsening.
> - Health education is a self-management tool in which individuals utilize print, video, electronic, and/or hardcopy materials to learn more about their disease so that they can improve their condition, keep their condition from worsening, and/or reduce the speed at which their symptoms worsen.
> - Lifestyle self-management occurs when individuals choose to make recommended changes in nutrition, physical activity, and/or other areas of life in order to support improvements in their illness and/or disease.

> **BOX 8.2** How Healthcare Administrators, Public Health Professionals, and Clinicians Can Serve as Partners with Physicians and Patients in Providing Self-Management Support
>
> - Self-management support may include referrals to community resources that bring together persons with common illnesses and diseases so that they can help and assist each other.
> - Self-management support may include running TV shows and/or videos in the waiting room to turn patients' minds toward behavioral change.
> - Self-management support may include healthcare insurance providers following the model of auto insurance providers and providing financial incentives to their members for excellent self-management practices.

case for their organization to provide highly effective self-management supports to the consumers whom they serve. These supports can assist patients in making their own behavioral choices. **Self-management support** refers to tools, materials, and training provided by healthcare institutions to assist individuals in maximizing their self-management activities. **BOX 8.2** provides more information about self-management support.

A number of scholars of public health have confirmed that the enhancement of knowledge regarding the prevalence and incidence, causes and correlates, and consequences of diseases and illness will sometimes trigger changes in behavior that can extend both the quantity and quality of life (Adams, 2010; Grady, 2014; Sarasohn-Kahn, 2012). Thus, self-management

support becomes an excellent tool for healthcare administrators, providers, and other professionals to promote to the institutions and patients whom they serve. Indeed, improved self-management is a critical tool for the exercise of choice behavior in a way that can ultimately reduce disparities in death rates.

▶ Use of Websites and Smartphone Apps to Support Self-Management

In some regards, the web is the single most important tool that can support physician–patient partnerships. Thus, we wholeheartedly recommend that patients use the web as a source of information to support self-management, *but it must be used carefully*.

Adages regarding the importance of knowledge are quite common. For example, "Knowledge is power" is an oft-cited truism. "He who knows not, and knows not that he knows not, is a fool—shun him (or her)" is another oft-cited adage. Such adages simply reference the fact that what humans know, or think that they know, has the potential to destroy, advance, and/or transform the human experience.

The pivotal role of knowledge is not merely observable at the macro level. Rather, knowledge is also transformative to the behavior and behavioral outcomes of individuals. Indeed, the nature of this relationship is historically observable by tracking the rapidity of change that has occurred since literacy traveled from the domain of those with power and became a tool for the democratization of human society. Accordingly, it is less than surprising that the growth of the Internet as a gateway to knowledge can have a critical impact upon the world of both consumers and providers and, as a result, health and healthcare disparities.

McColl-Kennedy et al. (2017) describe the impact of this change by suggesting that this new access to knowledge has shifted the field of health care from a unilateral human interaction in which a healthcare professional "tells" and the patient "complies" to a more interactive relationship. Stated differently, due to increased access to information and knowledge, consumers are now situated to partner with providers in shaping their healthcare treatment and outcomes. However, the potential benefits that may accrue from greater access to health information and knowledge cannot be simplistically actualized. Tonsaker, Bartlett, and Trpkov (2014) suggest that although multiple benefits can accrue to consumers in the use of the Internet for health information-seeking, consumers can also place themselves at risk by merely accepting as fact all and any information obtained when this tool is used. Accordingly, it becomes highly critical to explore the following question: "How can consumers utilize online health information in a way that supports the

maximization of their health outcomes and the minimization of healthcare disparities?"

Understand the Purpose of the Internet Search

Perhaps you have a pain in your left leg, or you have recently observed that one of your eyes appears smaller than the other. The immediate response of numerous consumers will be that of searching the web in order to identify the possible causes of such symptoms. However, before lifting up your smartphone and/or opening your tablet, computer, and/or other device to start a search, it might be helpful to first clarify the purpose of the proposed search.

Are you seeking information so that you can self-diagnose your problem? Or, do you simply want to increase your knowledge through your online search so that you can approach your physician as an individual who can now better describe his or her symptoms as professional input is sought? Patients may wish to clarify their purpose for accessing information before a search is initiated. A patient who actively acknowledges a specific purpose by saying, "I would like to simply increase my literacy regarding my current symptoms so that I can better converse with my provider," can then engage in a more targeted and useful search. It is important that consumers not seek information on the web in order to engage with their physicians from a conflictive or adversarial position. Consumers should not seek information with the goal of using it to frighten themselves or their friends and family by forming theories regarding a multiplicity of diseases that are associated with the symptoms the consumer is experiencing. In making the decision to access health information on the web, view it as a language exercise only; that is, your physician speaks "clinicalese" and you do not. By accessing information regarding your health symptoms online, you can prepare yourself to more accurately and effectively describe your symptoms to your provider using a common language that you both "speak." This can be referred to as "speaking health and healthcare terminology as a second language."

Utilizing Online Information for Symptom Clarification

Numerous consumer-based sites that focus on symptoms also embed search engines such as Google and Yahoo! in their websites. These consumer-oriented healthcare information sites distribute knowledge to consumers in seconds. **BOX 8.3** provides links to a number of consumer-focused health- and healthcare-related websites.

Numerous other diagnostic sites are also used by consumers to support self-management or prevention. Again, caution must be applied when such online tools are used. Semigran, Linder, Gidengil, and Mehrotra (2015) conducted an analysis of 23 symptom

---

BOX 8.3 Websites That Can Be Used for Symptom Clarification

AARP Symptom Checker (http://healthtools.aarp.org/symptomsearch)

Diagnose Me, Isabel Healthcare (https://symptomchecker.isabelhealthcare.com/suggest_diagnoses_advanced/landing_page)

HealthyChildren.org Symptom Checker (https://www.healthychildren.org/English/tips-tools/Symptom-Checker/Pages/default.aspx)

Mayo Clinic Symptom Checker (https://www.mayoclinic.org/symptom-checker/select-symptom/itt-20009075)

Patient Symptom Checker (https://patient.info)

Health Direct Symptom Checker (https://www.healthdirect.gov.au)

WebMD (https://symptoms.webmd.com/default.htm#/info)

---

checkers worldwide that allowed access by English speakers in the United Kingdom and other countries. The investigators found that an accurate diagnosis was offered in a mere 34% of cases. In order for the accuracy level to increase to 58%, 20 possible illness/disease diagnostic findings had to be offered. However, when these instruments were used for the purpose of recommending whether the consumer should seek professional medical advice and/or care, the accuracy rate increased to 80%. These finding suggests that consumers take a large risk when seeking and using symptom checkers as a substitute for seeking a physician's care. Other studies further confirm this finding. Mueller et al. (2017) performed a comprehensive literature review and analyzed 32 empirical research studies. These researchers found that approximately one-quarter to three-quarters of the participants in these studies used the web for the diagnosis of symptoms of illness and disease rather than for symptom clarification. The study also confirmed that many persons in the study appeared to have not yet visited a healthcare professional.

Why would consumers substitute a web search for a visit to a physician?

Well, the Mueller study found that some consumers had symptoms of which they felt embarrassed and/or which made them feel that they would be stigmatized by their physician. Additionally, a disproportionate number of users had prediagnosed their health symptoms as not being serious. Again, this research reconfirms the importance of only using the Internet to prepare for a visit to a physician as part of a patient's role in a physician–patient partnership since if used incorrectly, reliance on the internet can be harmful rather than helpful.

Physician–patient partnerships could actually be facilitated on primary care physicians' websites that allow patients to directly enter their symptoms into a diagnostic app at the time that an appointment is made. For example, Jutel and Lupton (2015) examined approximately 131 smartphone apps that were developed for the purpose of medical diagnosis. Directly available through the Apple App and Google Play stores, a number of these apps, although available to consumers, specifically target healthcare professionals who deliver clinical services. More than 64 such apps were found in the Apple App Store and 5 were found in Google Play. Approximately 36 of the apps identified targeted consumers, and 93 were directed toward helping clinicians. **BOX 8.4** lists a few of these medical diagnostic apps.

However, physicians and consumers must be cautious in how these apps are used. Both parties must clearly understand the degree of reliability that is attached to the responses provided when these apps are queried. Although apps and websites can be used to improve communication with trained physicians and to support overall self-management efforts, the message to consumers is a straightforward one: *never rely solely on the web for the diagnosis of disease and illness.*

Use of Medical Apps to Support Disease Prevention and Disease Management

A variety of medical apps have been created that can be distributed by public health professionals with the goal of reducing remediable health disparities. Apps and other informational technology can, as just mentioned, be effectively used to support prevention and/or to improve patient management of disease and illness. For example, many Americans have mental and/or behavioral health chronicities that can be supported through web-based and/or other technologies. Mobile apps are available that can be

---

BOX 8.4 Sample Medical Diagnostic Apps That Are Available to Both Physicians and Consumers

Common illnesses and diagnosis apps

Diagnosis Medical App (Google Play): This app features AI in a simulated Q&A format between a patient and the "physician." It holds information on over 1500 symptoms.

Disorders and Diseases Dictionary (Google Play): This free app is offline and includes features with which to look up symptoms, diseases, and treatment methodologies.

Diseases Dictionary (Google Play): This app includes descriptions of diseases and other illness as well as pharmacological agents and has a medical reference book and thesaurus available to users.

Disease Dictionary Offline 2017 (Apple): Offline and free, this app includes access to information regarding various symptoms, illness, disorders, and diseases. The listings contain detailed definitions and offer information regarding possible causes and treatment options.

Prognosis: Your Diagnosis (Google Play and Apple): Touts "over 600 case scenarios across 30 specialties."

Wiki Med—Offline Medicine Wikipedia (Google Play): This app is a medical dictionary with information including anatomy, pharmacological agents, sanitation, and other information put forth in an encyclopedic format. The app is available in many languages. A Wiki Med (Microsoft) Offline and free app is now available on devices with Windows 10.

Quick Medical Diagnosis & Treatment (Google Play and Apple): app contains an alphabetical listing that includes information on over 950 diseases and illnesses. The app is not free but does provide instantaneous access to important medical information that is regularly updated.

Medical Disease Dictionary (Google Play): Offline and free, this app is designed for use by healthcare professionals, clinicians, and other medical professionals. This app also includes information on available medications and other treatment remedies.

used to sustain recovery by delivering messages that allow individuals to restabilize when events have occurred that threaten their recovery. For example, mobile apps are available to support tobacco users during their moments of fragility. Mobile apps using sound and video can be downloaded and used to entice and/or motivate patients to choose to engage in physical activity. Indeed, diabetes mellitus, HIV/AIDS, hypertension, and other chronicities now have apps that consumers can download for free or at a fraction of the cost to assist them in the tedious task of disease management. **BOX 8.5** lists a few apps that current and/or future healthcare administrators, public health professionals, and clinicians may wish to integrate into their toolbox of items for use in reducing healthcare disparities through improved partnerships with consumers.

Again, a number of cautions must be directed to the public if such tools are used. Tseng (2017) suggests that because physicians, nurses, and/or other medical professionals are not usually involved in the design and development of healthcare apps, they must be used with caution. This is not to say that such apps are not currently regulated. Specifically, the Federal Drug Administration, the Office of Civil Rights, as well as the U.S. Department of Health and Human Services play various roles in protecting patients from the use of apps that are either unsafe and/or that distribute inaccurate information. However, patients must also engage in self-protection.

Telemedicine

Consumers are increasingly using web-based technologies to obtain preliminary diagnostic information before visiting their primary care physician and/or after a diagnosis of a chronic and/or acute condition. In addition, an increasing number of consumers are going online to obtain actual treatment via **telemedicine**. In 2001, Roine, Ohinmaa, and Hailey conducted a systematic literature review of 124 articles and performed a detailed

---

> **BOX 8.5**   Apps That Can Be Used for Disease Prevention and Disease Management
>
> ## Prevention-Oriented Apps
> Ask and Prevent Suicide
> CDC Bam!
> CDC Can I Eat This?
> CDC FluView
> CDC Heads Up Concussion Safety
> CDC Health Information at Your Fingertips,
> CDC 24/7
> CDC Ladder Safety
> CDC Milestone Tracker
> CDC Opioid Guidelines
> CDC Solve the Outbreak
> CDC STD TX Guide
> CDC TravWell
> CDC Vaccine Schedule
> Safe Driving Apps 2017
> Sprint's Drive Final App
> Yoga, Gym, Massage and More
>
> ## Disease Management Apps
> Allergy Alert
> Blood Pressure + Pulse Grapher
> Breast Disease Management
> Core Zone (for headaches)
> Diabetes Companion
> Diarrhea Drivers
> Glucose Buddy
> Go Meals (diabetes)
> Kidney Disease Management
> Living With (Cancer)
> My COPD
> My Pain Diary
> Ocular Disease Handbook

---

analysis of 34 articles on telemedicine. Based on this inquiry, the authors concluded that insufficient evidence existed for recommending the widespread use of telemedicine. Since that time, however, the use of telemedicine has grown exponentially, and a large body of literature confirms that it is accepted by consumers as a viable method for the support of their overall health. However, this is not to say that telemedicine is now in the maturity stage and should always be used by consumers. Wade and Smith (2017) argue that although a growing body of research has accrued, many of the studies are less than robust in their design. As a result, they argue that these research results cannot be used as evidence of the safety and effectiveness of the technology in supporting the self-management of illnesses and diseases such as those involving mental health, heart failure, and other diseases.

Nevertheless, a brief review of such medical efforts provides a glimpse of the increasing role of telemedicine as a web-based health tool that can be used as part of a patient–physician partnership. Commiskey, Afshinnik, and Cothren (2016) describe the process used for combining telehealth treatment with onsite treatment in order to provide hospitalized patients in rural areas with the advanced services needed. This unique type of partnership reduced the need to transfer stroke patients to larger and more specialized hospitals. D'andrea, Nedovic, and Calabro (2017) conducted research regarding telemedicine as a tool for the treatment of stroke, with the knowledge that the period of time from the onset of symptoms to the time of treatment is critical in the emergence of stroke disparities. This systematic literature review revealed that telemedicine is an effective tool that can be used to initiate the early treatment needed to reduce adverse outcomes.

Erten-Lyons et al. (2016) assessed patient and caregiver satisfaction with telemedicine services. The study revealed that the use of telemedicine brought benefits that current and future healthcare administrators can appreciate, in that it led to approximately 98.2% of all scheduled appointments being kept. Almost all of the patient–caretaker teams were complimentary of the care received, and 79% indicated that the telemedicine visits were convenient. However, a majority (68%) of the patients had a preference for a hybrid care schedule that included both onsite and online health care.

Kennedy et al. (2016) compared outcomes between telehealth and onsite treatment for persons with inflammatory arthritis. The analysis revealed no adverse outcomes for those who received web-based treatment. Likewise, Muller, Alstadhaug, and Bekkelund (2016) completed a similar study of patients with chronic headaches. Again, neither clinical outcomes nor patient satisfaction differed significantly across the participants in the study. Numerous other examples of positive views toward telemedicine can be cited. Despite the potential of telemedicine to reduce disparities, patients and providers should consider the guidelines shown in **BOX 8.6**.

Will insurance companies pay for patients to use telemedicine to improve the quality of their health care?

Many health insurance providers support telemedicine by providing 24/7 access to doctors and/or other medical professionals by phone or video as a part of their health promotion services. These services are convenient for the insured if they are traveling, at work, live far from medical facilities, do not have access to specialists at local clinics, or for who may be in hazardous areas during disasters or bad weather that prevent the immediate presence of medical personnel.

Virtual consultation can be accomplished in a number of ways. For example, the Telehealth Resource Center (n.d.) website states that a "live consultation" would involve the use of a computer or phone with video capability so that the patient and medical professional can talk face to face in real time. A "store-and-forward" consultation is one in which the patient captures a video or picture of the symptom and then sends it to the medical professional, who reviews it at a later time. With a "hybrid consultation," the medical doctor is on a video with the patient but may also be reviewing other information, such as x-rays and other diagnostic results that were sent before the video conference. Medical professionals, through these means, are able

BOX 8.6 Telemedicine Guidelines

1. The telemedicine treatment should be recommended by a patient's primary care physician. The primary care physician will be aware of clinical trials, demonstrations, etc., that are taking place that address the unique treatment needs of his or her patients.
2. A telemedicine program will require that patients, and their families, purchase the online equipment and/or software that is required by the program. At minimum, this will include:
   - An appropriate enterprise platform
   - A mobile app that is compatible with the platform used
   - High-speed home Internet that includes email
   - A computer or tablet that includes a camera
   - Other equipment
3. Before participating in a telemedicine program to support overall health care and self-management, patients must participate in training that instructs the patient and one or more family members about the purpose, design, operations, and data collection and evaluation associated with the program. Patient education must also include detailed information to prevent technical problems, etc.
4. After the first few sessions, the patient must confirm that the clarity of the equipment is sufficient for both the consumer and the provider to "read" each other's body language and facial expressions. Accurate patient–physician communication is critical.
5. Patients can use technology to support patient–physician partnerships by conducting research from journals and other scholarly sources and using a medical dictionary to be able to "translate" the findings so that they can be understood by a nonacademic reader.

to diagnose, treat, and prescribe medications or other treatments as needed for many nonemergency conditions. These types of consultations are best used for flu, allergies, rashes, bronchitis, suspected bug bites, bruises, sore throats, and similar symptoms.

Telemedicine is not used just for patient–provider consultations. Telemedicine technologies also now involve the provision of training and health care delivery. For example, Bhatt, Pourmand, and Sikka (2018) note that telemedicine drones have been used to deliver medications, defibrillators, and lab products and have been used as a tool in public health surveillance.

Is telemedicine different from telehealth?

Yes and no. The terms *telemedicine* and *telehealth* often are used interchangeably, and there is no one universally accepted definition for either term. However, **telemedicine** is generally defined as an electronic/computer-based consultation by a medical professional with the goal of diagnosing and/or recommending treatment for a condition or illness or evaluating the progress of treatment for a specific condition or illness. Telemedicine may also be used for second opinions, group consultations, and even in active medical procedures with other medical professionals who are distantly situated. In contrast, **telehealth** is often described as a nonclinical service that is provided through electronic means remotely to provide health education and training for end users and/or medical personnel, surveillance, caregiver support, and other areas. Banbury et al. (2018) lists mental health interventions and other support sessions as being viable telehealth offerings. Telehealth programs also have included self-management interventions and tracking and the collection of health data. Telehealth would also include the health-related apps discussed earlier.

▶ Health Disparities and the Major Causes of Death: Opportunities for Employing Self-Management in Reducing Disparities

The types of self-management behaviors and self-management support needed by a particular patient are very disease specific. As the data on the top 10 causes of death reveal, diseases of the heart are the primary cause of death for most racial/ethnic groups. Sharma et al. (2014) highlight the importance of personal behaviors and self-management practices for this unique disease, stating, "African Americans are disproportionately affected by heart failure . . . Much of the disparity can be blamed on modifiable risk factors" (pg. 301).

The critical role of personal variables in creating disparities in the area of heart disease is further confirmed by recent findings from the Jackson Heart Study (Min et al., 2016). This study found that even when *social determinants* of health, such as education and income, were incorporated into the analysis, the *personal factors*, such as insufficient physical activity, the presence of both overweight and obesity, and hypertension, supported the presence of disparities in the life prevalence of cardiovascular diseases.

Some would assert that the "disparity chain" may cause individual behaviors to be intermediated by higher levels of anger, stress, hostility and anxiety and that these accrue as disparity chain processes that intermediate food choices. However, Ogilvie et al. (2016) in a multiethnic study of these variables found no relationship between anger, stress, hostility, etc., and heart failure, except for those who reported themselves as having poor health at the study's onset.

Similarly, the opportunity to elevate self-management activities in order to reduce health disparities was demonstrated in a study by Spatz et al. (2016). Analyzing data from 1999 to 2013, the study discovered that even when counties were stratified by income, death rates from diseases of the heart were aligned with rates of hospitalization. Stated differently, if persons with diseases of the heart are able to self-manage their disease to such a degree that they are not hospitalized, the disparity in death rates from heart disease begins to close. Again, such findings suggest that despite the presence of social determinants of health, disparity reductions can be achieved.

You're starting to sound as if you're "blaming the victim"!

No, of course not. But at the same time, a premise that underlies the entirety of this text is that while humankind may have different degrees of constrained choices, humans can devalue themselves. They do this by not actively (and with intentionality) identifying and exercising those available choices that will move them closer to the achievement of their short- and/or long-term goals. Accordingly, the improvements in disease self-management are not a total solution to health disparities, but the maximization of available choices will surely "help." For example, diabetes and diabetes care are disease areas that require high levels of patient–physician partnering. When the level of required partnership is applied, improvements occur. LaVeist et al. (2009) performed logistic regression on diabetes prevalence data from the National Health Interview Survey and confirmed that, in the case of diabetes at least, *residency in environments that contained parallel risk factors were associated with similar diabetes prevalence rates for White Americans and African Americans.* Moreover, the REACH 2010 Charleston and Georgetown Diabetes Coalition documented that diabetes disparities can be completely eliminated. Through a comprehensive intervention that addressed not only self-management but healthcare system change as well, the investigators were able to totally eliminate prior disparities that had ranged from 11% to 28% (Jenkins et al., 2004). Note that the critical words in the previous sentence are "comprehensive intervention." A comprehensive intervention suggests that measures are needed to simultaneously address personal behaviors, socioeconomic determinants of health, environmental factors, and clinical-based variables. However, personal behaviors, given their greater controllability, become one strategy that can be supported by healthcare administrators, public health professionals, and clinicians in order to improve overall health.

▶ Other Strategies for Improving Patient– Physician Partnerships to Reduce Healthcare Disparities

Whether the morbidity is diabetes mellitus and/or another disease or illness, it appears that self-management practices that support health disparities reductions in one illness/disease may be useful in another. Stated differently, the current approach of developing single-disease interventions is costly and inefficient. Hypertension, diabetes mellitus, obesity, and heart disease can most efficiently and effectively be targeted through integrated interventions that simultaneously address each of these diseases. Substance abuse, mental health, and behavioral health issues that we, the authors, have labeled as physical activity aversion and unhealthy food addictions. can be simultaneously targeted through integrated interventions.

How do you define physical activity aversion and unhealthy food addictions?

Individuals who have been educated regarding the benefits of physical activity as a necessary prevention or self-management action can be defined as having a behavioral health problem that causes them to not act in their own self-interest. These have been labeled as physical activity aversion (refusal to exercise) and unhealthy food addictions (consistent consumption of unhealthy food and drinks).

Similarly, HIV, hepatitis, and other sexually transmitted disease (STDs) can be collectively targeted because they are closely linked in the disparities chain. This statement can be demonstrated by briefly reviewing a few of the major causes of death and disability from the framework of self-management.

Physician Visits and Monitoring/Screening

Even when populations experiencing health disparities have access to health care, poor self-management behaviors may lead to fewer primary care visits and fewer of the screenings that are necessary for medical monitoring. For example, Gary et al. (2004) identified a number of trends in an analysis of data on 1,106 adults with diabetes. Only 85% of African American diabetics in the study visited their physician four or more times annually. In contrast, 91% of White American diabetics made four or more visits to their physician annually. These differences were statistically significant ($p < .05$). Such data suggest that patients must support their own health in the patient–clinician partnership. The same study also found that only 56% of African Americans in the sample had received two or more HbA(1c) tests, and only 68% of white diabetics had had these vital tests. These differences were "real" because they were significant at the $p < .05$ level. (However, it is not clear whether the physicians failed to make the referrals and/or the referrals were made but the patients failed to comply.) Nevertheless, patient–physician partnerships cannot be effective unless physicians ensure that 100% of their patients are treated according to the diabetes practice guidelines.

What is an HbA(1c) test, and why is it important?

An **HbA(1c) test** is a glycated hemoglobin test that determines a person's blood glucose level. The test is designed to show the average level of blood glucose over the previous 3 months. High blood glucose levels are an indicator of diabetes mellitus.

Participation in such monitoring is particularly important to Asian Americans, Hispanic Americans/Latinos, and African Americans. This is because a higher percentage of African American diabetics who did have HbA(1c) tests were found to have poor glycemic control. Only 9.5% of white diabetics who took one or more HbA(1c) tests had poor glycemic control. These differences were significant at the $p < .001$ level. Given these data, it is less than surprising that the African Americans with diabetes made more emergency room visits (Gary et al., 2004).

This research suggests that several factors are important to self-management in general whether the disease is diabetes or another major cause of death. **BOX 8.7** describes activities that can be used to improve the overall healthcare experience for patients. Responsible parties for these activities (i.e., physicians, patients, etc.) have been identified in parentheses at the end of each statement.

As noted earlier, researchers have found that a large number of lifestyle factors are correlated with disparate health outcomes. Therefore, patient–physician partnerships and other interventions are needed across various subgroups and across diseases. For example, tobacco use rates among Native Americans living in the Southwestern states such as Arizona, New Mexico, etc., were higher than those living in the Northern Plains and/or Alaska (Mowery et al., 2017). Accordingly, access to tobacco use prevention and cessation programs are highly critical to this population as a part of the disruption of one aspect of the health disparities chain. Similarly, Alaskan Natives have very low knowledge levels of many common chronicities. Culturally engaging health education programs and materials are needed to address this aspect of the disparities chain.

Binge drinking is also disproportionately high (23.5%) among the Native American/Alaskan population (CDC, 2017a). Thus, linkages to alcohol/use/disorder programs are needed. Native Americans/Alaskan Natives are also more obese relative to all other subpopulations except Native Hawaiian/Pacific Islanders (CDC, 2017b). Native Americans/Alaskan Natives are more likely to report no physical activity relative to other groups and/or to meet exercise guidelines set by the nation's physical activity guidelines (CDC, 2017b). Thus, intensive interventions are needed in order to develop a basis for a campaign to promote improved self-management as a strategy to reduce currently observed health disparities among Native American/Alaskan Natives. Self-management and prevention behaviors will not occur automatically. Rather, populations experiencing health disparities must be encouraged and assisted to self-manage by their physicians as well as by public health professionals.

Women differ across subgroups in high-risk behaviors. Therefore, it is less than surprising that when these higher risks are present, some diseases and illnesses progress more rapidly. Some females are less likely to have been diagnosed with a chronicity because of differential access to medical care. Such data reveal a profound need for greater self-management education on the part of personnel in various health organizations in order for them to know the types of self-management supports that are needed.

Self-management efforts among pregnant women are critical in order to minimize the intergenerational transfer of health disparities. Fertility rates differ across racial/ethnic groups. However, differences also exist in access to the social capital needed for child-rearing. Strategies such as these can be applied across racial/ethnic groups. Thus, any newly recognized healthcare disparity subgroup will require new choice behaviors as their contributions to the reduction and elimination of healthcare disparities.

BOX 8.7 Key Elements of Effective Patient–Physician Partnerships

- Insurance coverage is vital for optimal care. (Patient)
- Scheduled regular primary care visits are essential. (Physician and patient)
- Understanding the importance of the required tests is necessary; that is, a diabetic should know what an HbA(1c) test is. If the disease is associated with the thyroid, the health disparity groups should know what the TSH (thyroid-stimulating hormone), TSI (thyroid-stimulating immunoglobulin), and TPO (antithyroid antibody) tests are. (Patient and physician)
- Physicians can ensure that their office administration provides appointment reminders and that consumers are referred to websites that include interesting videos to learn about the tests used to monitor their condition. (Physician and Healthcare Administrators)
- Awareness of the disparity chains that may exist between the various diseases is critical. It is often argued that only 20% of African Americans, 18% of Mexican Americans, and 13% of White Americans have zero risk factors for cardiovascular disease. However, hypertension, hypercholesterolemia, obesity, tobacco use, and diabetes comprise high-risk diseases for each of these populations. (Patients and physicians)
- Asians are at higher risk of a disease such as diabetes at lower body weight than other groups. However, Tolentino (2018) argues that not all diabetes treatment differentials for Asians are incorporated into the diabetes practice guidelines. Additionally, according to Tolentino, physicians must exert a stronger effort to be aware of how their treatment must be modified for subgroups. (Physicians)
- Healthcare administrators, public health personnel, and clinicians can help support reductions in health disparities by urging their organizations to invest in a case manager who checks not only for co-occurring diseases in the medical histories of patients, but who also collects data on the socioeconomic needs of patients. (Physicians and Healthcare Administrators)
- Case management interventions can support greater self-management by linking consumers to the broader community resources needed to improve other aspects of the health disparity chain. (Patients and physicians)
- Patients may be particularly receptive to the case management approach because power remains with the individual in driving his or her self-management efforts rather than putting his or her health in the hands of external individuals. (Patients and physicians)
- Critical to a self-management effort is the use of a checklist that informs patients of the protocols that should be applied by the provider for each of their chronicities. The patient can then remind the physician of procedures that were not completed. (Patients)
- The healthcare administrator, public health professional, and/or clinician can assist in the institutionalization of such protocols in his or her organization. (Physicians and Healthcare Administrators)
- Self-management supports can be customized by a healthcare institution to meet the unique needs of each subgroup. For example, the self-management needs of consumers will differ by age, health status, sex, and, of course, by race/ethnicity, as well as other factors. (Physicians and Healthcare Administrators)
- Native Americans and Alaskan Natives are at greater risk for diabetes, cardiovascular disease, cancer, and HIV. Accordingly, their medication adherence practices may require more supports than other racial/ethnic groups. (Patients and physicians)
- Self-management efforts must be integrated with improved primary prevention by public health professionals. (All healthcare personnel)

Chapter Summary

The literature on the need for behavioral changes among health disparity populations is definitive. Across subgroups, these individuals must improve their dietary practices. Much higher levels of physical activity are also needed. A systematic effort must be made to augment health knowledge. Yet, physicians must also partner in these efforts. The progress of chronicities such as diabetes, obesity, and/or hypertension must be monitored by the physicians and the patients. Required physician visits must be scheduled by the physician and kept by the patient. Patients must be empowered to take ownership of their care and, when necessary, appropriately and politely question the treatment regimen. Physicians must interface with patients in a way that encourages communication. Notes should be taken by patients on incidents with healthcare professionals that suggest patient bias and letters sent to the appropriate oversight individuals and/or institution. Physicians must self-monitor their own behaviors and engage in self-improvement. Additionally, the language of each disease must be learned and understood. Adherence and the application of standard care must be monitored and reported to appropriate agencies by the physicians. Through these strategies, patient–physician partnerships can be used to discontinue some of the multisystem disparities chains that germinate and sustain health disparities.

Review Questions and Problems

1. Assume the role of a healthcare administrator, a public health professional, or a clinician. Using information learned in this chapter, describe in 500 or more words how you can support change as a strategy to decrease the contribution of personal behaviors to disparate outcomes.

2. Compile a list of the clinical tests that are used to diagnose and track each of the 10 major causes of death.
3. Write an original review of the literature on health disparities or health care by income.
4. As you are aware, clinicians sometimes feel superior to healthcare administrators. Construct a chart that includes clinical language and definitions for each of the major causes of death so that as a current or future healthcare administrator you can better converse with clinicians.

Key Terms and Concepts

behavioral change contract A patient-centered process of change whereby the patient agrees to adhere or not adhere to certain behaviors and the benefits or repercussions of doing so.

HbA(1c) test A glycated hemoglobin test that determines a person's blood glucose level. The test is designed to show the average level of blood glucose over the previous 3 months. High blood glucose levels are an indicator of diabetes mellitus.

self-management The adoption of behaviors that maximize treatment outcomes and minimize the progression of a disease.

self-management supports Tools, materials, and training provided by healthcare institutions to assist the individual in the maximization of their self-management activities.

telehealth Remote provision of nonclinical services through electronic means to provide health education and training for end users and/or medical personnel, surveillance, caregiver support, and other areas.

telemedicine Use of telecommunications technologies to provide remote diagnosis and treatment of patients.

References

Adams, R. J. (2010). Improving health outcomes with better patient understanding and education. *Risk Management and Health Care Policy, 3,* 61–72.

Banbury, A., Nancarrow, S., Dart, J., Gray, L., & Parkinson, L. (2018). Telehealth interventions delivering home-based support group videoconferencing: Systematic review. *Journal of Medical Internet Research, 20*(2), e25. doi: 10.2196/jmir.8090

Bhatt, K., Pourmand, A., & Sikka, N. (2018). Targeted applications of unmanned aerial vehicles (drones) in telemedicine. *Telemedicine Journal and E Health.* doi: 10.1089/tmj.2017.0289

Centers for Disease Control and Prevention. (2017a). American Indians/Alaskan Natives and tobacco use. Retrieved from https://www.cdc.gov/tobacco /disparities/american-indians/index.htm

Centers for Disease Control and Prevention. (2017b). Summary health statistics: National Health Interview Survey, 2016. Retrieved from http://www.cdc.gov /nchs/nhis/shs/tables.htm

Commiskey, P., Afshinnik, A., Cothren, E., Gropen, T., Iwuchukwu, I., . . . Gaines K. (2017). Description of a novel telemedicine-enabled comprehensive system of care: Drip and ship plus drip and keep within a system of stroke care delivery. *Journal of Telemedicine and Telecare, 23*(3), 428–436.

Cordoba, E., & Aiello, A. E. (2016). Social determinants of influenza illness and outbreaks in the United States. *North Carolina Medical Journal, 77*(5), 341–345.

D'andrea, M., Nedovic, D., Calabro, G. E., Delon, M., Ricciardi, W., & de Waure, C. (2017). The impact of telemedicine in reducing onset to treatment time in the management of acute stroke. *European Journal of Public Health, 27*(suppl 3). https://doi.org/10.1093 /eurpub/ckx189.091

Erten-Lyons, D., Lindauer, A., Mincks, K., Silbert, L., Lyons, B., . . . Kaye, J. (2016). Alzheimer's Care Via Telemedicine for Oregon (ACT-ON), Phase II: A pilot study of to-the-home dementia care via telemedicine. *Neurology, 12*(7), Supplement, P1186–P1187. doi: https://doi.org/10.1016/j.jalz.2016.07.134

Gardner, B. (2018). Habit formation and behavior change. *Oxford Research Encyclopedia of Psychology.* Oxford: Oxford University Press. http://psychology.oxfordre. com/view/10.1093/acrefore/9780190236557.001.0001 /acrefore-9780190236557-e-129. doi:10.1093/acrefore /9780190236557.013.129

Gardner, B., Lally, P., & Wardle, J. (2012). Making health habitual: The psychology of 'habit-formation' and general practice. *British Journal of General Practice, 62*(605), 664–666.

Gary, T. L., McGuire, M., McCuley, J., & Brancati, F. L. (2004). Racial comparisons of health care and glycemic control for African American and white diabetic adults in an urban managed care organization. *Disease Management, 7*(1), 25–34.

Girgis, L. (2017). How to give bad news to your patients, Physicians Practice, Modern Medicine Network. http://www.physicianspractice.com/difficult-patients /how-give-bad-news-your-patients.

Grady, P.A., & Gough, L.L. (2014). Self-management: a comprehensive approach to management of chronic conditions. *American Journal of Public Health, 104*(8), e25-e31. doi: 10.2105/AJPH.2014.302041

Jenkins, C., McNary, S., Carlson, B.A., King, M.G., Hossler, C.L., Magwood, G., . . . Ma'at, I. (2004). Reducing disparities for African Americans with diabetes: Progress made by the REACH 2010 Charleston and Georgetown diabetes coalition. *Public Health Report, 119*(3), 322–330.

Jethwani, K., & Sperber, J. (2017). Who gives the right to empower patients. *New England Journal of Medicine.* NEJM Catalyst, https://catalyst.nejm.org/gives-right-patient-empowerment/.

Jutel, A., & Lupton, D. (2015). Digitizing diagnosis: a review of mobile applications in the diagnostic process. *Diagnosis, 2*(2), 89–96. doi: https://doi .org/10.1515/dx-2014-0068

Kennedy, C. A., Warmington, K., Flewelling, C., Shupak, R., Papachristos, A., . . . Hogg-Johnson, S. (2017). A prospective comparison of tele-medicine versus in-person delivery of an interprofessional education program for adults with inflammatory arthritis. *Journal of Telemedicine and Telecare, 23*(2), 197–206. doi: 10.1177/1357633X16635342

LaVeist, T. A., Thorpe, R. J., Galarraga, J. E., Bower, K. M., & Gary-Webb, T. L. (2009). Environmental and socio-economic factors as contributors to racial disparities in diabetes prevalence. *Journal of General Internal Medicine, 24*(10), 1144–1148. doi: 10.1007 /s11606-009-1085-7.

McColl-Kennedy, J. R., Snyder, H., Mattias, E., Witell, L., Helkkula A., Hogan, S. J., & Anderson, L. (2017). The changing role of the health care customer: Review, synthesis, research agenda. *Journal of Service Management, 28*(1), 2–33.

Min, Y., Anugu, P., Butler, K., Correa, A., Hartley, T., . . . Winters, K. (2016). Abstract P084: Cardiovascular disease burden in African Americans: The Jackson Heart Study. *Circulation, 133*(suppl. 1).

Monden, K. R., Gentry, L., & Cox, T. (2016). Delivering bad news to patients, proceedings. *Baylor University Medical Center, 29*(1), 101–102.

Mowery, P. D., Dube, S. R., Thorne, S. L., Garrett, B. E., Homa, D. M., & Henderson, P. N. (2015). Disparities in smoking-related mortality among American Indians/ Alaska Natives. *American Journal of Preventive Medicine, 49*(5), 738–744.

Mueller, J., Jay, C., Harper, S., Davies, A., Vega, J., & Todd, C. (2017). Web use for symptom appraisal of physical health conditions: A systematic review. *Journal of Medical Internet Research*, 19(6), e202. doi: 10.2196 /jmlr.6755

Muller, K. I., Alstadhaug, K. B., & Bekkelund, S.I. (2016). Telemedicine in the management of non-acute headaches: A prospective, open-labelled non-inferiority, randomised clinical trial. *Cephalagia*, 37(9), 855–863.

National Center for Health Statistics. (2017). Health, United States, 2016: With Chartbook on Long-term Trends in Health. Hyattsville, MD.

Ogilvie, R. P., Everson-Rose, S. A., Longstreth, W. T., Rodriguez, C. J., Diez-Roux, A. V., & Lutsey, P.L. (2016). Psychosocial factors and risk of incidents of health failure: The multi-ethnic study of atherosclerosis. *Circulation and Heart Failure*, 9(1), e002243.

Pomey, M. P., Ghadiri, D. P., Karazivan, P., Fernandez, N., & Clavel, N. (2015). Patients as partners: A qualitative study of patients' engagement in their health care. *PLOS One*, 10(4), e0122499.

Roine, R., Ohinmaa, A., & Hailey, D. (2001). Assessing telemedicine: A systematic review of the literature. *Canadian Medical Association Journal*, 165(6), 765–771.

Sarashon-Kahn, J. (2012). A role for patients: the argument for self-care, *American Journal of Preventive Medicine*, 44:1,1 pp. 516–518, https://doi.org:10.1016/j.amepre .2012.09.019

Semigran, H. L., Linder, J. A., Gidengil, C., & Mehrotra, A. (2015). Evaluation of symptom checkers for self-diagnosis and triage: Audit study. *British Medical Journal*, 351:h3480. doi: 10.1136/bmj.h3480

Sharma, A., Colvin-Adams, M., & Yancy, C.W. (2014). Heart failure in African Americans: Disparities can be overcome. *Cleveland Clinic Journal of Medicine*, 81(5), 301–311.

Spatz, E.S., Beckman, A. L., Wang. Y., Desai, N.R., & Krumholz, H.M. (2016). Geographic variation in trends and disparities in acute myocardial and infarction: Hospitalization and mortality by income levels, 1999–2013. *JAMA Cardiology*, 1(3), 255–265.

Stewart, M. A. (1995). Effective physician–patient communication and health outcomes: A review. *Canadian Medical Association Journal*, 152(9), 1423–1433.

Telehealth Resource Center. (n.d.). Types of telemedicine specialty consultation services. Retrieved from https:// www.telehealthresourcecenter.org/toolbox-module /types-telemedicine-specialty-consultation-services.

Tolentino, S.M. (2018). Disparity notes for primary care physicians who treat Asians with diabetes. Unpublished paper, UNLV, Dept. of Health Care Administration and Policy.

Tonsaker, T., Bartlett, G., & Trpkov, C. (2014). Health information on the Internet: Gold mine or minefield? *Canadian Family Physician*, 60(5), 407–408.

Tseng, D. (2017). Study shows medical apps for chronic disease management have significant quality issues. iMedicalApps. Retrieved from https://www.imedical apps.com/2017/05/medical-apps-chronic-disease -management/#

Wade, J., & Smith, C. A. (2017). Research methods and methodology in telemedicine. *Journal of Telemedicine and Telecare*. 23(9), 757–758.

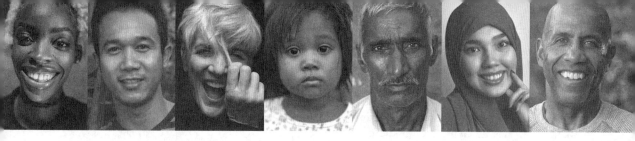

CHAPTER 9

Disparities in Primary, Specialty, and Tertiary Healthcare Markets

"…there are disparities in the health care children receive even after they're in our hospitals."

—**Casey Lion**, MD, MPH, Pediatrician, Seattle Children's Hospital and
Research Center for Child Health, Behavior and Development

LEARNING OBJECTIVES

After reading this chapter, learners will be able to:

- Summarize research on disparities in one or more disease areas that are specific to primary care healthcare providers.
- Identify some of the types of disparities that occur in specialty care.
- Compare and contrast treatment outcomes for selected illnesses and diseases treated by tertiary care providers.

▶ Introduction

In 2015, healthcare providers had medical encounters with more than 80% of all adults in the United States (National Center Health Statistics, 2016a). In the same year, U.S. residents made 990.8 million visits to physicians in their offices to obtain diagnostic and/or therapeutic services. Approximately 51.0% of these visits were made to primary care physicians and their clinical and administrative teams. Most of these healthcare consumers were seeking general examinations, progress visits, postoperative visits, pharmaceutical solutions to their illnesses and/or diseases, and/or counseling. Interestingly, 29.9% of all patients presented with hypertension as a chronic condition during their visit, making hypertension the disease most often encountered by primary care physicians.

The patients who visited healthcare providers in 2015 were not only served by physicians, but also by nurse practitioners, certified nurse midwives, registered nurses, advance practice nurses, physician assistants, and other clinicians. Healthcare services were delivered in physicians' offices, outpatient hospital units, and other practice sites that are managed by healthcare administrators (National Health Statistics, 2016b). Additionally, many of the patients had been exposed to public health information campaigns and other interventions designed to promote health improvements. This chapter introduces a variety of health disparity "case studies" by identifying some of the service points at which physicians may have unintentionally supported health disparities despite efforts of patients to engage in behavioral change and self-management.

▶ Health Disparities in Primary Care: The Case of Hypertension

Physicians and other clinical personnel rely upon clinical guidelines to direct the care provided to their patients. As new evidence emerges, new directives are provided to primary care and other physicians. For example, Ioannidis (2018) summarizes changes in the diagnosis and treatment of hypertension, the most common disease encountered by primary care physicians. These clinical guidelines will probably result in highly inflated disparities in the prevalence and incidence of hypertension in American society.

Why might this be the case?

In 2017, the clinical guidelines for the statistical measure of hypertension were revised downward (Whelton et al., 2018). Once established as a blood pressure greater than 140/90 mm Hg, **hypertension** is now officially identified as a chronic disease in persons with a blood pressure greater than 130/80 mm Hg. In lowering the floor for this disease, some analysts have proclaimed that approximately 46% of adults will now require treatment. The proportion for key subpopulations will be even higher. Similarly, under the new guidelines, physicians and their teams are explicitly mandated to work in partnership with their patients so that patients share in the effort to control the levels of this highly dangerous disease via improved disease management efforts.

Why was this change made?

As mentioned, research efforts are constantly under way to improve the quantity and quality of life for humankind in the area of health. One such study, the Systolic Blood Pressure Intervention Trial (SPRINT), National Heart, Lung, and Blood Institute (2017) and the Sprint Research Group (2015), demonstrated that death rates from the many hypertension-related illnesses and diseases could be significantly decreased by beginning treatment at the lower threshold and by increasing the number of pharmaceutical products used in the treatment of hypertension from 1.8 to 2.8 medications (Sprint Research Group, 2015).

Is hypertension an area of health care that has been characterized by treatment differentials?

Yes. Kendrick, Nuccio, Leiferman, and Sauaia (2015) in an analysis of survey data from physicians, nurse practitioners, and physician assistants found that although these primary care physicians embodied the belief that subgroup disparities existed with regard to hypertension, only one-third of respondents acknowledged the existence of disparities in hypertension care by race/ethnicity in their own practices. In contrast, more than 40% of the respondents agreed that overall disparities in care by socioeconomic status existed in their practices. Although these primary care physicians were reluctant to acknowledge disparities in their own practices, a substantial body of literature has documented disparities for a variety of subgroups. Gu, Bart, Paulose-Ram, and Dillon (2008), using data from the National Health and Nutrition Examination Survey (NHANES), 1999–2004, identified disparities in hypertension healthcare treatment in both female and African American populations. Even though the practice guidelines in place at that time did not recommend differential treatment by gender, differences in care by gender were observed. As a result, males were 14.06% more likely to achieve blood pressure control. However, the testing of the intervention is ongoing.

Cognizant of disparities in the treatment of hypertension by primary care physicians, a number of interventions have been implemented to improve care. Hong et al. (2018) report on an initiative called Project ReD CHiP (Reducing Disparities and Controlling Hypertension in Primary Care). This initiative uses care coordination and self-management as intervention tools. The authors concluded that the ReD CHiP was a cost effective initiative.

Do disparities exist in the prevalence of hypertension?

Yes. Lackland (2014) found that although disparities exist across subgroups, the widest disparities are between Americans of European and African descent. Differences occur not only with regard to prevalence rates, but disparities also occur in terms of age at onset, achievement of hypertension control, and incidence of disability due to hypertension-related conditions such as stroke, kidney failure, etc.

Important research is also emerging regarding unique factors associated with the higher prevalence and incidence rates of hypertension in certain subgroups. Tung et al. (2018) found, based on a sample of 14,799 patients, that persons who lived in neighborhoods with

the highest levels of violent crime were 25% more likely to be hypertensive and 53% more likely to be obese than those who lived in areas with lower crime rates. Thus, hypertension is a perfect case study for examining disparities in primary care. Moreover, such asymmetries are far from benign. Hypertension mediates health outcomes such as strokes, blood clots, blocked arteries, enlarged heart, fatal heart attack, aneurysms, coronary artery disease, enlarged left heart, dementia, kidney failure, kidney scarring, and other conditions.

How much of these disparities are related to behavior rather than from lower-quality health care?

It is difficult to provide a definitive answer to this question. It is possible, for example, that some providers have incomplete knowledge of how clinical guidelines must be adjusted for this very high-risk population—African Americans. Although physicians, nurses, and other direct service personnel are well trained in the treatment of hypertension, the knowledge gained from health disparity research has not been thoroughly disseminated to primary care clinicians. Lunn and Sanchez (2011) address this issue by recommending that academic health centers begin providing education to providers specifically on how to improve outcomes for health disparities populations. VanderWielen et al. (2015) suggest that medical schools have already integrated limited information regarding healthcare disparities into medical education but that this is an area in which improvement is needed. Smith (2007) emphasizes training of nurses as a strategy to reduce healthcare disparities. Phillips and Malone (2014) recommend the infusion of a higher proportion of culturally concordant nurses into the healthcare field in order to reduce disparities.

Such voids in education on health disparities suggest that health administrators, public health personnel, and clinicians must be equipped to exercise vigilance in the healthcare institutions in which they serve. It also increases the importance of healthcare administrators creating supports that will lead to greater disease self-management as a disparity prevention and/or reduction strategy.

Are you saying that physicians and other providers may not be adequately prepared to provide the needed differentiations in care?

This is certainly a possibility. Clinical care providers all know, of course, that vascular abnormalities related to the renin-angiotensin-aldosterone system serve as the physiological mechanism for the pathological changes in blood vessel walls that are associated with hypertension. However, few, if queried, would know that the correlates of hypertension transcend such factors.

Could you explain this "clinicalese"?

The **renin-angiotensin-aldosterone system**, or *RAAS system*, is the hormone system that regulates blood pressure and fluid balance. If this system is overactive, blood pressure will be too high. Renin, which is an enzyme released primarily by the kidneys, stimulates the formation of angiotensin in blood and tissues, which, in turn, stimulates the release of aldosterone from the adrenal cortex.

In describing the RAAS system, we hope to convey that hypertension is a complex disease that may have a variety of causes. For example, in addition to the commonly cited lifestyle elements, some evidence suggests that depression and other psychosocial factors may serve as intermediating variables in determining not merely the onset of hypertension, but its progression after treatment begins as well. Likewise, some studies have found that time urgency/impatience and hostility are also significant predictors of hypertension over the long run.

I thought you said that the practice guidelines are differentiated by race/ethnicity?

Yes, the practice guidelines do include evidence-based directives for modifying treatment for health disparity groups, but they

may be incomplete. In recent years, an abundant body of research has accrued that has addressed the extreme prevalence of hypertension among different subgroups. For example, Wassink et al. (2017) identified darker skin color as mediating hypertension, diabetes, obesity, and health risks among Latinos and African Americans. Similarly, Dent et al. (2017), in an examination of 130 African Americans, also found linkages between skin tone in physical health outcomes such as hypertension and in mental health. Research has included descriptive studies that have sought to confirm inter- and intra-ethnic trends in hypertension prevalence rates.

Ancheta (2014), for example, analyzed not merely hypertension but also waist circumference, body mass index, and blood lipids as risk factors for cardiovascular disease among Cambodian, Vietnamese, Filipino, and Chinese females in Florida. They found significant differences ($p < .05$) in the distribution of risk factors intraethnically. In particular, Cambodians and Vietnamese women had levels of hypertension that were comparable to the Filipinos in this study although their body mass index was much lower.

Epidemiological research that explains the different patterns in the incidence of hypertension has also been completed. For example, Fagard et al. (2009) completed research on hypertension that reminds health-care professionals of the importance of not allowing hypertension disparities to subordinate attention to patterns that may transcend subgroup differences. Specifically, Fagard et al., in a meta-analysis of four studies conducted in Europe, discovered that hypertensive patients with significant ($p < .01$) differences between the values of the systolic blood pressure (BP) ratio by night and day had a very high risk of death and/or a serious cardiovascular problem. This finding appears to be universally applicable. Balfour et al. (2015) highlights the fact that the prevalence rates of hypertension are high across almost all ethnic groups. At the time of

Balfour's study, the hypertension prevalence rates were 25% for subgroups native to the Americas and Canada, 37% for persons native to Hawaii and/or the Pacific Islands, 44% for non-Hispanic persons of African descent, 39% among Americans from Asia, and 42% among persons of Latin descent. Programs such as the Hispanic Community Health Study of Latinos, Healthy People 2020, the Million Hearts Initiative, the REGARDS initiative, and other efforts are examples of specialized interventions that have been launched in order to reduce hypertension disparities with varying degrees of success. Yet, a paucity of scientific literature on the inclusion of psychosocial interventions in the treatment of resistant hypertension among specific subgroups remains. Moreover, even less research exists that embraces the psychosocial intermediaries within the broader context of the patient–clinician relationship. Britt-Spells, Slebodnik, Sands, and Rollock (2016) found, for example, a positive relationship between perceptions of discrimination and depression. Thus, depression may coexist with the physiological mechanisms that elevate blood pressure. Such an approach may improve treatment efficacy given a growing body of psychiatric evidence which suggests that hostility, anxiety, depression, aggression, and other mental dysfunctions may be differentially distributed across America's racial/ethnic subgroups. For example, Macintyre, Ferris, Goncalves, and Quinn (2018) have revived the argument that socioeconomic factors adversely affect mental health and, as a result, may affect hypertensive disparities.

Healthcare clinicians are, of course, taught that hypertension is associated with the genesis of a wide range of other forms of cardiovascular disease. As mentioned, hypertensive Americans are far more likely than their normotensive friends and family members to experience strokes, ischemic heart disease, peripheral vascular disease, and, of course, renal impairment (National Center for Health Statistics, 2016c). Unfortunately hypertensive

patients are often asymptomatic resulting in perhaps millions of insured Americans not seeking treatment.

Healthcare providers may even contribute to disparities at this point in the disparities chain. Even when those with health insurance present for routine checkups, healthcare providers may miss opportunities to provide information that can improve treatment options (Lin et al., 2017). Moreover, when hypertension is identified, the severity of the side effects of antihypertensive medications may impact treatment choices and compliance (Brown & Bussell, 2011). Healthcare professionals may also support nonadherence by not being aware that such medications do not affect all subgroups equally (Tedia et al., 2016). In addition, physicians might even prescribe medications that the patient cannot afford (Iuga & McGuire, 2014).

Thus, in spite of the knowledge of physicians, nurses, and other clinicians about the potential impact of hypertension upon the cardiovascular system, a number of disparity-related factors that can confound the processes of diagnoses and treatment may not have been included in their training.

Healthcare administrators, public health professionals and clinicians can recommend the use of self-management supports (Hallberg, 2015). Self-management supports can help those with more serious elevations of blood pressure and objective signs of cardiovascular damage such as heart disease, stroke, and so on to reduce their risks of stroke and/or renal failure through frequent monitoring and improved medication adherence. Indeed, more frequent monitoring of blood pressure is recommended under the revised practice guidelines.

Medication-Related Disparities with Regard to Hypertension

Providers use the most recent Joint National Committee on Prevention, Detection, Evaluation, and Treatment of High Blood Pressure

(JNC) guidelines to continue to investigate the boundaries and limitations of pharmacological agents such as thiazide diuretics, beta blockers, calcium channel blockers, renin inhibitors, angiotensin-converting enzyme inhibitors (ACEs), and angiotensin II receptor blockers (ARBs) (Weinberger, 1990). Alexander et al. (2018) provide a comprehensive summary of medications currently used for the treatment of hypertension. However, these drugs are not equally effective across all subgroups (Whelton et al., 2018).

Other health disparities also operate in this disease area. Indeed, the manufacturer of losartan specifically states in the instructions that accompany the packaging that the medication may be less effective with African Americans. Yet, losartan is routinely prescribed to African Americans. In addition, Rao (2007) also discusses the differential hypertension medication needs of African American patients with high blood pressure. Specifically, these researchers suggest that hypertensive African Americans may wish to first follow a regimen that includes following the Dietary Approaches to Stop Hypertension (DASH) diet and the consumption of a diuretic to see if there are positive changes in their hypertension status. However, in the event that improvements are not realized with this formula, the addition of a calcium channel blocker, angiotensin-converting enzyme (ACE) inhibitor, angiotensin II receptor blocker (ARB), or beta blocker can then be added to the regimen.

African Americans are not the only subgroup that have been identified with hypertension drug disparities. For example, Cheung et al. (2014) conducted a study of the effectiveness of various hypertensive drugs with Asians. The conclusion drawn from the clinical trials was: "New National Institute for Clinical Excellence guidelines suggested the use of ACE inhibitors or ARBs as the first line treatment for essential hypertension. However, a higher incidence of dry cough with ACE inhibitor was reported in Asian populations. Therefore, ARB may be more suitable for Asian patient

with hypertension" (pg. 450). Rodriguez et al. (2016) examined the use and results of anti-hypertensive medications with Latinos from the mainland United States and those from Puerto Rico relative to other participants in the SPRINT clinical trials. The study noted comparable rates of medication adherence, lower mean rates of hypertension medications, and lower rates of blood pressure control. Thus, it was not clear whether the prescribed anti-hypertensive medications were less effective and/or whether the number and/or combinations used led to differential results.

In contrast, Hayslett et al. (2001), in a now dated study on hypertension control in American Indians from North and South Dakota, Arizona, and Oklahoma, found that when single therapies were used, diuretics were most effective in achieving blood pressure control but the highest levels of control occurred among hypertensives who were prescribed a diuretic and an ACE inhibitor. This study did not report side effects.

When patterns of hypertension treatment effectiveness are analyzed by sex, disparities are also revealed. Gu et al. (2008) sought to assess the equal applicability of National Practice Hypertension Treatment Guidelines by sex since these guidelines recommended nondisparate treatment approaches for males and females. Nevertheless, differences in application of the recommended guidelines occurred by gender. The analysis revealed significant differences in anti-hypertensive medication use patterns by gender. Specifically, more women used these medications. Differences also existed in the type of medications prescribed. Specifically, women were significantly ($p < .08$) more likely to be prescribed diuretics and angiotensin receptor blockers. However, women were significantly less likely to be treated with three or more drugs. Finally, women were significantly less likely to achieve blood pressure control once they were treated.

Other examples could be cited. However, this case study clearly demonstrates that primary care physicians need much more support if they are to be able to reduce health disparities in hypertension and/or in other primary care areas. First, this case study suggests that there is a greater need to prepare clinicians in general for the treatment of subgroups during their medical training. Second, the case study suggests that Practice Guidelines may require greater attention to the inclusion of clinical trial data regarding the use of medications across subgroups.

As mentioned, disparities in health outcomes among some subgroups may require more monitoring because providers are not yet trained to analyze the differential impact of modern pharmacological solutions by subgroup. As a result, ongoing monitoring is particularly important because the number of adverse effects is negatively correlated with medication adherence in various subgroups (Brown & Bussell, 2011).

How Healthcare Administrators and Public Health Professionals Can Better Support Healthcare Providers in Preventing Disparities in the Treatment of Hypertension

As this discussion indicates, although clinicians may follow the current clinical guidelines in the care of all healthcare consumers, research findings on the treatment needs of subgroups may be still scattered across journals. Thus, healthcare administrators working in partnership with public health professionals may wish to implement policies that include the use of disparity apps. While there are a number of health apps available to healthcare providers and physicians (mHealth, Epocrates, UpToDate, Medscape, etc.) few, if any, include data or information on health disparities. Disparity apps would deliver health disparities information regarding certain illnesses and diseases via a physician's smartphone and/or tablet with instantaneous results to the user's query. Disparity apps can be updated annually to ensure that state-of-the-art knowledge is available for integration into the care provided.

Healthcare administrators can also require disparity analyses to be completed on a yearly

basis in order to track the quality of health care provided. **BOX 9.1** lists questions that could be included in healthcare disparity analysis for patients with hypertension.

Overworked healthcare providers will, of course, become overwhelmed if healthcare administrators recommend approaches that only focus upon physician management strategies. Both prevention and self-management support can be provided to address key control variables, including body weight, salt intake, and level of physical activity, through public health partnerships. An established body of research indicates nutritional interventions that consist of a diet based upon fruits, vegetables, and reduced-fat dairy products result in the most significant reductions in blood pressure levels (Schwingshakl et al., 2017). Moreover, blood pressure values among minorities tend to respond even more favorably to such dietary interventions as compared to nonminorities. For example, Vollmer et al. (2001) report on the effectiveness of the DASH diet across subgroups. However, because the impact of dietary measures may be even greater for various subgroups, Siervo et al. (2015), based upon a comprehensive review of findings from multiple databases, found that, "Changes in both systolic and diastolic BP (blood pressure) were greater in participants with higher baseline BP or BMI (body mass index)" (pg. 14). As is known, racial/ethnic and gender subgroups in the DASH clinical trials had higher baseline BPs and BMIs. The critical role of nutritional interventions across subgroups is also confirmed by the fact that Tiong et al. (2008) reported positive outcomes for Malaysian and Filipino hypertensives.

In addition, healthcare administrators can create zero-tolerance policies for unfounded clinical care differences in their organizations. This is important because a considerable body of knowledge suggests that provider care varies by race/ethnicity and other categories of patients. Doyle (2015) reports on one study of minority patient care over the time period 2005 to 2013. Analyzing data on wait times, these

---

BOX 9.1 Sample Questions for a Healthcare Disparities Analysis for Hypertensive Consumers

- Are beta blockers and ACE inhibitors or other medications being used less frequently with minority patients?
- Are the responses of racial/ethnic groups to these agents definitely positive?
- Does a subgroup, such as Asian Americans, respond more favorably to calcium antagonists as opposed to ACE inhibitors?
- Can diuretics and beta blockers lead to responses that match those obtained through the use of calcium antagonists for Asian Americans?
- Are there disproportionate responses among treatment modalities for Latinos?
- How effective are nonpharmacological approaches for the control of hypertension among those populations experiencing health disparities?
- Does the highly publicized DASH (Dietary Approaches to Stop Hypertension) nutritional program affect blood pressure rates of adult Americans with baseline blood pressure rates of greater than 160 mm Hg systolic and 80 to 95 mm Hg diastolic? (These levels are more characteristic of some subgroups than for others.)
- How effective are interventions based on the most recent clinical trials when data are analyzed across subgroups?
- When the bivariate data analyses are performed, are previously unidentified subgroup disparities revealed?

---

researchers found that minority Americans spent significantly more time in physician offices. Ly et al. (2010), identified longer lag times before obtaining an appointment, longer wait times before seeing a physician, and differential rates of service satisfaction between patients of European descent and other patients.

Some differential treatment may occur at an indirect level among providers. For example, physician interactions that are more concordant with Latinos and African Americans include longer visits and personal patient-centered interactions. Martin et al. (2013), in a study of 39 primary care practices in Baltimore, Maryland, found that, "…positive physician affect and longer visits were significantly associated with high-patient trust…for African American patients" (pg. 156). Saha et al. (2003) found that when patients were Asian and/or Latino, patient satisfaction was even lower than for African Americans or Americans of European descent. In contrast, Geraghty et al. (2007) found a direct relationship between the length of a visit to a primary care physician and patient satisfaction

for patient subgroups with muscoskeletal disorders, depression, and other conditions that were not directly related to race/ethnicity or gender. This is consistent with earlier research by Lin et al. (2001) who also confirmed higher patient satisfaction based upon time spent with his or her primary care physician.

Yet, primary care physicians may be unaware that this is the case. And more physician time is costly! However, these cost implications can be ameliorated by supplementing physician interactions with trained community health workers who can provide the education, counseling, monitoring, and overall client support that physicians cannot cost-effectively provide. For example, Natale-Pereira, Enard, Nevarez, and Jones (2011) recommend the use of patient navigators. Patient navigators addend the care provided by the physician and other staff by engaging in relationship-building with patients as they assist them in going through the sequential processes needed to receive treatment. Similarly, healthcare administrators whose organizations use case management to link consumers with structured community-based programs can enhance blood pressure control. O'Neill et al. (2014) describe the positive outcomes that accompanied the use of a collaborative case management hypertension intervention at a Veterans Affairs Medical Center at an undisclosed location in the Midwest.

Moreover, the benefits of case management in the treatment of hypertension transcend the area of health disparities. Weinberger (1990), for example, in an article written several decades ago, describes the racial differences in the outcomes associated with the use of various high blood pressure medications. Ozpancar et al. (2017) conducted a clinical trial and also recorded positive antihypertension benefits for case management. Indeed, a recurring theme is that it is imperative that healthcare administrators ensure that their institutions play a greater role in supporting self-management among various subgroups.

Thus, a practice such as asking patients to monitor their blood pressure on a more frequent basis and sharing their data with their physician for feedback can possibly lead to improved blood pressure control (McManus et al., 2018; Bengtsson et al., 2016).

Is there any research to support this notion?

While no clinical trials supportive of this recommendation have been completed, empirical research does support the testing of this hypothesis. Kluger and DeNisis (1996) completed a meta-analysis of studies on feedback interventions.

What is a meta-analysis, and what are feedback interventions?

Feedback interventions are a tool used in management in which supervisors provide positive and negative input to workers regarding their workplace performance. A *meta-analysis* collects statistical findings from multiple studies on a common theme and statistically combines them so that findings can be reanalyzed based upon a larger, yet, statistically compatible sample. The objective of feedback interventions is to improve performance. The results of this study revealed that while feedback did improve worker performance overall, it also reduced worker performance in more than one-third of the cases. These investigators also identified three causal mechanisms through which feedback affects performance. First, feedback can improve the learning of how a task should be completed and why. Feedback can also increase and/or decrease the individual's motivation to improve their performance. Last, feedback can allow the individual to better understand the sub-processes that must be completed in order for the overall tasks to be more efficiently performed.

The argument can therefore be advanced that primary care physicians who treat hypertension, diabetes, chronic kidney disease (CKD), and other chronic diseases are positioned to input data from lab results and patient visits into predictive analytical software that provides a probability of a major health crisis based upon the patient's "performance." For example, a hypertensive patient who does not adhere to his or her medication regimen and does not follow the physician-recommended lifestyle changes would be provided a "performance score" with each 3-month visit. This performance score would be calculated by a program that embodies an algorithm based upon data from other patients. This "performance score," if given to the chronically ill patient at each of their quarterly visits, may have the power to improve their self-management. That is, knowing that the probability of a stroke or heart attack has increased or decreased as a result of one's self-management efforts may catalyze positive change from quarter-to-quarter.

But who is in the position to mandate such changes?

The number of solo medical practices has now declined. Kane (2017) cites data from the American Medical Association's Physician Practices, Benchmark Survey. These data reveal that 52.9% of physicians currently work in a practice that is owned by a hospital, a physician group, a managed care organization, or other entity. These arrangements provide an excellent opportunity for healthcare administrators, public health professionals, and clinicians to test the use of predictive analytics in assessing and in providing patients' self-management performance.

▶ Health Disparities in Pediatrics

Primary care specialties include family practitioners and general-level internal medicine practitioners such as those who treat hypertension and other diseases. General pediatricians also provide primary care. Thus, one can explore another primary care area by asking, "Do healthcare disparities exist in pediatric care?"

A number of investigators have identified disparities in pediatric care. For example, Langellier, Chen, Bustamente, Inkelas, and Ortega (2016) analyzed data from the 2006–2011 National Health Interview Survey to examine healthcare access and utilization among children age 17 or younger in the United States by race/ethnicity. They found that Latino children were significantly less likely to receive primary care services than their White American counterparts. Additionally, these differentials did not vanish when the data were held constant across education and income.

Was this because of discrimination?

The study cited was not designed to identify the reason for these disparities.

Are there any studies that identify direct and/or indirect bias with regard to the pediatric population?

Our team did not seek such research. However, Goyal et al. (2015) performed logistic regression to analyze whether differences existed in access to pain medication for

children admitted to emergency departments for appendicitis. This study found significant undertreatment of pain by race/ethnicity *even when the pain was severe.* Additionally, Sabin et al. (2015) found that physicians who assessed Native American/Alaskan Native children regarding their weight and/or obesity demonstrated indirect bias. Thus, there are a number of areas that healthcare administrators, public health professionals, and/or clinicians may wish to address regarding indirect bias and the pediatric population.

Was the purpose of this study to identify bias or to "root out" bias?

Completing research to identify bias and/or to root out bias is, from the perspective of the authors, dysfunctional to improvements in the human condition. As mentioned repeatedly, health care, whether delivered by a biased and/or unbiased health care provider system, only determines a small percent of health outcomes. Accordingly, the critical questions are: (1) Do health disparities exist? (2) Where and within what groups, subgroups, intersectoral groups do disparities exist? (3) What are the immediate and distal "causes" of these disparities? (4) How can any remediable disparities identified be reduced and/or eliminated in a way that the health outcomes of all of humankind is also advanced? A research focus on bias minimizes this larger purpose.

Does differential pain management only affect primary care physicians who are pediatricians?

Many studies have confirmed that differential pain management is not limited to pediatrics or even to primary care. Green et al. (2003) completed a comprehensive literature review of scholarly articles on research that were data-based rather than case studies. They found that, whether for primary, specialty, and/or tertiary care, pain had been historically undermanaged for racial/ethnic subgroups. They found this to be true in every single setting from emergency rooms to surgery units. These practices not only varied within healthcare settings, but also across disease areas.

Did these differences in pain management exist for cancer also?

Yes. These differences were identifiable throughout the healthcare system.

In your view, did these pain practices lead to the disproportionate burden of the opioid crisis upon Whites?

Some would argue that this is, indeed, the case. Our team would suggest that an approach to health disparities that was more broad-based could have predicted the adverse potentiality in these pain management practices and prevented the emergence of the current opioid crisis.

What does more recent literature indicate regarding differentials in pain management?

Hoffman et al. (2016) confirmed the highly critical role that ontological beliefs can play in the quality of health care that medical practitioners deliver. Specifically, this study, which was completed by a team of researchers consisting of a psychologist, a family practitioner, and a public health scholar, discovered that a number of physicians and medical students who engaged in pain management undertreatment practices literally held ontological beliefs *which assumed that racial/ethnic differences between Whites and African Americans are biological in nature and, as a result, the same level of pain management is unnecessary.*

Wow, That's Terrible!

It is absolutely dysfunctional to the creation of change that advances humankind to view this research judgmentally. Rather, our mention of this study simply allows current and future clinicians the opportunity to introspect and transform their own ontological beliefs.

Can we return to pediatric care?

Yes. Noble et al. (2015) demonstrated the criticality of initiating health and healthcare

disparity interventions early in the disparities chain by impacting life mediators such as education and income. Specifically, these researchers found that, independent of race/ethnicity, even small differences in income are reflected in differences in brain development among children aged 3 to 20 years. The authors found that familial income is exponentially related to the total area of the brain structure of children of all racial/ethnic groups. Thus, even small differences in familial income were reflected in large differences in the overall area of the brain surface.

Why is this important?

It is important because these differences in brain area occur in the parts of the brain that affect knowledge acquisition through reading, language use and development, and that support thinking, reasoning, and decision making.

Healthcare disparities that affect brain development ultimately limit access to education—one of the most important forms of social capital available to humankind. The study by Noble et al. (2015) revealed that poverty can create permanent brain damage in children in ways that may affect their acquisition of the skills needed to negotiate their life outcomes.

Pediatricians have contact with parents far before teachers do. Pediatricians and other primary care physicians are positioned to inform parents of findings such as these. They are also positioned to educate parents regarding the role of adverse childhood experiences (ACEs) that may impact healthy individuals once they reach adulthood. ACEs are events that happen in the lives of children from birth to 18 that can negatively affect the child. For example, data from the Centers for Disease Control and Prevention reveal that the risk of suicide has actually increased for high school youth as a whole and that different patterns of racial/ethnic disparities have emerged over the decade since 2005. Suicide risks in youth are oftentimes related to adverse childhood experiences. Perez et al. (2016), using data from 64,239 multiethnic Florida male and female youth, confirmed that adverse childhood experiences are linked with risk of suicide. However, they also identified the pathways that lead from adverse childhood experiences to suicidality as including poor academic performance and other problems in the school experience. In addition, based upon the child's personality, behavioral issues such as high levels of impulsive behavior and aggressive actions can generate scenarios that result in the risk of suicide in adolescents and youth. Yet, in most cases, as mentioned, an absolute informational disconnect appears to exist between the children's teachers and counselors, and pediatricians and parents relative to these risks and their linkages. Indeed, because of the disciplinary boundaries between the public health community, clinicians, and administrators of healthcare institutions that serve children, adolescents, youth, and their parents, the highly threatening aggregate and disparate risks described in **TABLE 9.1** remain unaddressed.

TABLE 9.1 Changes in Suicide Risks Among High School Students in 2005 and 2015 by Race/Ethnicity Ranked from Highest-to Lowest-Risk Group

Category #1: Percentage of YBRSS Youth Felt Sad or Hopeless Ranked from Highest to Lowest

Rank	Race/Ethnicity	2005 (%)	2015 (%)	% Change
1.	Multiple Race American Youth	37.4	38.8	+1.04
2.	Hispanic American Youth	36.2	35.3	−2.48
3.	American Indian/Alaskan Native Youth	30.8	34.9	+13.31
4.	Asian American Youth	28.8	22.9	−20.48
5.	Black/African American Youth	28.4	25.2	−11.26
6.	White American Youth	25.8	28.6	+10.85
All Youth		28.5	29.9	+4.91

Category #2: Seriously Considering Suicide				
1.	Multiple Race American Youth	27.1	26.6	−1.84
2.	American Indian/Alaskan Native Youth	23.4	20.9	−10.68
3.	Hispanic American Youth	17.9	18.8	+5.02

4.	White American Youth	16.9	17.2	+11.32
5.	Asian American Youth	15.9	17.7	+11.13
6.	African American Youth	12.2	14.5	+18.85
All Youth		16.9	17.7	+4.73

Category #3: Made a Plan About How They Would Attempt Suicide

1.	Multiple Race Youth	26.4	19.6	−25.75
2.	Hispanic/Latino Youth	14.5	15.7	+8.27
3.	American Indian/Alaskan Native Youth	13.8	17.4	+26.08
4.	Asian American Youth	13.3	13.8	+3.7
5.	White/Caucasian Youth	12.5	13.9	+11.2
6.	Black/African American Youth	9.6	13.7	+47.2
All Youth		13.0	14.6	+12.3

Category #4: Attempted Suicide One or More Times During the 12 Months Before the Survey

1.	American Indian/Alaskan Native Youth	17.6	15.0	−14.77
2.	Multiple Risk Youth	14.6	15.2	+6.16
3.	Hispanic/Latino Youth	11.3	11.3	0
4.	Black/African American Youth	7.6	8.9	+17.1
5.	White/Caucasian Youth	7.3	6.8	−6.84
6.	Asian American Youth	6.9	7.8	+13.04
All Youth		8.4	8.6	+2.38

(continues)

TABLE 9.1 Changes in Suicide Risks Among High School Students in 2005 and 2015 by Race/Ethnicity Ranked from Highest to Lowest Risk Group *(continued)*

Category #5: Attempted Suicide That Resulted in an Injury

Rank	Race/Ethnicity	2005 (%)	2015 (%)	% Change
1.	American Indian/Alaskan Native Youth	5.5	4.0	−27.27
2.	Hispanic/Latino Youth	3.2	3.7	+15.62
3.	White/Caucasian Youth	2.1	2.1	0
4.	Black/African American Youth	2.0	3.8	+90
5.	Multiple Race Youth	2.0	4.7	+135
6.	Asian American Youth	1.9	1.5	−21.05
All Youth	Total All Youth	2.3	2.8	+21.73

Constructed by authors using data from Centers for Disease Control and Prevention, High School Youth Risk Behavior Survey, 2005 and 2015.

As Table 9.1 reveals, collective efforts are needed between pediatricians, public health personnel, health care administrators, educational personnel, and parents in order to reduce the experiences of youth that have resulted in a greater risk of suicide over the last ten years. Specifically, the percent of all youth surveyed in the 2015 Youth Behavioral Risk Surveillance Survey who felt sad and hopeless had increased by 4.91% over the course of one decade. While these risks decreased for Hispanic/Latino youth (−2.48%), Asian American youth (−20.48%), and African American youth (−11.26%), they increased for multiple race youth (+1.04%), American Indian/Alaskan Native youth (+13.31%), and White/Caucasian youth (+10.85%). It is also clinically significant that more than 25.8% of all youth experienced feelings of hopelessness during 2005 and nearly 30% felt hopeless in 2015. Many of the youth

surveyed in 2015 are now sitting in classrooms in colleges and universities nationwide without such feelings being addressed by those who are the guardians of their future.

Similarly, a 4.73% increase occurred in the percentage of high school youth who were seriously considering suicide over the 2005–2010 decade. Again, while some improvements in risks occurred for multiple race (+1.84%) and American Indian/Alaskan Native youth (+10.68%), increases took place in the percentages of all youth in the sample who had seriously considered suicide. Of even greater concern, a 12.3% increase occurred over baseline in the percent of youth who had made a suicide plan. Overall, a 2.38% increase took place in the percent of youth who actually attempted suicide. This increase was largely driven by the increase in Asian American (+13.04%) and African American youth (+17.1%) who attempted suicide in 2015. Finally, there was a 21.73% increase in the percent of youth who injured themselves through an unsuccessful suicide attempt. Yet, it is doubtful that this growing crisis among America's youth and young adults who were still in high school in 2015, has yet been recognized among healthcare providers. This crisis may not be apparent to members of the healthcare community due to the absence of cross-disciplinary, multidisciplinary, and transdisciplinary teams who work with pediatricians and primary care physicians who embrace the preventative as well as the curative.

▶ # Disparities in Specialty Care: The Case of Cancer

A number of researchers have advanced the argument that the American healthcare system is overpopulated by specialists (Ameringer, 2018; Dalen, Ryan, and Alpert, 2017; Gabriel, 1996). This issue is bypassed in this section. Rather, the query that is addressed is, "What types of healthcare disparities have been observed in a specialty area of health care, specifically with regard to cancer?"

Siegel, Miller, and Jemal (2018) describe a number of differentials in the prevalence and incidence of cancer. They determined that in 2017 more than 1.6 million new cases of cancer were diagnosed. However, when the time period is expanded from 1991 to 2014, U.S. residents experienced a 28% decrease in cancer deaths. In the absence of interventions by physicians specializing in cancer treatment, and public health professionals seeking to prevent the initiation of cancers, the number of cancer deaths would have included more than 2 million more lives lost.

This study also revealed that although the incidence rate of cancer was 20% higher in males than females, and cancer death rates were 40% higher for males than females, women had a much higher incidence of some cancers than males. For example, the incidence of thyroid cancer was 200% higher for women than for men. However, all subgroups have a reason for celebration despite the existence of such differences because overall cancer rates decreased.

Why do unfavorable disparities exist between males and females?

Carè et al. (2018) hypothesize that differences between cancer types and deaths may be biologically based rather than the outcome of disparate health care. However, the growth of research on this topic can improve cancer outcomes for all subgroups. It is important to note that males are at greater risk of a cancer incident and a cancer death.

Are there any disparities in how oncologists deliver cancer care?

Chang, Huang, and Wu (2018) cite research that revealed differential outcomes for some subgroups in the diagnosis, treatment, and survival of patients with pancreatic cancer. However, in their study of 2,103 patients treated for pancreatic cancer at Kaiser Permanente in Southern California, these researchers found no disparities in terms of diagnosis, treatment, and post-treatment outcomes associated with pancreatic cancer. Neal et al. (2015) further expand knowledge of this relationship. These researchers remind analysts that the relationship between time of diagnosis and cancer outcomes is not always linear. Specifically, this relationship varies by the type of cancer and whether the cancer has manifested itself via symptoms at the time of diagnosis. Thus, the existence of differential outcomes in health care can certainly be reduced or eliminated by the healthcare institution.

Are you saying there were no racial/ethnic differences in cancer treatment for this organization?

Yes, the data reveal a 100% absence of significant differences in pancreatic cancer treatment for Kaiser Permanente. The patient panel included all racial/ethnic groups. No differences existed in the rate of the diagnosis, or in the time to an oncology consultation, or in the time to surgery by racial/ethnic group. Although there were a few differences in survival rates, these may have been associated with slight differences in the patient's choice of treatment. Chang, Huang, and Wu (2018) credited the use of an integrated healthcare model for these outcomes.

Has research assigned differentials in cancer survival to later diagnoses?

Yes, some research has found that differences in the time of diagnosis significantly affect cancer survival. For example, Homan et al. (2016) analyzed 2010 data and found direct linkages between time of diagnosis and years of survival for persons with breast cancer. Independently of such factors, Nautsch et al. (2018) found differences in the time of cancer diagnosis by race/ethnicity. Cristi and Grunfeld (2013), Mehnert et al. (2013), and Phillips et al. (2013) also found that disparities exist by race/ethnicity in fear of cancer recurrence after it is in remission. However, citing studies that reflect disparities without some analysis of the causes can promote subtribalism. Moreover, the complete or near-complete characterization of existing disparities can be overwhelming to health care professionals seeking to address remediable patterns.

What do you mean by this?

Consider the following example. HIV/AIDS is typically treated by specialists, not primary care providers. HIV/AIDS is also a disease to which stigma is attached, and stigma is often associated with lower-quality health care. Levinson et al. (2018) conducted a study examining the care of 57 HIV-infected females with cancer. These patients were disproportionately African American. As previously discussed, quality of care is higher for a disease when it is delivered in a way that is consistent with the practice guidelines for that specific disease. This study found that 49% of these women did not receive care for their vulvar, cervical, ovarian, and endometrial cancers that was consistent with the practice guidelines. Simply by reviewing the descriptive data, one would immediately hypothesize that these circumstances reflected stigma and discrimination by the specialty providers who provided the treatment. However, this was definitely not the case.

There were two main reasons that 28 of the women in the study group did not receive care that was compliant with the practice guidelines for their diseases. First, the practice guideline treatments proved toxic to some of the women. Second, other patient-based variables disallowed these specialty-care physicians from administering the treatments that were recommended in the practice guidelines. Not a single instance of the descriptive data findings were sourced in negative human behavior among the providers who delivered the care!

▶ Disparities in Tertiary Health Care: The Case of Kidney Transplantation

Hypertension was utilized as a case example of how disparities can occur in primary care treatment. As mentioned, hypertension was used as the disease of choice because it is the single most widely treated disease by primary care physicians. Pediatric care was also discussed as a demonstration of how disparities can be operative among physicians who deliver primary care services. Cancer care was briefly reviewed as a case study of specialty care. In this section, transplantation surgery has been selected as a case study for the examination of how disparities can characterize tertiary health care.

Tertiary care represents a third level of care by providers. Whereas primary care is the portal into the clinical care component of the American healthcare system, tertiary care can be viewed as the last segment of care that is available to the patient. Accordingly, tertiary care is the most complex level of care that can be provided. In this section, kidney transplantation surgery is used as a case study for the understanding of how disparities can characterize this third level of care.

Because hypertension was used as the case study for primary care physicians, it makes sense to discuss kidney transplantation and end-stage renal disease in a discussion of tertiary care. Chronic kidney disease and end-stage renal disease (as well as other variables) are causatively linked to hypertension and diabetes. Thus, it somehow seemed appropriate to examine disparities in one of these two areas.

▶ Kidney Transplantation: A Case Example of Tertiary Care Disparities

The year was 1954. Although the first tier of immunosuppressants had yet to be produced, Dr. Joseph Murray of Peter Bent Brigham Hospital in Boston, driven by the dream of elevating the human condition, completed the first kidney transplant (Nagy, 1999; Hatzinger, Statsny, Gruzmacher, & Sohn, 2016). In so doing, a disease that was normally associated with a continued life expectancy of less than 1 year without dialysis was radically transformed. Since that time, via continued improvements in surgical techniques and in pharmaceutical products to prevent the rejection of the transplanted kidney, a new field of tertiary medicine has grown and thrived. However, in some respects, the area of tertiary medicine that is known as organ transplantation is characterized by an infrastructure that can easily breed disparities.

Why would you say that?

Despite the fact that federal, state, and local governments help finance health care, the American healthcare market is, nevertheless, primarily market-based. Thus, because the demand for transplantation services exceeds supply, the healthcare marketplace for kidney transplantation is characterized by extreme shortages. The demand for kidneys and other organs far exceeds the supply. Accordingly, it is less than surprising that researchers have identified a number of disparities that exist in this unique segment of the American healthcare marketplace.

UNOS, the United Network for Organ Sharing, an organization established by the National Organ Transplant Act in 1986, administers the small, nonprofit marketplace that connects available organs from donors with patients in need of an organ. A part of this effort includes continuous data collection, tracking, storing, analysis and efforts to distribute organs according to established guidelines.

Because all humans have two kidneys, shouldn't these disparities be easy to address?

It would seem so. But currently this marketplace is highly dependent upon deceased donors who signed an organ transplantation card and held a discussion about their decision with their families before their death.

But don't patients receiving kidneys from live donors have better outcomes?

Yes. Patients receiving kidneys from live donors do have higher rates of survivorship. Maggiore et al. (2017), for example, state that "Kidney transplantation with living donor organs is associated with longer graft and patient survival compared with deceased donor organs," (pg. 216). Other researchers in this unique area of tertiary physician care have had similar findings. However, Maggiore et al. (2017) also highlight the fact that risks of kidney donorship to the donor may be higher than initially anticipated. Moreover, the potential risks of live kidney donorship are disparately distributed. Subpopulations who have higher prevalence rates of hypertension and diabetes are also at greater risks from serving as living donors. Accordingly, it is less than surprising that racial/ethnic differences exist in the proportion of minority donors who are willing to donate a kidney to a relative. In fact, over recent years, there has actually been a decrease in the percentage of Latinos and African Americans who donate a kidney to a family member (Jay & Cigarroa, 2018). Thus, there is a relatively greater reliance on deceased donors.

Does research reveal that intragroup behaviors are creating disparities in the area of kidney transplantation?

Intragroup behaviors have been identified as an important variable. For example, Purnell, Luo, and Cooper (2018), in a study comparing 1995–1999 and 2010–2014 time periods, documented that White Americans experienced a 62.86% increase in family members and others deciding to donate a kidney to persons who had been on the wait-list for 2 years, whereas Asian Americans experienced only a 9.8% increase in live donorship rates. Moreover, decreased rates in live kidney donorship occurred among Latinos and African Americans. Approximately 12.24% fewer Latinos decided to give their family member a kidney from 1995 to 2014. For African Americans, the decrease was 14.7%. However, it is important to point out that even in 1995, only 3.4% of this group decided to provide a kidney to their family member after they had been on the wait-list for 2 years. This rate of "gifting" was only 48.47% as high as the 7% rate that existed for their white counterparts at that time.

What does this mean in terms of healthcare disparities?

It suggests a need for public health professionals to conduct research to identify why such patterns exist. Simultaneously, clinicians must complete greater follow-up so that a larger pool of data is available on the impact of live donorship upon donors. Henderson and Gross

(2017) suggest that insufficient research may now exist regarding the long-term impact of live kidney donorship in the data. Once this research is completed, educational campaigns can be launched that address the benefits of live donorship to family members, the risks to the donor, and other issues that may affect live donorship rates.

Should these campaigns only target Latinos and African American because their rates are the lowest?

Absolutely not. Even the 11.4% rate for the Caucasians who do serve as live kidney donors is quite low. Thus, the campaign must be targeted to all groups with messages embedded that simultaneously address the hesitancies of all groups that were identified in the research and the biological risks that longer-term research will reveal.

Do kidney transplantation specialists support disparities in this tertiary area of medicine?

Kidney transplantation embodies many physician-based disparities. Malek, Keys, Kumar, Milford, and Tullius (2010) identified the following disparities:

- Racial/ethnic minorities are provided less access to transplantation as an option by their nephrologists.
- Racial/ethnic minorities are more likely to be excluded by their nephrologists from the kidney wait-list.
- Some nephrologists believe that providing a kidney to minorities is wasteful because graft rejection rates are higher among these groups once a transplant occurs.
- Some nephrologists are hesitant to assign a kidney from a deceased donor to a minority because they embody an ontology that leads to the belief that transplantation will not extend the length of life for minority groups.
- Some nephrologists do not equally evaluate racial/ethnic subgroups to determine their suitability for transplantation.

- Some nephrologists embody an ontology that does not see some racial/ethnic subgroups as willing to commit to the treatment adherence levels needed to support a successful kidney transplantation.
- Rural subgroups are less likely to be wait-listed than their urban counterparts because some nephrologists believe that they cannot get to the transplantation center in a timely fashion.
- An array of biomedical factors affects the kidney matching process for nephrologists.
- The cost of medications after transplantation occurs is more burdensome to lower-income versus higher-income subgroups.

Taken together, one sees that systemic variables within the organ transplantation system interact with biomedical differentials and socioeconomic variables to create disparities in this unique tertiary care market.

▶ Some Notes on Reducing Disparities in Primary, Specialty, and Tertiary Care

This chapter used several examples to demonstrate the operation of disparities among primary care, specialty care, and tertiary care physicians. Disparities in hypertension treatment, pediatric care, cancer care, and organ transplantation were discussed. Across these and other health areas, it was recommended that the most current practice guidelines should always be closely followed for all consumers. Medications that minimize the number and severity of adverse events should be prescribed based on current treatment guidelines. Because of the comprehensiveness of disparity research, providers may benefit from smartphone apps that allow them to quickly access research that is specific to the health disparity population being

served for a specific disease area. Independently of the disease area, the entire provider staff must ensure that the patient–clinician interaction is mutually satisfactory. Similarly, frequent electronic monitoring with counseling and consultation is needed. The healthcare provider must ensure access to, as well as compliance with, all prescribed medications. Nonadherence should prompt research to determine whether a specific medication generates differential side effects in persons from selected subgroups. The use of self-management supports to patients at home to ensure better medication compliance and behavioral change is a critical and often overlooked aspect of effective disparity outcomes disease management. Indeed, primary care physicians may wish to implement the use of behavioral "prescriptions" that are written on the same pads as pharmacological prescriptions. This will enable providers to encourage patients to adopt a lifestyle that promotes increased physical activity and proper nutrition, as well as to avoid poor health habits, such as smoking, inactivity, and excessive alcohol consumption.

Even when healthcare administrators, public health personnel, and clinicians seek to provide leadership in implementing such practices, the process will be difficult. This is because medical practices are not normally organized nor financially supported to offer comprehensive management strategies even when such strategies may be effective in controlling disparities in clinical care.

To maximize adoption of the recommended strategies, the healthcare administrator must be able to demonstrate that it is a win-win situation for their institution. In particular, cost-effectiveness must be proven. The use of e-strategies can be effective relative to health care and cost-effectiveness. For example, few physicians are even aware that physician-driven psychological interventions may be highly effective. Yet, sufficient research exists to support a case for the use of such an approach. Stress, hostility, etc., are included in the health disparity chain that supports many illnesses and diseases. Indeed, contemporary tribalism generates stress across all subgroups. Such circumstances may have health consequences. Similarly, while depression is not directly correlated with illness and disease, it can intermediate healthcare needs by promoting poor dietary intake, poor medication compliance, and other factors. Thus, as this chapter indicates, strategies are available to reduce disparities in the area of health care in general. Both providers as well as patients must increase their familiarity and use of such strategies. Additionally, there is an urgent need for participation in the knowledge economy to produce new knowledge regarding health disparities in selected primary, specialist, and tertiary care areas. Hopefully, this new knowledge can serve as ingredients for new strategies of remediation.

Chapter Summary

Health disparities reductions are critical in health care. Koebniek et al. (2012) reveals that the sociodemographics of the consumers served by Kaiser Permanente closely resemble the diverse sociodemographic patterns of Southern California. Thus, nationwide, healthcare practitioners are serving a *population of subpopulations* with varying needs. Arnett, Thorpe, Gaskin, Bowie, and LaVeist (2016) reveal that medical mistrust as a result of past experiences and reported experiences in medical care already affect the use of healthcare resources. Zestcott, Blair, and Stone (2016) also explore the presence of subgroup bias in healthcare disparities. While this chapter has delved into only a few selected areas of healthcare, it has sought to demonstrate the criticality of healthcare professionals partnering with educators, employers, psychologists, and other disciplines in seeking solutions that can remedy, in whole or in part, unidentified and/or

partially identified problems that can easily be bypassed if the "lenses" used by health disparity researchers are not broadened.

Medical care providers comprise the very core of the American healthcare system. Accordingly, this chapter has sought to support collective efforts to generate disparity reduction without the use of a framework that supports fragmentation of the public's trust.

Review Questions and Problems

1. This chapter focused on hypertension, pediatric care, cancer, and kidney transplantation as case studies of disparities in primary, specialty, and tertiary health care. Create a healthcare disparities reduction plan that you could present to a group of primary, specialty, or tertiary care providers on a topic of your choice.
2. Research and describe at least two examples of the side effects of pharmacological solutions used in the treatment of various cancers by subgroups.
3. Complete a detailed research on disparities in pain management, and relate your findings to the current opioid crisis.
4. Design a promotional campaign to increase or decrease live kidney donorship among a specific subgroup.

Key Terms and Concepts

hypertension A chronic disease in persons with a blood pressure greater than 130/80 mm Hg.
renin-angiotensin-aldosterone system The hormone system that regulates blood pressure and fluid balance. If this system is overactive, blood pressure will be too high.
tertiary care A third level of care by providers. It can be viewed as the last segment of care that is available to the patient. Accordingly, it is the most complex level of care that can be provided.

References

Alexander, M. R., (2018). Hypertension medication, the heart.org Medscape, https://emedicine.medscape.com /article/241381-overview

Ameringer, C. F. (2018). US Health Policy and Health Care Delivery: Doctors, Reformers and Entrepreneurs. Pg. 6. Cambridge University Press: Cambridge CB2 8BS, UK.

Ancheta, I. B., Carlson, J. M., Battie, C. A., Borja-Hart, N., Cobb, S., & Ancheta, C. V. (2015). One size does not fit all: cardiovascular health disparities as a function of ethnicity in Asian-American women. *Applied Nursing Research,* 28(2), 99–105. https://doi.org/10.1016 .japnr.2014.06-001.

Arnett, M. J., Thorpe, R. J. Jr., Gaskin, D. J., Bowie, J. V., & LaVeist, R. A. (2016). Race, medical mistrust and segregation in primary care as usual source of care: Findings from the exploring health disparities in integrated communities study. *Journal of Urban Health,* 93(3), 456–467.

Balfour, P. C., Rodriguez, C. J., & Ferdinand, K. C. (2015). The role of hypertension in race-ethnic disparities in cardiovascular disease. *Current Cardiovascular Risk Reports,* 9(4) 18, doi:10.1007/s12170-015-0446-5.

Bengtsson, U., Kjellgren, K., Hallberg, I., Lindwall, M., & Taft, C. Improved blood pressure control using an interactive mobile phone support system. *Journal of Clinical Hypertension,* 18(2), 101–108.

Britt-Spells, A. M., Slebodnik, M., Sands, L. P., & Rollock, D. (2018). Effects of perceived discrimination on depressive symptoms among black men residing in the United States: A meta-analysis. *American Journal of Men's Health,* 12(1), 52–63.

Brown, M. T., & Bussell, J. K. (2011). Medication adherence: WHO cares? *Mayo Clinic Proceedings,* 86(4), 304–314, doi:10.4065/mcp.2010.0575

Carè, A., Bellenghi, M., Matarrese, P., Gabriele, L., Salvioli, S., & Malorni, W. (2018). Sex disparity in cancer: Roles of microRNAs and related functional players. *Cell Death & Differentiation,* 25(3), 477–485.

Centers for Disease Control and Prevention, High School Youth Risk Behavior Survey, 2005 Results. https:// nccd.cdc.gov/youthonline/App/Results.aspx

Centers for Disease Control and Prevention, High School Risk Behavior Survey, 2005 Results. https://nccd.cdc .gov/youthonline/App/Results.aspx

Chang, J. I., Huang, B. Z., & Wu, B. U. (2018). Impact of integrated healthcare delivery on racial and ethnic disparities in pancreatic cancer. *Pancreas,* 47(2), 221–226. Doi:10.1097/MPA.0000000000000981.

Cheung, T. T., & Cheung, B. M. (2014). Managing blood pressure control in Asian patients: Safety and efficacy of losartan. *Clinical Interventions and Aging,* 19(9), 443–450, doi:10.21471/CIA/S39780.

Cristi, J. V., & Grunfeld, E. A. (2013). Factors reported to influence fear of recurrence in cancer patients: A systematic review. *Psycho-Oncology,* 22(5), 978–986. http://dx.doi.org/10.1002/pon.3114.

Dalen, J. E., Ryan, K. J., & Alpert, J. S. Where have the generalists gone? They became specialists, then subspecialists. *The American Journal of Medicine, 130* (7), 766–768. http://dx/doi.org/10.1016/j.amjmed.2017 .01.026.

Dent, R. B., Hagiwara, N., Stepanova, E. V., & Green, T. L. (2017). The role of feature-based discrimination in driving health disparities among Black Americans. *Ethnicity and Health,* 6, 1-16, doi:10.1080/13557858, 2017.1398314.

Doyle, K. (2015). Race and employment tied to U.S. clinic wait times, Reuters, Health News. Mon, Oct. 5, 2015//9:50 a. m., EST. https://www.reuters.com/article /us-health-access-race/race-and-employment-tied -to-u-s-clinic-wait-times-idUSKCN0RZ1XF20151005

Fagard, R. H., Thijs, L., Staessen, J. A., Clement, D. L., DeBuyzere, M. L., & DeBacquer, D. A. (2009). Night–day blood pressure ratio and dipping pattern as predictors of death and cardiovascular events in hypertension. *Journal of Human Hypertension,* 23(10), 645–653, 2009. Doi.10.1038/jhh.2009.9

Gabriel, S. E. (1996). Primary care: Specialists or generalists. *Mayo Clinic Proc. 71,* 415–419.

Geraghty, E. M., Franks, P., & Kravitz, R. L. (2007). Primary care visits length, quality, and satisfaction for standardized patients with depression. *Journal of General Internal Medicine,* 22:(12), 1641–1547, doi:10.1007/s111606-007-0371-5.

Goyal, M. K., Kupperman, N., Cleary, S. D., Teach, S. J., & Chamberlain, J. M. (2015). Racial disparities in pain management of children with appendicitis in emergency departments. *JAMA Pediatrics,* 169(11), 996–1002. Doi:10.1001/jamapediatrics.2015.1915.

Green, C. R., Anderson, K. O., Baker, T. A., Campbell, L. C., Decker, S., Fillingim, R. B. . . . Vallerand, A. H. (2003). The unequal burden of pain: confronting racial and ethnic disparities in pain. *Pain Medicine,* 4(3), 277–294.

Gu, Q., Burt, V. L., Paulose-Ram, R., & Dillon, C. F. (2008). Gender differences in hypertension treatment, drug utilization patterns, and blood pressure control among U.S. adults with hypertension: Data from the National Health and Nutrition Examination Survey (NHANES), 1999–2004. *American Journal of Hypertension,* 21(7), 789–798. Doi.10.1038/ajh.2018.185

Hallberg, I., Ranerup, A., & Kjellgren, K. (2016). Supporting the self-management of hypertension: Patients' experiences of using a mobile phone-based system. *Journal of Human Hypertension,* 30(2), 141-146. Doi:10.1038/jhh.20a5.37.

Hatzinger, M., Stastny, M., Grützmacher, P., & Sohn, M. (2016). The history of kidney transplantation, *Urologe A,* 55(10), 1353–1359.

Hayslett, J. A., Eichner, J. E., Yeh, J. L., Wang, W., Henderson, J., Devereaux, R. B., Welty, T. K., Fabsitz, R. R., Howard, B. V., & Lee, E. T. (2001). Hypertension treatment patterns in American Indians: The strong heart study. *American Journal of Hypertension, 14*(9 Pt 1), 950–956.

Henderson, M. L., & Gross, J. A. (2017). Living organ donation and informed consent in the United States: Strategies to improve the process. *The Journal of Law, Medicine and Ethics, 45*(1), 66–76, https://doi.org/10.1177/1073110517703101

Hoffman, K. M., Trawalter, S., Axt, J. R., & Oliver, M. N. (2016). Racial bias in pain assessment and treatment recommendations, and false beliefs about biological differences between blacks and whites. *Proceedings of the National Academy of Sciences of the USA, 113*(16), 4296–4301. Doi.10.1073/pnas.1516047113.

Homan, S. G., Kayani, N., & Yun, S. (2016). Risk factors, preventive practices, and health care among breast cancer survivors, United States, 2010. *Prevention of Chronic Disease.* Doi:10.5888/pcd13.150377

Hong, J. C., Padula, W. V., Hollin, I. L., Hussain, T., Dietz, K. B., Halbert, J. P., Marstellar, J. A., & Cooper, L. A. (2018). Care management to reduce disparities and control hypertension in primary care: A cost-effectiveness analysis. *Medical Care, 56*(2), 179–185.

Ioannidis, J. P. (2018). Diagnosis and treatment of hypertension in the 2017 ACC/AHA guidelines and in the real world. *JAMA, 319*(2), 115–116.

Iuga, A. O., & McGuire, M. J. (2014). Adherence and health costs. *Risk Management and Healthcare Policy, 7*, 35–44. Doi:10.2147/RMHP.S19801

Jay, C. L., & Cigarroa, F. G. (2018). Disparities in live donor kidney transplantation: Related to poverty, race or ethnicity? *JAMA, 319*(1), 24–26.

Kane, C. K. (2017). Police Research Perspectives. Updated data on physician practice arrangements: Physician ownership drops below 50 percent. American Medical Association, 2017.

Kann, L., McManus, T., Harris, W. A., Shanklin, S. L., Flint, K. H., Hawkins, J . . . Zaza, S. Centers for Disease Control and Prevention (2016). Youth Risk Behavior Surveillance, United States, 2015. *MMWR Surveillance*, June 2016, *65*(6), 12–13.

Kendrick, J., Nuccio, E., Leiferman, J. A., & Sauaia, A. (2015). Primary care providers' perceptions of racial/ethnic and socioeconomic disparities in hypertension control. *American Journal of Hypertension, 28*(9), 1091–1097.

Kluger, A., & DeNisi, A. (1996). The effects of feedback interventions on performance: A historical review of meta-analysis and a preliminary feedback intervention therapy. *Psychological Bulletin, 119*(2), 254–284. Doi:10.1037/0033-2909.119.2.254.

Koebnick, C., Langer-Gould, A., Gould, M. K., Chao, C., Iyer, R. L., Smith, N., & Jacobsen, S. J. (2012). Do the sociodemographic characteristics of members of a large,

integrated health care system represent the population of interest? *Permanente Journal, 16*(3), 37–41.

Lackland, D. T. (2014). Racial differences in hypertension: Implications for high blood pressure management. *American Journal of the Medical Sciences, 348*(2), 135–138.

Langellier, B., Chen, J., Bustamante, A., Inkelas, M., & Ortega, A. (2016). Understanding healthcare access and utilization disparities among Latino children in the United States. *Journal of Child Health Care, 20*(2), 133–144.

Levinson, K. L., Riedel, D. J., Ojalvo, L. S., Chan, W., Angarita, A. N., Fader, A. N., & Rositch, A. F. (2018). Gynecologic cancer in HIV-infected women: Treatment and outcomes in a multi-institutional cohort. *AIDS, 32*(2), 171–177.

Lin, C-T., Albertson, G. A., Schilling, E. M., Cyan, E. M., Anderson, S. N., Ware, L., & Andersen, C. J. (2001) Is patients' perception of time spent with the physician determines of ambulatory patient satisfaction. *Journal of American Medical Association Internal Medicine, 161*:11, 1437–1442. Doi:10.100a/archinte, 161.11.1437.

Lunn, M. R., & Sánchez, J. P. (2011). Prioritizing health disparities in medical education to improve care. *Academic Medicine, 86*(11), 1343.

Ly, D. P., & Glied, S. A. (2010). Disparities in service quality among insured adult patients seen in physicians' officers. *Journal of General Internal Medicine, 25*:4, 357–362, doi:10.1007/s11606-009-1231-2.

Macintrye, A., Ferris, D., Gonçalves, B., & Quinn, N. (2018). What has economics got to do with it? The impact of socioeconomic factors on mental health and the case for collective action. *Palgrave Communications, 4*(1), 10.

Maggiore, U., Budde, K., Keemann, U., Hilbrands, L., Oberbauer, R., Oniscu, G. C., Pascual, J., Sorensen, S. S., Viklicky, O., & Abramouragi, D. (2017). Long-term risks of kidney living donation: Review and position paper by the ERA-EDTA DESCARTES working group. *Nephrology Dialysis Transplantation, 32*:2, 216–223, https://di.org.10.1093/No1/gfw429.

Malek, S. K., Keys, B. J., Kumar, S., Milford, E., & Tullius, S. G. (2010). Racial and ethnic disparities in kidney transplantation. *Transplant Informational, 24*(5), 419–424.

Martin, K. D., Roter, D. L., Beach, M. C., Carson, K. A., & Cooper, L. A. (2013). Physician communication behaviors and trust among black and white patients with hypertension. *Medical Care, 51*:2, 151–157. Doi:1.1097/MLR.0b013e31827632a2.

McManus, R. J., Mant, J., Franssen, M., Nickless, A., Schwartz, C., Hodgkinson, J . . . Hobbs, F. D. R. Efficacy of self-monitored blood pressure, with or without telemonitoring, for titration of antihypertensive medication (TASMINH4): An unmasked randomized controlled trial. *The Lancet. 391*(10124), 949–959.

Mehnert, A., Koch, U., Sundermann, C., & Dinkel, A. (2013). Predictors of fear and recurrence in patients one year after cancer rehabilitation: a prospective study. *ActaOncologici 52,* 1202-109, http://dx.doi.org/10.3109/0284186x.2013.765063,

Nagy, J. (1999). A note on the early history of renal transplantation: Emerich (Imre) Ullmann. *American Journal of Nephrology, 19*(2), 346–349.

Natale-Pereira, A., Enard, K. R., Nevarez, L., & Jones, L. A. (2011). The role of patient navigators in eliminating health disparities. *Cancer, 117*(S15), 3541–3550.

National Center for Health Statistics. (2016a). Summary Health Statistics Tables for U.S. Adults. National Health Interview Survey, 2015, Table 4. Hyattsville, MD.

National Center for Health Statistics. (2016b). National Ambulatory Medical Care Survey: 2015 State and National Summary Tables, Table 19. Hyattsville, MD.

National Center for Health Statistics. (2016c). *Health, United States, 2015: With special feature on racial and ethnic health disparities.* Hyattsville, MD.

National Heart, Lung, and Blood Institute (2017). Systolic blood pressure intervention trial (SPRINT) Overview. https://www.nhlbi.nih.gov/news/systolic-blood-pressure-intervention-trial-sprint-overview.

Nautsch, F., Ludwig, J. M., Xing, M., Johnson, K. M., & Kim, H. S. (2018). Racial disparities and sociodemographic differences in incidence and survival among pediatric patients in the United States with primary liver cancer: A Surveillance, Epidemiology, and End Results (SEER) population study. *Journal of Clinical Gastroenterology, 52*(3), 262–267.

Neal, R. D., Tharmanathan, P., France, B., Din, N. U., Colton, S., Fallon-Ferguson, J., . . . & Emery, J. (2015). Is increased time to diagnosis and treatment in symptomatic cancer associated with poorer outcomes? *British Journal of Cancer, 112* (Suppl 1), S92–S107, doi:10.1038/bjc.2015.48.

Noble, K. G., Houston, S. M., Brito, N. H., Bartsch, H., Kan, E., Kuperman, J. M., . . . Sowell, E. R. (2015). Family income, parental education and brain structure in children and adolescents. *Nature Neuroscience, 18*(5), 773–778.

O'Neill, J. L., Cunningham, R. L., Wiitala, W. L., & Bartley, E. P., (2014). Collaborative hypertension case management by registered nurses and clinical pharmacy specialists within the patient aligned care teams (PACT) model. *Journal of General Internal Medicine, 29*(Suppl 2), 675–681. Doi:10.1007/s11606-014-2-774-4.

Ozpancar N., Paryaw, S. C., & Topau, B. (2017). Hypertension management: what is the role of case management? Revista Da Escold de Enfermage. *Journal of School of Nursing, University of Sao Paulo, 51*:e03291, DIA:http://dx.doi.org/10.1390/S1980-110x2017016903291.

Perez, N. M., Jennings, W. G., Piquero, A. P., & Baglivio, L. 2016. Adverse childhood experiences and suicide attempts: The mediating influence of personality development and problem behaviors. *Journal of Youth and Adolescence, 45*(8) 1527–1545.

Phillips, J. M., & Malone, B. (2014). Increasing racial/ethnic diversity in nursing to reduce health disparities and achieve health equity. *Public Health Reports, 129* (Suppl 2), 45–50.

Phillips, K. M., McGinty, H. L., Gonzalez, B. D., Jim, H. S. L., Small, B. J., Minton, S., . . . Jacobs, P. (2013). Factors associated with breast cancer worry 3 years after completion of adjuvant treatment. *Psycho-Oncology, 22*, 936-939. http://dx/doi.org/10.1002/pon.3010.

Purnell, T. S., Luo, X., & Cooper, L. A. (2018). Kidney transplantation in the United States from 1995 to 2014. *JAMA, 319*(1), 49–61.

Rao, S., Cherukui, M., & Mayo, H. G. (2007). What is the best treatment for hypertension in African Americans? *Journal of Family Practice, 56*(2). 149–57.

Rodriguez, C. J., Still, C. H., Garcia, K. R., Wagenknecht, L., White, S., Bares, J. T., . . . & Contreras, G. (2016). Baseline blood pressure control in Hispanics: Characteristics of Hispanics in systolic blood pressure intervention trial (SPRINT). *Journal of Clinical Hypertension, 19*(2) 116–125. https://doi.org/10.1111/jch.12942.

Sabin, J. A., Moore, K., Noonan, C., Lallemand, O., & Buchwald, D. (2015). Clinicians' implicit and explicit attitudes about weight and race and treatment approaches to overweight for American Indian children. *Child Obesity. 11*(4), 456-465,

Saha, S., Arbelaez, J. J., & Cooper, L. A. (2003). Patient-physician relationships and racial disparite sin the quality of health care. *American Journal of Public Health, 93*(10), 1713–1719, doi:10.2105/AJPH.93.10.1713.

Schwingshackl, L., Saumani, A., Hoffman, G., Schwedhelm, C., & Boeing, H. (2017). Impact of different dietary approaches on blood pressure in hypertensive and pre-hypertensive patients: protocol for a systematic review and network meta-analysis. *BMJ Open, 7*(4), http://doi.org/0.117:e1436bmjo-2016-014736.

Siegel, R. L., Miller, K. D., & Jemal, A. (2017). Cancer statistics, 2017. *CA: A Cancer Journal for Clinicians, 67*(1), 7–30.

Siervo, M., Lara, J., Choudhary, S., Ashorie, A., Oggionia, C., & Mathers, J. D. (2015). Effects of the Dietary Approach to Stop Hypertension (DASH) diets on cardiovascular risk factors: A systematic review and meta analysis. *British Journal of Nutrition, 113*:1, 1–15.

Smith, G. R. (2007). Health disparities: What can nursing do? *Policy, Politics, & Nursing Practice, 8*(4), 285–291.

Tedia, Y. G., & Bautista, L. E. (2016). Drug side effect symptoms and adherence to antihypertensive medication. *American Journal of Hypertension, 29*(6), 772-779. https://doi.org/10.1093/ajh/hpv185.

Tiong, X. T., Shahirah, A. N., Dun, W. C., Wong, K. Y., Fong, A. Y. Y., Sy, R. G., . . . Venkataraman, K. (2018). The association of the dietary approach to stop hypertension (DASH) diet with blood pressure, glucose and lipid profiles in the Malaysia and Philippines populations. *Nutrition, Metabolism and Cardiovascular Diseases*, doi:10.1016/jnumecd, 2018.04.014.

Tung, E. L., Wroblewski, K. E., Boyd, K., Makelarski, J. A., Peek, M. E., & Lindau, S. T. (2018). Police-recorded crime and disparities in obesity and blood pressure status in Chicago. *Journal of the American Heart Association, 24*(7). https://doi.org./10.1161/JAHA.117.008030

VanderWielen, L. M., Vanderbilt, A. A., Crossman, S. H., Mayer, S. D., Enurah, A. S., Gordon, S. S., & Bradner, M. K. (2015). Health disparities and underserved populations: a potential solution, medical school partnerships with free clinics to improve curriculum. *Medical Education Online, 20*,1–4.

Vollmer, W. M., Sacks, F. M., Ard, J., Appel, L. J., & Bray, G. A. (2001). Effects of diet and sodium intake on blood pressure subgroup analysis of the DASH sodium trial. *Annals of Internal Medicine, 135*(12), 1019–1028.

Wassink, I., Perreira, K. M., & Harris, K. M. (2017). Beyond race/ethnicity: Skin color and cardiometabolic health among blacks and hispanics in the United States. *Journal of Immigrant and Minority Health, 19*(5), 1018-1026. doi: 10.1007/s10903-016-0495-y.

Weinberger, M. H. (1990) Racial differences in antihypertensive therapy: Evidence and implications. *Cardiovascular Drugs Therapy, 4*(Suppl 2), 379–392.

Whelton, P. K., Carey, R. M., Aronow, W. S., Casey, D. E. Jr., Collins, K. J., Dennison H. C.,… Wright, J. T. Jr. (2017). ACC/AHA/AAPA/ABC/ACPM/AGS/APhA/ASH /ASPC/NMA/PCNA guideline for the prevention, detection, evaluation, and management of high blood pressure in adults: A report of the American College of Cardiology/American Heart Association Task Force on Clinical Practice Guidelines. *Hypertension. 72*, 1–487.

Whelton, P. K., Carey, R. M., Aronow, W. S., Casey, D. E. Jr., Collins, K. J., Dennison, H. C., . . . Wright, J. T. Jr. (2018). 2017 ACC/AHA/AAPA/ABC/ACPM /AGS/APhhA/ASPC/NMA/PCNA guideline for the prevention, detection, evaluation, and management of high blood pressure in adults: A report of the American College of Cardiology/American Heart Association Task Force on Clinical Practice Guidelines. *Journal of the American College of Cardiology, 71*, e127–e248.

Williamson, J. D., Whelton, P. K., Wright, J. T., Rocco, M. V., Reboussin, D. M., Rahman, M., . . . Ambrosia, W. T. (2015) A randomized trial of intensive versus standard blood pressure control. *New England Journal of Medicine, 373*(22), 2103-16. Doi:10.1056/NEJMOA 15119391 Epub 2015. Nov. 9

Zestcott, C. A., Blair, I. V., & Stone, J. (2016). Examining the presence consequences, and reduction of implicit bias in health care: A narrative review. *Group Processes & Intergroup Relations, 19*(4), 528–542.

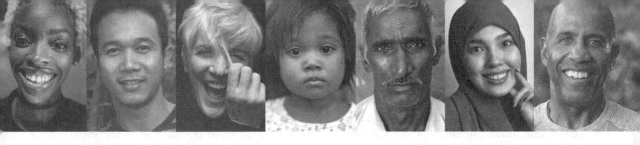

CHAPTER 10

Hospitals and Healthcare Disparities

"Healing is a matter of time, but it is sometimes also a matter of opportunity."

—**Hippocrates (c. 460–377 BC)**, an ancient Greek physician, the "father of medicine"

LEARNING OBJECTIVES

After completing this chapter, each learner will be able to:

- Summarize data on the current status of the hospital industry.
- Analyze factors relating to the changing role of hospitals in the American healthcare system.
- Use current and past scholarly studies to review and synthesize the type of disparities that can be observed in some hospitals.
- Explain the importance of using quantitative management skills in order to identify and explain the nature of Hospital Compare disparities and other problems in hospitals that disproportionately serve health disparity populations.

▶ Introduction

In 2014, approximately 5,627 registered hospitals were operating within the U.S. healthcare system. By 2016, this number had dropped to 5,534, representing a 1.65% decrease in just 2 years (American Hospital Association, 2018). A **registered hospital** is one that has listed itself with the American Hospital Association (AHA), has met all accreditation standards of the Joint Commission on the Accreditation of Healthcare Organizations (JCAHO), and is certified under Titles 18 and 19 of the Social Security Act. Title 18 of the Social Security Act includes regulations regarding Medicare, and Title 19 pertains to those regarding Medicaid. In addition, a hospital must have at least six inpatient beds and meet other requirements.

Approximately 4,926 hospitals (87.5% of all hospitals) were defined as community hospitals in 2014. By 2016, this number had dropped slightly to 4,840 (87.46%) of all hospitals. **Community hospitals** are public institutions that provide acute or short-term care. They may provide general services and/or treatment for highly specialized illnesses and diseases. As the dominant form of hospitals within the United States, approximately 2,849 (51.48%) of community hospitals operate as nonprofits and 1,035 (21.38%) are structurally positioned to maximize profits (AHA, 2018).

In addition to community hospitals, 209 hospitals are directly owned and operated by the federal government. Approximately 397 hospitals are for persons whose mental health needs require institutionalization. Eighty-eight hospitals are for persons with illnesses and diseases that require continual or long-term care. Ten hospitals are institutional facilities such as prison hospitals, college acute care facilities, and so on. Collectively, U.S. hospitals had 902,202 beds on any given day in 2014. By 2016, this number had dropped to 894,574, a decrease of 0.85%. Approximately 34,878,887 hospital admissions were made in 2014, dropping to 33,424,253 in 2016, a decrease of 4.17% (AHA, 2018).

This chapter seeks to determine whether disparities exist in the operation of these institutions. Such an exploration is important given that approximately $991.5 billion was spent on hospital care in 2016, a 7.56% increase over the amount spent in 2014 (National Center for Health Statistics, 2016).

▶ The Role of Hospitals in the American Healthcare System

The role of hospitals in the American healthcare system has changed over time. From 2014 to 2016, data reveal a continuing trend of transformation in the role that hospitals play in the American healthcare system. While hospitals continue to serve as the largest single source of national healthcare expenditures in the United States, the shift from a retrospective to a prospective payment system that occurred as part of the 1983 change in hospital reimbursements has generated restructuring and shrinkage in the size of the hospital industry in the United States.

What do you mean by "retrospective" and "prospective" payments?

Hospitals, like other components of the U.S. healthcare system, first deliver services and then are reimbursed for the costs of the services delivered. The amount of reimbursement is based on a predetermined, fixed amount; thus, it is a **prospective payment**. However, until 1983, hospital services were not pre-priced. Hospitals delivered the service, decided on a price, and then billed Medicare and Medicaid after services were delivered. Thus, the term **retrospective payment** was used.

So, in 1983 this practice was discontinued?

Yes. As a current or future healthcare professional, you probably are aware that Medicare and Medicaid were both created in 1965 as amendments to the Social Security Act of 1935. In 1983, another amendment was made, the Social Security Act of 1983. This amendment shifted reimbursement from a retrospective to a prospective system. Under the prospective system, core prices for hospital services and/or groups of hospitals services were pre-established based upon diagnosis-related groups (DRGs). This reimbursement shift was also accompanied by the use of greater restraints upon the number of days spent in the hospital for a selected diagnosis.

As one reviews data on hospital occupancy rates, it becomes clear that patient care at acute hospitals has declined. This decline has occurred for a variety of reasons. First, the exponential growth in medical technology has eliminated the need for overnight hospital stays for many procedures. Steiner, Karaca, Moore, Imshaug, and Pickens (2018) reported that of 17.2 million hospital visits in 2014, approximately 57.8% occurred without an overnight hospital stay. Moreover, highly invasive surgeries that were once performed on an overnight basis were done as outpatient procedures. For example, 78.5% of surgeries involving the skin and/or breast and 95.6% of tonsillectomies were all completed on an ambulatory basis (Steiner et al., 2018). Second, the alterations in reimbursement methodologies have interacted with other variables to decrease demand for overnight services. For example, a female's decision regarding whether maternity care will be in a hospital or a birthing center can be influenced by financial considerations as well as personal preferences. Third, some evidence suggests that the general public has a preference for outpatient care. Izugami and Takase (2016) report that, based upon past patient experience, some patients may prefer ambulatory care. Accordingly, many treatments once completed on an overnight basis are now being delivered on an outpatient basis (Steiner, 2018).

▶ Hospitals and Healthcare Disparities

A number of studies suggest that if hospitals in different geographic areas serve patients with different health risks, healthcare disparities will be observable. Barnett, Hsu, and McWilliams (2015), based upon a sample of approximately 8,067 Medicare patients, found that hospital readmission rates, a primary measure of healthcare quality, do differ across various hospitals for different subgroups. However, most of these disparities in hospital readmission rates were directly explainable because of differences in the health status of patients at the time of the initial admission. Accordingly, when subgroup disparities in hospital readmissions occur, they can also be associated, in part, with the type of illness and/or disease for which the patients were hospitalized. Merkow et al. (2015) found, for example, that overall readmission rates for surgical site infection were as high as 28.8% for hysterectomy and 36.4% for a lower extremity vascular bypass. Thus, to the degree that a particular subgroup is overrepresented in

these types of surgeries, the aggregate data will reveal a pattern of disparate care. Phibbs and Lorch (2018) further contributes to the notion that rather than subgroups being provided the worst care while hospitalized, at least some percentage of any documented disparities in outcomes are due, in part, to other factors. For example, the rate of preterm infant births is higher among African Americans and Latino Americans than among their White American and/or Asian American counterparts. Differences in preterm birth rates reflect themselves in differential infant mortality rates (Schindler, Koller-Smith, Lui, Bajuk, & Bolisetty, 2017).

As a result, subgroup differences in infant mortality rates may exist during hospitalization. But, even these findings require scrutiny. Yes, it is true that current data (CDC, 2018) indicate that in 2016, approximately 9% of births to women of European descent in the United States occurred before 37 weeks of pregnancy relative to 14% of babies born to women of African descent. However, even these numbers differ significantly by geographic area. In high poverty states such as Mississippi, White American women have preterm birth rates of 11.6% relative to 10.4% for Hispanic American women.

So, are you saying that when disparities occur in hospital care, they appear to have causes other than direct or indirect discrimination?

We are suggesting that when a disparity is observed in hospital care, the hospital administrators may wish to engage in causal analysis. For example, these administrators may ask, "Do such trends represent a poorer quality of hospital care, earlier differentials in the disparities chain, or other factors?" Using data from hospitals in New York City, Howell, Egorova, Balbierz, Zeithlin, and Hebert (2016) found that 40% of the disparities in mortality and morbidity between African American and White American preterm babies and 30% of that between Hispanic and White American preterm babies were directly related to the choice of the hospitals selected.

In still another study of disparities in hospital care, the authors sought to determine whether differentials exist in hospital care for hospitalized patients receiving palliative care. Worster et al. (2018), cognizant of past research that has shown subgroup differences in access to hospital care and to pain medication, sought to determine whether such differences exist when the inpatient palliative care service was provided in an urban academic medical center. Utilizing data from 3,207 Asian Americans, African Americans, Latino Americans, Native Americans, White Americans, and other patients served from March 2006 to April 2015, the analysts found no disparities in services at this hospital in any phase of palliative care. This suggests once again that relative to hospital care, sophisticated and robust analyses are needed to untangle causation. For example, it can be that hospitals that serve various subgroups serve patients with vast differences in the determinants of health outcomes. Such pre-existing variables are then reflected in the measured quality of care. Additionally, differentials in the types of health insurance may relate to quality of care since reimbursement disparities exist by insurance type. However, it appears that differentials in hospital care may be less likely to reflect implicit or explicit bias.

For example, Hasnain-Wynia et al. (2007) conducted research which suggests that disparities in hospital care may be driven more by the quality of the overall care delivered by the hospitals elected than by implicit and/or explicit bias of those persons who deliver the care. These researchers utilized data from the Hospital Quality Alliance Inpatient Quality of Care Indicators for 123 hospitals. This allowed access to a sample size of 320,970 patient files. The findings were quite interesting. It appears that because hospital care is typically driven by well-defined clinical protocols that apply to virtually all components of the care process, single individuals in hospitals, even if they hold implicit and/or explicit biases are not positioned to heavily influence the quality of care. However, systemic adherence to clinical processes of care differ across hospitals. Thus, it is less

than surprising that these investigators found that disparities in subgroup care within the 123 hospitals studied was related to the quality of the hospital where care was sought. However, when the outcomes of the services provided involved more person-to-person care than a chain of technically guided clinical processes of care, minority and non-minority patient differentials in care existed. Specifically, for services in which one-on-one patient counseling was required, the care varied by subgroup.

So, are you saying that when a large number of persons are involved in hospital care who are required to follow well-defined protocols, the margin-of-error for subgroup bias is reduced. Therefore, if one received care in a hospital that is more adherent to these processes of care, significant disparities in outcome will not occur. However, if subgroups disproportionately select hospitals that are less adherent to established processes of care, health disparities by subgroup will occur?

We are suggesting that hospital administrators thoroughly analyze their data to assess the relationship between their quality ratings and the clinical, demographic and socioeconomic characteristics of their patients as well as their service delivery protocols. To demonstrate the importance of such an analysis, let's perform a very, very, simplistic statistical exercise. Let's determine whether there is an association between the percentage of 1- and/or 2-star hospitals in a state and the socioeconomic characteristics of the population from whom these patients are drawn.

▶ Analyzing the Relationship Between Hospital Choice and Hospital Disparities

As is always true, in order to test a hypothesis, we must have one.

So what hypothesis will we use?

The hypothesis is:

H_0: There is no association between the percentage of hospitals with lower Hospital Compare ratings (1 or 2 stars) and the percentage of the population in that state who are minority, impoverished, and who have four-year college degrees or higher.

H_1: H_0 is false.

I'm a bit confused. Why would we formulate this particular hypothesis?

If we can demonstrate a relationship between the demographic and socioeconomic context and overall measured hospital quality in each state, we can then adjust Hospital Compare quality ratings to reflect such associations. Even more importantly, better support can be provided to all hospitals and their patients.

So, what are the independent variables and what is the dependent variable we will use?

The number of hospitals in each state with a 1- or 2-star overall Hospital Compare quality rating is our dependent variable. The percentage of the population in each state who are minority, impoverished, and who have four-year college degrees or higher are the independent variables.

So, where do we find the data on "Hospital Compare" ratings by state? By the way, what is Hospital Compare?

While a number of organizations collect data on the performance of the healthcare organizations in which healthcare administrators, public health officials, and clinicians work, one of the most respected is the Centers for Medicare and Medicaid Services (CMS). CMS collects quality measurement data on hospitals that are Medicare and/or Medicaid certified through Hospital Compare (https://www.medicare.gov/hospitalcompare/). This data collection effort began in December 2002.

How is the quality of the Hospital Compare data?

CMS's Hospital Compare data is the most respected dataset on hospital care outcomes.

Nevertheless, like all datasets, it has its limitations. First, the data are limited because they do not include all of the 5,000+ hospitals in the United States. In fact, only 3,000+ are included. Second, a number of analysts have argued that Hospital Compare data have other limitations. Data collection instruments must meet various standards of validity (determinations of whether the data measure that which it purports to measure) and reliability (the ability of the data instrumentation to deliver the same results across the same users). Some analysts have argued that the Hospital Compare data collection system may embody fragilities in one or both of these areas. Hu et al. (2016) asserts that Hospital Compare may embody some weaknesses in the measures used for the assessment of hospital quality. Jha (2016), in an analysis of quality as measured by the risk of unnecessary mortality, found that 1-star and 5-star hospitals have no differences in terms of the risk of death when the size of the hospital, the hospitals' status as a teaching or not a teaching hospital, and other factors are taken into consideration. Tsugawa, Jena, Figueroa, Blumenthal, and Jha's (2017) research included highly unique findings that have direct implications for the measurement of hospital quality. Indeed, one unique finding has never been included in any health quality measurement model. This variable is the sex of the physicians. These authors found significantly lower 3-day mortality rates, and 30-day readmission rates between 1,583,028 elderly patients treated by female rather than male internists.

Despite findings such as these, however, Hospital Compare is highly respected and is considered as the premiere dataset for use as an aggregate measure of hospital quality. Thus, 2015 Hospital Compare data were used to compile a listing of the percentage of hospitals in each state with ratings of 1 or 2 overall stars.

What were the independent variables, and where was these data acquired?

The U.S. Bureau of the Census collects data on the number and percentage of minorities in each state, the percentage of the population who are impoverished, and the percentage of the population who have 4-year college degrees of higher. **TABLE 10.1** below presents the results of the data search.

So, how do we analyze the data to see if there is a relationship? Do we hire a statistician?

Before a health administrator, public health professional, and/or clinician would move to

TABLE 10.1 The Relationship Between the Percentage of Poorly Performing Hospitals and Key Socioeconomic and Demographic Variables, 2015				
Dependent Variable[a]		**Independent Variables**		
% Hospitals with Lower Ratings (1 or 2 stars)		**% Minority[b]**	**% Impoverished[c]**	**% 4 or More Years of College Education[d]**
No.	**State**	**Y**	**X_1**	**X_2**	**X_3**
1	Alabama	3%	33.7%	18.8%	23.5%
2	Alaska	18%	37.6%	10.2%	28.0%
3	Arizona	26%	43.5%	18.2%	27.5%
4	Arkansas	10%	26.4%	19.3%	21.1%
5	California	40%	61.3%	16.3%	31.4%
6	Colorado	0	30.9%	12.7%	38.1%
7	Connecticut	15%	30.8%	10.5%	37.6%
8	Delaware	0	36.1%	12.0%	30.0%
9	District of Columbia	72%	64.4%	18.0%	54.6%
10	Florida	45%	43.9%	16.5%	27.3%
11	Georgia	17%	45.4%	18.4%	28.8%
12	Hawaii	8%	77.1%	11.2%	30.8%
13	Idaho	0	16.9%	15.5%	25.9%
14	Illinois	15%	37.5%	14.3%	32.3%
15	Indiana	4%	19.5%	15.4%	24.1%
16	Iowa	0	12.6%	12.5%	26.7%
17	Kansas	5%	23.0%	13.6%	31.0%
18	Kentucky	5%	14.4%	18.9%	22.3%
19	Louisiana	4%	40.5%	19.8%	22.5%

20	Maine	0	6.1%	13.9%	29.0%
21	Maryland	34%	47.0%	10.0%	37.9%
22	Massachusetts	17%	25.7%	11.6%	40.5%
23	Michigan	12%	24.1%	16.7%	26.9%
24	Minnesota	2%	18.3%	11.3%	33.7%
25	Mississippi	15%	42.6%	22.5%	20.7%
26	Missouri	7%	19.8%	15.6%	27.1%
27	Montana	4%	13.0%	15.2%	29.5%
28	Nebraska	3%	19.2%	12.7%	29.3%
29	Nevada	69%	48.0%	15.5%	23.0%
30	New Hampshire	0	8.6%	8.9%	34.9%
31	New Jersey	46%	42.8%	10.8%	36.8%
32	New Mexico	34%	60.8%	21.0%	26.3%
33	New York	50%	43.2%	15.7%	34.2%
34	North Carolina	5%	35.8%	17.4%	28.4%
35	North Dakota	10%	13.0%	11.5%	27.7%
36	Ohio	9%	19.7%	15.8%	26.1%
37	Oklahoma	12%	32.7%	16.7%	24.1%
38	Oregon	4%	22.8%	16.5%	30.8%
39	Pennsylvania	16%	21.9%	13.5%	28.6%
40	Rhode Island	9%	25.5%	14.2%	31.9%
41	South Carolina	6%	36.1%	17.9%	25.8%
42	South Dakota	0	16.8%	14.1%	27.0%
43	Tennessee	16%	25.3%	17.6%	24.9%
44	Texas	15%	56.2%	17.3%	27.6%
45	Utah	3%	20.5%	12.3%	31.1%
46	Virginia	13%	36.6%	11.5%	36.3%
47	Vermont	8%	6.4%	11.5%	36.0%
48	Washington	13%	29.2%	13.3%	32.9%
49	West Virginia	24%	7.5%	18.0%	19.2%

(continues)

50	Wisconsin	0	17.6%	13.0%	27.8%
51	Wyoming	13%	15.5%	11.5%	25.7%

TABLE 10.1 The Relationship Between the Percentage of Poorly Performing Hospitals and Key Socioeconomic and Demographic Variables, 2015 *(continued)*

[a] Hospital Consumer Assessment of Healthcare Providers and Systems and the Centers for Medicare & Medicaid Services. HCAHPS Star Ratings. Distribution of HCAHPS Summary Start ratings by State, January 1 – December 31, 2015 (October 2016 Public Reporting) http://www.hcahpsonline.org/en/hcahps-star-ratings/

[b] Census Bureau. (2015). American Fact Finder. American Community Survey. ACS Demographic and Housing Estimates. 2011–2015 American Community Survey 5-Year Estimates. https://factfinder.census.gov/faces/nav/jsf/pages/community_facts.xhtml#

[d] Census Bureau. (2015). American Fact Finder. American Community Survey. ACS Demographic and Housing Estimates. 2011–2015 American Community Survey 5-Year Estimates. Educational Attainment for 2015 by State. Retrieved from https://factfinder.census.gov/faces/nav/jsf/pages/community_facts.xhtml#

hire a professional statistician to complete a more sophisticated analysis that can be used to better assess healthcare disparities related to their hospital and/or their facility, these data can be analyzed as exploratory research in order to better understand the relationship between lower hospital healthcare quality ratings in race/ethnicity, poverty, and education.

So, how do we complete such an analysis?

We utilize an online statistical calculator to run a multiple regression with three independent variables. A few online calculators that can be used to complete this exercise are listed in **BOX 10.1**.

Why are readers continually encouraged to engage in research analysis of this type?

It is particularly important for hospital administrators and others to have elementary skills in this type of analysis. This is because lower-performing hospitals are penalized based upon their Hospital Compare data. Yet, methodologies for ranking hospitals do not adjust for patient characteristics, or community differentials, or other factors that may possibly affect ratings. Yet, it is critical to do so since, as said, hospitals are financially penalized for "low" Hospital Compare ratings.

So what do we do next?

Enter the data directly into the online calculator. Now go back and check each number to

BOX 10.1 Selected Online Calculators That Can Be Used to Run a Regression with Three Independent Variables

- Free Statistics Calculators, Version 40, Calculator: F-Value and P Value for Multiple Regression, https://www.danielsoper.com
- Multiple Linear Regression; https://home.ubalt.edu/ntsbarsh/Business-stat/otherapplets/MultRgression.htm
- How to Run a Multiple Regression in Excel, https://www.wikihow.com/Run-a-Multiple-Regression-in-Excel
- Multiple Linear Regression, https://www.shoder.org
- Multiple online regression calculated regression. Structural_analyser.com
- Multiple Linear Regression. (MLR) Equata Calculator-Easy Calculator, https://www.easycalculation.com/statistics/multiple-regression.php

confirm that the entries are error-free and then touch the right buttons. You will "end up" with a table that looks something like **TABLE 10.2**.

What does all this mean?

As a healthcare administrator, you need the skills to be able to interpret these findings so let's go step-by-step.

TABLE 10.2 Summary Output

Regression Statistics

Multiple R	0.64072337
R square	0.41052643
Adjusted R Square	0.37290046
Standard Error	0.13585868
Observations	51

ANOVA	df	SS	MS	F	Significance F
Regression	3	0.60415646	0.20138549	10.9107196	1.4778E-05
Residual	47	0.86750629	0.01845758		
Total	50	1.47166275			

	Coefficients	Standard Error	t Stat	P-Value	Lower 95%	Upper 95%
Intercept	−0.4133992	0.19099369	−2.1644653	0.03554127	−0.7976289	−0.01291695
X_1	0.5037069	0.13671933	3.68424068	**0.000592 ***	0.2286631	0.77875071
X_2	1.14640933	0.77217768	1.48464448	0.14431446 **	−0.4070118	2.69983045
X_3	0.81964498	0.40041388	2.04699443	**0.04623***	0.01411616	1.62517381

*$P<0.05$; **$P<0.01$; ***$P<0.001$
X_1: % Minority; X_2: % Impoverished; X_3: % 4 yrs or more college

- Multiple R: 0.64072337 – The Multiple R is similar to the R in a correlation coefficient. However, multiple R in a multiple regression tells us the degree to which changes in our independent or predictor variables (% minority, % impoverished, and % of the population with 4 or more years of college) are associated with the change in the dependent variable (the % of hospitals with 1 or 2 star overall ratings). While this figure is written as a decimal, it is most often converted to a percentage for purposes of interpretation.

So, this tells us....

Well, the multiplier tells us that the differences in the percentage of hospitals with 1- or 2-star ratings across the 50 states (and DC) is *moderately associated* with the differences in the three key disparity-related independent variables—the % minorities in each state, the % of persons who are in poverty, and the % of persons with 4 or more years of college.

Why do you use the modifier, "moderately"?

The value of R is always between +1 and −1. The .64 is positively associated with the change in the % of lower quality hospitals in the country. Thus, as the % of the three independent variables increase in value, the % of hospitals with 1 or 2 star ratings increase.

We describe this as a *moderate-strong relationship* based upon a statistical guideline that tells us that if R is 0.70, the relationship is strong, if it is 0.50, it is moderate, if it is 0.30, the relationship is weak, and if it is zero, there is no relationship.

Okay, what does the R square tell us?

- R square = 0.41052643
- The R square tells us that 41.05% of the variability in the percentage of 1- and 2-star rated hospitals is explained by the three independent variables. It is what is called a "goodness-of-fit" measure for linear regression.

So, is this good or bad?

As future and/or current healthcare professionals, we know that numerous other factors determine the quality rating in each hospital in each state. Accordingly, the 41.05% of the variation that is determined by patient-level characteristics is extremely encouraging for it suggests that we have identified three important factors. However, we still must ask, "If we add or subtract variables, would our R square change?" In other words, we can seek to adjust the R square.

- Adjusted R square = 0.37290046
- The adjusted R square reflects the number and nature of the independent variables. There are only three independent variables. Independent variables are also called predictor variables. Let's say that we wanted to try to improve the "fit" of the model and add the mean number of residents in each state per hospital as a predictor variable.

How did you choose mean number of residents in the state per hospital?

If the number of persons living in an area is quite high per hospital, patients can be easily underserved. For example, the U.S.

Department of Health (2016) Report, Rural Hospital Participation, reveals that only 34% of rural hospitals experience financial penalties for spreading hospital-acquired infections relative to 49% of urban hospitals. This is probably because each health care professional serves fewer patients. The number of hospitals per capita population is therefore based upon research. Rural hospitals also perform better in other areas. If this variable were added, the adjusted R square would most likely change again since the adjusted R square reflects the number and quality of independent variables.

- The standard error = 0.13585868
- The **standard error** is used to estimate the degree of distance of each state's outcome from the mean values for all states. For example, in our initial data tables, for the States of South Dakota, Wisconsin, Delaware, Colorado, Iowa, Idaho, Maine, and New Hampshire, there is no association between the dependent and independent variables because these states have zero percent low performing hospitals. Yet, in California (40%), the District of Columbia (72%), Florida (45%), Maryland (34%), New Jersey (46%), New Mexico (34%), Nevada (69%), and New York (50%), the mean proportion of underperforming hospitals is quite high. The standard error helps to summarize the degree of variation that each state's data fall from the average for all states. The + or − 0.13585868 reveals that there is considerable variation in the states.

Is that "bad"?

Because the standard error is a measure of dispersion of variation in the model, we know that there is wide variation, but we must interpret everything together to determine whether our overall model suggests that there is a relationship between the percentage of lower-quality hospitals in a state and the selected demographic and socioeconomic variables.

- ANOVA table

  As you may or may not remember from your basic statistics course, **ANOVA** stands for analysis of variance. Accordingly, the calculations described in the ANOVA simply attempt to integrate the variations per state in each of the independent variables and the dependent variables. So let's interpret each component of the ANOVA table.

- Regression
  - Consider the initial hypothesis.
  - H_0: There is no association between the percentage of hospitals in a state with a 1- or 2-star Hospital Compare rating and the percentage of the population in that state who are minority, impoverished, and who have four-year college degrees or higher.
  - H_1: H_0 is false.
  - Now let's write this as a straight line.
  - $Y = \alpha + \beta X_1 + \beta X_2 + \beta X_3 + \varepsilon$
  - Where Y = the percentage of lower quality hospitals in the state
  - βX_1 = The percentage of minorities in the state
  - βX_2 = The percentage of the population with incomes at or below the federally defined poverty level in each state
  - βX_3 = The percentage of the population with college degrees
  - Alpha (α), the intercept of a regression line, is the height on y when x = 0. Beta (β), the slope of the regression line, can also refer to as the average change in y associated with a one unit change in x. In order for the null hypothesis to be true, beta (β), the coefficient of each X must be equal to zero. Epsilon (ε), a standard deviation of y for a fixed x, is included to imply that y itself is subject to uncertainty.

In order to test whether these coefficients are equal to zero, the ANOVA F-test for multiple regression is calculated by the online statistical calculator that was used.

As a part of this ANOVA F-test, the values below are calculated:

- The SS or sum of the squares.
- The MS or mean square.

You forgot to tell us what we mean by the degrees of freedom.

The **degrees of freedom** tell us by how much a value can vary given the number of values that are fixed.

- The F statistic is calculated by the statistical calculator using a formula that is a ratio.

Do we really have to know all of this to interpret the output of the analysis?

You actually do not, but we introduce these terms to simply improve your ability to better understand the type of data analysis that is common in disparity research.

So, what is the minimum that we need to know? Stated differently, what are the findings?

Observe the signs of the coefficients and the numbers calculated as the *p*-values in the last part of the output from the statistical calculator. Notice that the coefficients are not zero! Therefore, these coefficients tell us that a percentage change in each of the independent variables is associated with a change in the percentage of 1- or 2-star rated hospitals in each state. Specifically, the data analysis gives us three critical pieces of information.

1. When the % of the population that is minority in a state is higher, the % of lower-quality hospitals is higher. Moreover, the relationship is highly significant ($p < .000592$).
2. When the % of the population that is impoverished increases in a state, the number of "lower-quality" hospitals increases. However, the increase is not of a magnitude as to be considered significant ($p < 0.14431446$).

3. When the % of the population with four years or more of college in a state is higher, the percentage of "lower quality" hospitals is significantly higher ($p < 0.04627257$).

So, as a healthcare professional working in a hospital, these are the three things I would need to be able to discuss from this original exercise on disparities in hospital care?

Yes, those are the points you would want to remember.

I'm still a little confused. Could we discuss these findings a bit here?

These findings are quite provocative because they suggest the need for more research. This is very important given that hospitals are being financially penalized based upon their Hospital Compare data. These findings suggest that the percentage of hospitals with a 1- or 2-star rating is higher in states with higher minority populations. The question becomes, "Are these healthcare institutions receiving lower Hospital Compare scores because their patient base includes a higher percentage of minorities and these groups may have very different baseline conditions at admission that lead to disparate outcomes?" Yet, if these hospitals are financially penalized without additional analysis their capacity to serve these higher need minority populations would further decrease!!! Additionally, as all healthcare professionals are aware, Medicaid payments for medical care are below the rates paid to private insurance companies. Accordingly, hospitals that serve a greater percentage of Medicaid patients may also have a higher proportion of 1- and 2-star ratings because the lower payments they receive cause them to "cut corners." However, this exercise was not designed to address this issue.

Given their importance, how sound are these findings?

In order for a linear regression analysis of the type used here to be considerable as "sound," several assumptions must be met. For example, there must be evidence that the relationship between the variables can be expressed by a scatterplot along which the variables resemble a straight line and not a curved line. These data meet that assumption. There are other equally important requirements which will not be discussed here for purposes of simplification. However, one of the strongest arguments that could be used to render findings meaningless is the argument that minority status, poverty, and education are correlated with each other. We call this **multicollinearity**. There are several statistical measures that can be used to check for multicollinearity.

So, was this analysis checked for multicollinearity?

Yes, it was. We calculated something called a **Variance Inflation Factor (VIF)**. If the VIF is greater than a certain amount, it suggests that multicollinearity is possibly affecting the findings. Our analysis revealed no collinearity among the pairs of predictors. Moreover, we use this example in order to encourage healthcare professionals to continually engage in knowledge creation.

So, given that we can preliminarily take these findings seriously, is there any evidence that there is a threat that may decrease access to care in communities that serve large percentages of minorities?

CMS is aware of the contrariety implicit to this dilemma. Dickson (2017) summarizes some of the debate and the proposed resolution to such circumstances. This writer mentioned that the 21st Century Cures Act that was passed in 2016 may offer some relief since this legislation asks CMS to adjust for patient-level factors in the determination of hospital admission penalties.

So, since other analysts are aware of this problem our analysis doesn't really add anything to the debate does it?

This analysis does add to the debate because it demonstrates several factors that have not been included in current discussions of the penalties currently facing hospitals. First, the current debate on the impact of penalties focuses upon impoverished low-income and minority communities. Our analysis reveals that the direct relationship between the proportion of persons in poverty in a state is not significantly associated with the proportion of "lower-rated" hospitals in the country as a whole. Rather, the issue appears to be a stronger threat to future hospital care for communities with higher numbers of minorities in general. Indeed, the data revealed that West Virginia is the only state without a high percentage of minorities which has a high proportion of hospitals with 1- or 2-star ratings.

Second, this very simple analysis also reveals that a dual marketplace exists in hospitals as healthcare institutions. This brief, highly simplistic analysis can be interpreted to mean that persons with four years or more of college do not, on average, patronize hospitals with 1- or 2-star Hospital Compare ratings. In the analysis, as the percentage of persons with a four-year or higher college degree increased in a state, the percentage of lower hospital star ratings also increased. This suggests that hospital marketplaces are becoming stratified so that persons with four years of college or higher, a group with higher income, a group that has a lower probability of illness and disease, and a group that may conduct more research and analysis when hospitalization is needed, do not patronize the same facilities as health disparity subgroups.

Addressing Current and Prospective Needs of 1- and 2-Star Hospitals

As the discussion thus far demonstrates, healthcare disparities in hospitals may be institutionally based, and/or sourced in patient/staff interactions. In order to assess whether the latter appears to be correct, one healthcare institution that serves large numbers of health disparity populations was used as a case study.

For the sake of not tarnishing its reputation, we will call this institution Urban Medical Center X. Urban Medical Center X is a teaching hospital that is located in a city with a population that exceeds 611,000 persons and is located in a county with approximately 831,128 persons (U.S. Bureau of the Census, 2017). The Bureau of the Census data for the year 2015 also reveal that the population of this urban city has continually declined since 2014 when it served as home to 614,000 individuals, and 2010 when 621,000+ persons called the city home. This city has a slightly lower population of persons age 18 and over and of persons age 65 and over than the nation as a whole. Relative to race/ethnicity, this urban area has a population that is 27.7% White American, 4.8% Latino American, 2.4% two or more races, 1/10 or 1% Native Hawaiian/Pacific Islander, 3/10 or 1% Native American, and 63.0% African American. Approximately 9.3% of the population speak a language other than English in the home, and 53% of the population are female relative to 50.8% of the county as a whole.

Relative to education, this urban area is an interesting one. While it has nearly as many persons with a college degree (29.7%) as the nation as a whole (30.3%), it has far fewer high school graduates (83.5%) than the country as a whole (87%). It also has a lower proportion of the population who are in the workforce (61.7%) than is true nationwide (63.1%). Of particular relevance to the hospital care marketplace, this urban area has a greater proportion of the population under age 65 who have a health disability—11.9% versus 8.6%. Approximately 23.1% of the population of this city were impoverished versus 12.7% of the nation from 2012 to 2016. However, despite such a profile, the same proportion (89.9%) of individuals had health insurance as was true nationwide at the time that these data were collected (2011–2015).

Thus, a first step that healthcare administrators at hospitals with low Hospital Compare ratings may wish to do is to compare the demographics and socioeconomic characteristics of the city or county which they serve in order to identify whether statistically significant differences exist in the social determinants of health in their service area. However, more detail is needed than that which is provided here. Facts such as the number of retail liquor stores, marital status of the population, percentage of the population who have been jailed and/or imprisoned, profile data from the CDC Risk Factor Surveillance data, data from the Department of Health, risks associated with residency near landfills, air quality, and other environmental risks, and other data are needed that may be reflected in baseline health status. So, it is critical that hospitals with 1 or 2 overall stars implement their own self-assessment.

Second, Urban Medical Center X must harvest data from within that allows it to statistically characterize the percentage of its population who have a higher risk, of hospital-acquired urinary tract infections, bloodstream infections as well as methicillin-resistant *Staphylococcus aureus* (MRSA), vancomycin-resistant enterococcus (VME) and/or other infections. Thus, the analysis requested by the hospital administrator must describe the number and characteristics of persons served utilizing an instrument such as that in **TABLE 10.3**.

By analyzing whether the hospital had a higher frequency and percentage of patients in the categories in Table 10.3, it becomes possible for a lower-rated hospital to demonstrate that higher re-infection rates do not simply reflect poor hygiene by medical staff and/or the improper insertion of IV drips, drain tubes, catheters, and/or other equipment. Rather, these infections can reflect patient characteristics such as those outlined.

However, it is also critical that the hospital conduct an open and honest assessment of its customer service practices. Internal and external bias against culturally and/or economically diverse groups is nonmythical. Blair, Steiner, and Hanraner (2011) discuss implicit bias based on race/ethnicity. Fitzgerald and Hurst (2017) identified bias against other subgroups.

Moreover, Havekes, Coenders, Dekker, and Van Der Lippe (2014) confirm that even within racial/ethnic subgroups, explicit and implicit bias against lower income groups exists. Within hospitals, such sentiments may reveal themselves in the Hospital Compare Star Ratings based upon areas such as communications with nurses and physicians. Similarly, a disdain for economically impoverished patients can reveal itself in lowered rates of responsiveness of the hospital staff, poorer pain management and a failure to provide adequate information regarding medications, a less-than-clean physical environment, a failure to maintain a quiet environment on the wards, and in other behaviors.

For example, despite its status as a nationally ranked medical center by *U.S. News & World Report* in the areas of general medicine, hospital size, and the quality of its nursing staff, Urban Hospital X, like many large hospitals that address the unique ambulatory and hospitalization needs of urban populations, is in urgent need of qualitative and quantitative interventions that can advance its customer service ratings.

The customer service interventions needed extend across a number of areas. Based upon a brief assessment of need using postings in Health Grade, 23% of past patients reporting to this site indicated unmet needs in the area of physician and nurse communication. Similarly, 41% identified customer service needs in another communication area—explanations provided by staff. Relative to facility needs, approximately 47% of respondents cited an absence of quiet at night as a customer service need and 37% experienced insufficient cleanliness and other problems in their hospital rooms. Clinically, approximately 33% of admitted patients who responded to the Health Grade survey made note of problems in pain management. Because these findings are from such a small sample size, they are, of course, inconclusive.

However, online comments from other sites seemingly triangulate these areas of customer service need. For example, Google's 200+ customer service reviews on Urban Hospital

TABLE 10.3 Identifying Risk Factors Associated With Vulnerability to Hospital-Acquired Infection

Risk Category	Length of Stay (1)	Type of Surgery (2)	Length of the Surgery (3)	Anti-biotics Given (4)	Type of Wounds (including burns) (5)	Patients' Length of Residency in High Risk Care Units		
						Intensive Care Unit (ICU) (including neonatal intensive care unit) (6)	Critical Care Units (7)	Other Special Care or High-Risk Hospital Units (i.e., long-term acute care, special care unit, burn unit, etc.) (8)
1. Premature Babies of any age								
2. Persons age 65–74								
3. Persons age 75–85								
4. Persons 85+								
5. Frail elderly of any age								
6. Persons with medical conditions such as diabetes								
7. Persons with compromised immune systems including: Persons treated with chemotherapy Persons treated with steroids Persons treated with HIV and other								

NOTE. This table is intentionally left blank as a sample instrument for adoption by hospitals.

X also include a litany of comments by past patients who are discontented with services received. In fact, 64 or 32% of the 200 customers who entered remarks rated Urban Hospital X as a 1- or 2-star facility based upon their customer service experience. Glassdoor, a service for *employee reviews*, indicated that 36% of respondents would not recommend Urban Hospital X to a friend. This suggests that internal employee needs may be complicit in the creation of weaknesses in patient service. That is, dissatisfied staff oftentimes deliver less than standard customer service.

Additional data also revealed a need for improvements in customer service by clinical staff. Specifically, Urban Hospital X's nursing staff may require training in infection control. As of March 31, 2017, the rate of bloodstream infections was 16% higher than the mean for the nation's other 3000+ hospitals for which CMS collected data. Catheter-associated urinary tract infections were 20% higher than those that existed nationwide. Surgical site infections exceeded the nation's average by 38% and MRSA infections were 43% higher than nationwide. *C. difficile* infections were 18% higher. Accordingly, Urban Hospital X's Hospital Administration has an urgent need to preempt future poor ratings by providing training to promote greater adherence to medical guidelines in each of these areas.

Interestingly, a statistical contradiction exists between Urban Hospital X's patient satisfaction with customer service as posted on informal online sites and the information gathered through the CMS's Hospital Compare. Hospital Compare website transmits a portrait of a facility in which 86% of the patients asked were satisfied with the cleanliness of their room, and 85% were pleased by the solitude and quietness of their rooms at night. Moreover, 89% were pleased with the service and attitude of the hospital staff. As the data discussed earlier indicate, these numbers are significantly higher than the informal online ratings. This finding suggests that the Hospital Compare data may embody sampling errors.

Hospitals need to routinely reconcile their formal and informal quality assessments. Thus, given the preliminary data, there exists a mild to urgent need for interventions that reduce the divergence between the online customer reports and those in the formally collected Healthcare Effectiveness Data and Information Set (HEDIS), Hospital Consumer Assessment of Healthcare Providers and Systems, CDC National Healthcare Safety Network, CMS QIO Clinical Data Warehouse, and data collection via the CMS Certificate and Survey Provider Enhanced Reporting (CASPER) system.

In addition, data internal to Urban Hospital X may reveal that some "customer service problems" are actually sourced in "system" needs. For example, like all hospitals, Urban Hospital X probably collects data on its nursing unit activities. If so, Urban Hospital X could conduct a performance rating flow process analysis based upon the observed time in minutes versus the standard time to complete activities such as patient assessment, care planning, treatment, medication administering, collecting blood/lab specimens, and other duties. Lower performance ratings of nurses in the core 20 areas included in their performance ratings can generate a pathway that leads to differential customer satisfaction. Likewise, what appears to be poor customer service can, in many cases, be explained by the illnesses and diseases and medical needs of Urban Hospital X's patients. Based on Urban Hospital X's daily census, nursing duties will and should exceed those which are standard. For example, a hospital with a lower daily census will record higher nursing performance ratings than those with a higher census. This is because, as most hospital administrators are aware, the service delivery guidelines require that *occupied beds be changed by a nursing professional, while empty beds can be changed by a non professional.*

Customer service complaints have also been levied against emergency room staff at Urban Hospital X. However, improvements in customer service by reducing wait time in an emergency room will be highly dependent on the proportion of patients who, after patient entry and triage, must have blood drawn. A high proportion of patients who require that blood be drawn generate service delays at several key points. First, the specimen must wait for an MD's order. Second, after the order entry, the specimen must be labeled and packaged. Third, after the actual lab analysis, the lab must verify the findings and enter them into the internal patient system for the appropriate patient. Fourth, the lab analysis must then be sent back to the ER for physician review and termination of the lab order. This process can, of course, be shortened. Nevertheless, if a high proportion of emergency room patients require this service, delays will occur that lengthen queues in emergency departments. The hospitals should analyze their operational procedures to determine steps needed to reduce process waste and improve customer service in this area. Given the complexities involved in providing true customer service that extends beyond asking staff to behaviorally "be nice" to all customers independent of the diversity of those being served, the most effective customer service interventions can be crafted only after an assessment of need.

Why were such detailed recommendations provided?

It is important that hospitals that serve large number of subgroups not be unfairly penalized via the use of methodologies of quality measurement that do not properly stratify and analyze the data. Yet, it is critical these same hospitals confront and address actual quality needs so differential subgroup hospital care does not occur. CMS's 2018 National Impact Assessment of CMS Quality Measures Report (2018) specifically addresses the need to better integrate both client mix issues and the behavior of clinical staff into an understanding of hospital outcomes. It is critical that future and/or current hospital professionals advance the use of innovative strategies to measure the quality of their services to health disparity populations.

You've discussed health disparities and quality of hospital care issues. What about disparities in emergency room care?

▶ Hospitals and Healthcare Disparities: Emergency Departments

In some respects, the very role that emergency rooms play in the American healthcare system generates a point in the disparity chain for differential outcomes. Chen, Cheng, Bennett, and Hilbert (2015), for example, found that the assertion that hospital emergency departments have, in some respects, become the outpatient solution for many health disparity populations appears to be true. In an analysis of more than 6,592,501 emergency department visits in the state of South Carolina over the period 2005–2010, these researchers found that 76% of visits were for nonurgent reasons. Moreover, Medicaid patients and African Americans were over-represented among those whose emergency department visits were for nonurgent reasons.

Although hospitals have expanded their level and types of outpatient services, many of these very important facilities now find themselves with another "outpatient" problem. This is the phenomenon of "crowding" in their emergency department services. As the research cited above indicates, disparities exist in the nature and type of patients who are impacted by emergency room crowding. Barish, Mcgauly, and Arnold (2012) argue that despite the decline in usage of hospitals for overnight stays, the use of emergency departments for outpatient care has accelerated thereby creating the very serious problem of emergency room crowding.

Why has this occurred?

Barish et al. (2012) suggest that two key factors have prompted Americans in need of health care to seek it from emergency departments. First, the absence of a system of universal access to healthcare services has been a strong causal factor. The logic is quite linear. While the value structure of Americans does not support a public sector–based universal access healthcare system, federal law has implicitly made emergency departments the one component of the healthcare apparatus that is *mandated* to provide universal access. Hospital emergency departments are required by law to deliver needed healthcare services to all patients who present themselves, regardless of their insurance status or ability to pay.

What federal legislation "opened wider the doors" of emergency departments to the uninsured as well as the insured?

The initial legislation that mandated the provision of essential care was the Emergency Medical Treatment and Active Labor Act (EMTALA). The EMTALA was voted into law in 1986. Although this law was well meaning in its intent, a multitude of variables at play in the disparity chain has led to circumstances that create disparate levels of healthcare quality for selected subgroups who seek care from emergency departments.

Specifically, there is an overrepresentation of low-income Americans in emergency care. Thus, the question becomes, "How does the disparity chain lead to low income?" The processes that are in the disparity chain that produce low income are far, far more complex than is normally assumed. Consider this research-based example: Braveman et al. (2015) literally found an oftentimes overlooked relationship that exists between being low income as an adult and being born preterm. Moreover, this relationship between poverty and preterm birth exists for all subgroups. Braveman et al. (2015), in a sample of approximately 10,400 American women of both African and European descent, found that no differences existed in the increased

rate of preterm births of lower income women in the sample. But, a preterm birth can lead to low income for children of any race/ethnicity because it initiates a disparity chain that results in low-income status as an adult. Odd, Evans, and Emond (2016) discovered that because preterm infants actually enter school earlier than would have been the case based upon their due date, they, on average, academically perform below their full-term counterparts. Such an outcome is not benign. A study by the University of Warwick (March 9, 2016) reported on research which revealed that these academic problems in school subsequently increase the probability that as adults, these preterm children will have lower income. Thus, this research suggests that the disparity chain operates in such a fashion that a preterm child is at greater risk of low income and/or joblessness. Joblessness, of course, can result in uninsured status. Uninsured status can then increase the representation of this subgroup—adults who were born preterm—in the emergency department of hospitals.

But, aren't African American women more likely to have a preterm birth?

Apparently, the key causal factor in the risk of a preterm birth is low income rather than race/ethnicity.

How can emergency room-quality disparities be avoided?

Disparities can never be eliminated and/or reduced if their nature or causes are not identified and analyzed. Thus, hospital emergency departments require the application of quantitative management tools of analysis. **BOX 10.2** emphasizes the intimate relationship between healthcare disparity reductions and the use of quantitative tools.

If a patient is admitted as a result of an emergency room visit, the health disparity chain at play in hospitals is extremely complex. As noted, disparities in health care may occur as a result of disparities in insurance

---

BOX 10.2 How Quantitative Management Can Be Applied to Create Long-Term Decreases in Quality Losses in Hospital Emergency Departments

1. Healthcare administrators can conduct a quantitative analysis of emergency department data in order to answer the following questions:
   - How many patients frequented the emergency room over a given period? What percentage of the encounters were for primary care? For acute care?
   - How many emergency room visits led to hospital admissions during each quarter?
   - What were the characteristics of the patients in each of the above categories relative to demographics, socioeconomic variables, rural/urban status, zip codes, insurance status, disease and illness status, and by other variables?
   - What were patient outcomes in terms of the emergency room wait times? What percentage of visits resulted in wait times that exceeded the recommended limit? Did these outcomes differ by subgroup?
   - What percentage of all patients and various subgroups were "boarded" for 48 hours or more while they waited for an inpatient bed?
   - What percentage of patients left without seeing a physician? Did the proportions differ by subgroup?
   - What was the percentage of deaths that occurred among high-risk patients?
   - What was the mean number of patients who were seen by a physician?
   - What percentage of patients were redirected to alternate institutions and/or providers?
   - What were the periods of time when the emergency department was most likely to be overbooked?
2. Based on the findings to these questions, healthcare administrators, clinicians, and other staff can then apply the appropriate queuing analysis to identify optimal trade-offs between capacity and service delays for the emergency room.
3. After selecting the best queuing model, healthcare administrators can then decrease the healthcare quality losses that occur in emergency departments by simply applying other state-of-the-art quantitative management tools.

---

status. Englum et al. (2016), based on data from the 2010 National Trauma Data Bank, used a multivariable regression model to determine whether insurance status intermediated the length of a hospital stay for consumers whose lives had been threatened by trauma. To avoid comparing "apples to oranges," the study matched consumers from a set of 884,493 persons by variables such as the severity of injury, age, sex, and other factors and the existence of other medical conditions to determine if there were differences in length of stay (LOS). The data revealed that disparities did exist in hospital stays by insurance status even if the hospital visit involved trauma. As would be expected, the LOS was shortest for consumers who were uninsured (0.3 days).

Uninsured status is higher for some subgroups than for others. Barnett and Berchick (2017) indicated that in 2016, while 91.2% of the overall population had healthcare insurance, 7% of impoverished children under age 19 were uninsured relative to only 5% of children who were not impoverished. Likewise, Hispanic Americans had uninsured rates of 16% versus 6.3% for White Americans, 7.6% for Asian Americans and 10.5% for African Americans. These subgroups may differ by geographic region, sex, race/ethnicity, and even by mental health status. Yet, when hospital stay data were analyzed by subgroups, an interesting outcome emerged (Englum et al., 2016). Specifically, consumers with private insurance, a group that included a greater proportion of White Americans and Asian Americans and higher-educated and higher-income groups, were *less* likely to have the optimal LOS for their injuries compared to those who had public insurance (Medicaid or Medicare). Publicly insured persons had the longest LOS (0.9 days). However, this study did not examine whether those patients with the longest lengths of stay had the best outcomes. Nevertheless, healthcare administrators in hospitals may wish to track data and complete an assessment of the LOS at their facility and health outcomes in order to ensure that the optimal LOS is provided across patient subgroups.

Additionally, greater dialogue may be required between the hospital, the insurance sector, and the general public. Some members of the public favor repealing the Affordable Care Act (ACA). Indeed, many Americans were excited when the requirement that states expand Medicaid was "struck down" by the U.S. Supreme Court. However, health disparities regarding access to hospital care is an intimate part of the disparities ladder relative to having the optimal length of hospital stay because persons in expanded Medicaid states are more likely to have longer lengths of stay (Anderson et al., 2015).

Akinyemiju, Jha, Moore, and Pisu (2016) found that those states that did *not* expand Medicaid had the highest number of persons who were uninsured as well as the highest number of persons with multiple illnesses and diseases. This suggests that healthcare administrators of hospitals in these states have an even greater need to explore the relationship between LOS and healthcare outcomes.

What states did not expand Medicaid?

The 19 states that chose not to expand Medicaid include Alabama, Florida, Georgia, Idaho, Kansas, Maine, Mississippi, Missouri, Nebraska, North Carolina, Oklahoma, South Carolina, South Dakota, Tennessee, Texas, Utah, Virginia, Wisconsin, and Wyoming (Garfield, Damico, Stephens, and Rouhani, 2016).

▶ Consequences of Healthcare Disparities in Hospitals

Whether disparities in hospitals occur in the emergency room or after admission, such circumstances can have serious outcomes. For example, as mentioned, the issues of disparities in readmission rates can have serious consequences for hospitals because Medicare now applies financial penalties for readmissions. It is imperative that every single hospital administrator ensure that an annual and/or quarterly multivariate analysis is completed that uses the age, sex, and diagnostic status of the patient and other explanatory variables. This is important since Barnett, Hsu, and McWilliams (2015), using data from 2009 to 2012, found 22 independent patient-based variables that can clinically account for readmission rates. These variables were disparately distributed within the patient base of higher admission hospitals. Hospital leadership who are unaware of this study may find themselves being unfairly penalized. The variables were those associated with hospitals that are more welcoming to health disparity populations, including patients with lower levels of education, fewer financial resources, lower levels of physical functioning, higher probably of rating their own health as fair to poor, greater problems with the activities of daily living and/or the instrumental activities of daily living, more mental health dysfunctions, and other traits, etc. Again, hospitals serving subgroups with differential needs may be penalized for higher rates of readmissions if the statistical model used to assess readmissions is improperly characterized.

What do you mean by "improperly characterized"?

A statistical model that includes most of the independent variables needed to "explain" the dependent variable, or behavior, is a well-characterized model.

Is this always the case, or do some disparities in hospital care actually reflect poorer quality of care for some subpopulations?

Some disparities do actually exist, in part, because of poorer-quality care. Accordingly, it becomes even more important for hospitals to conduct their own statistical analyses so that they can identify and correct remediable disparities.

Isn't it is also important for them to analyze their data so that they will know whether they should not be penalized?

Yes, of course, but it is important for many other reasons. Rangrass, Ghaferi, and Dimick (2014), based on data from the 2007–2008 Medicare database, conducted an analysis using 173,925 Medicare beneficiaries who had received coronary artery bypass graft (CABG). They discovered that minority Medicare beneficiaries experienced death after this procedure 33% more often than did their White counterparts. However, when socioeconomic variables and hospital quality were included in the statistical model, the disparity in death rates dropped to 16%. Nevertheless, this 16% disparity suggests a need for remediation.

Are there other examples of hospital disparities?

Many more examples of disparities can be identified. For example, Zhang et al. (2016) analyzed data for both Medicare patients and veterans who were admitted to a hospital to receive total knee arthroplasty to determine whether racial/ethnic differences in care could be identified. Their analysis found that Asian Americans, Native Americans, Latino Americans, and persons who classified themselves as mixed race had: (1) lower rates of knee surgery,

(2) less access to hospitals that performed this surgery on a routine basis, (3) higher death rates, (4) a higher incidence of complications, and (5) worse outcomes than their White American counterparts. Moreover, such disparities worsened over the time period examined. Although these findings are unfortunate, we cannot apply a value judgment. The key issue is identifying the causes and correlates of these circumstances and then to work together collectively to address every point in the disparity chain that produced such outcomes.

Healthcare disparities across subgroups of patients in hospitals are not merely a problem within the United States. Rather, it is a global problem. For example, Wang et al. (2015) compared data on 36,921 patients in hospitals in Scotland, 29,187 patients from hospitals in Hong Kong, and 162,464 patients from hospitals in China. They found that persons with multiple diseases or illnesses were, as would be expected, more likely to be admitted to hospitals in all three countries than was the case with their counterparts with only one severe illness. However, they discovered that in Scotland, persons who were poor and had multiple medical conditions were 62% more likely to be admitted to the hospital than their non-poor counterparts. In contrast, in China, persons with the greatest income constraints were only 58% as likely to receive acute hospital care as their highest-income counterparts.

A very different pattern of inequalities emerged in Hong Kong hospitals. It appears that the system of stratification in Hong Kong operated in such a way that income segregation occurred in the hospitals. Public hospitals were 68% more likely to serve as the institutions that delivered care to poor persons with multiple morbidities. This socioeconomic group was only 18% as likely to be admitted to the private hospital care system.

What does this study imply?

The study by Wang et al. (2015) suggests that not only within the United States but also worldwide, there is a need for individuals to subordinate tribalistic loyalties to the "good of humankind." Humankind is strengthened, not weakened, by the "gifts" that are embodied in each individual. Thus, social investment in the capital goods of health and education across all subgroups benefits all who inhabit the planet.

Are findings such as these the reason that some subgroups exhibit "medical mistrust" of hospitals, their physicians, and/or the health-care system as a whole?

It seems so. Davis, Bynum, Katz, Buchanan, and Green (2013) conducted an analysis regarding cancer screenings that revealed that Hispanic Americans patients were more likely to exhibit mistrust in medical personnel which negatively affected the likelihood of the patients undergoing cancer screenings. Additionally, Armstrong, McMurphy, Ravenell, and Putt (2007) found that there were lower levels of trust in physicians among patients of African descent and Hispanic patients than their White American counterparts. However, these researchers also found varying reasons for the low trust levels. The analysis indicated that socioeconomic status, location, and other factors could be operative.

Interestingly another study by Boulware, Cooper, and Ratner (2003) revealed that most of the subgroups examined trusted hospitals. However, they were less likely to trust their physicians. Although the overall sample was relatively small (118 persons), this study also found that while approximately 70% of respondents trusted their hospitals, only 28% trusted their healthcare insurance plans. When the data were stratified between African American and White respondents, no significant ($p > .05$) differences existed with regard to trust of hospitals, but African American patients were less likely to trust their physicians. Medical mistrust in physicians by patients of African descent was also found in a study by Sewell (2015). The study revealed that Hispanics and African Americans did harbor more mistrust of physicians, but for different reasons. But, the study also found that both subgroups had higher trust issues regarding

the physicians' medical knowledge, experience, capability, and moral principles than did their White American counterparts.

Despite what you say about wanting to broaden the field of disparities, you continue to focus upon race/ethnicity! Why?

This tendency to focus on race/ethnicity is due, in part, to the fact that so much secondary data exist on these subgroups. However, a number of studies have examined hospitalization disparities for other groups. Ailey, Johnson, Fogg, and Friese (2015), in an exploratory study of disparities between persons with intellectual disabilities and persons without such conditions, identified extreme differences in outcomes for patients with and without intellectual disabilities treated by academic hospitals. They found that in academic hospitals, persons with intellectual disabilities were 100% more likely to have complications from surgery and nearly 300% more likely to have complications if they were admitted through the emergency room. These patients were autistic, displayed behaviors that could be assessed as aggressive, and/or had cerebral palsy or a respiratory disorder. Note that the study embodied a descriptive design and not a causal one; thereby, we cannot "explain" these findings.

Are there any studies that reveal no disparities at all in hospital care? Those of us who are new to the field of health care need hope!

Yes, a number of disparity studies have found absolutely no disparities. Parikh et al. (2015) in a study of 1,128 patients who received care for breast cancer at an academic medical center that was highly inclusive obtained very interesting results relative to increased mortality. Absolutely no statistically significant differences in mortality rates occurred by race/ethnicity or public versus private insurance status.

So, there was absolute equality in mortality rates?

No, but this study revealed that other subgroup characteristics were operative. Specifically, relationship status was associated with higher death rates among cancer patients. Patients who were single were 136% more likely to have increased mortality. As would be expected, patients older than age 70 were 288% more likely to experience increased mortality. Last, as would also be expected, patients who had stage 4 breast cancer were 71.81% more likely to have increased rates of mortality. This study suggests that more research is needed on the role of relationship status in the mortality chain.

Anything else on disparities in hospitals?

In addition to the hospital disparities already discussed, some researchers have found ethnic/racial and age disparities in rehospitalization rates. *Qualis Health*, a Medicare Quality Improvement Organization (QIO), conducted a study on hospital readmission rates (based on rehospitalization within 30 days of initial discharge) in the state of Washington. The Qualis Report (2016) found that in 9 of the 16 communities targeted in the study, Medicare patients who identified as being Native American experienced higher rates of readmissions than most other racial/ethnic groups in these communities. In one of the communities, the data revealed that the readmission rate for Native American patients was approximately 700% higher than the rate for Asian American patients, the group that experienced the least number of readmissions for that specific community. Moreover, Native American patients in nine of the communities experienced rehospitalization rates that were 107% higher than those of the racial/ethnic group in each community with the least number of readmissions. The study also stated that many different causes were possibly operative that led to such readmission disparities. Again, it is critical that hospital administrators have the statistical literacy to work closely with statisticians in planning research studies that analyze the causes of such trends.

Brooks-Carthon, Lasater, Rearden, Holland, and Sloane (2016) found that older African American patients from 253 hospitals throughout California, New Jersey, and Pennsylvania had an 18% greater probability of hospital readmission within 30 days of discharge. However, further analyses revealed that the point in the health disparity chain that was most directly related to this outcome was differential attention by the nurses. This study indicates that hospital healthcare administrators should analyze differences in nursing care when their quality data differ by subgroup.

▶ Disparities in Nursing Care

Indeed, it is not possible to discuss disparities in hospital care without examining nursing care. This is because historically nursing has been disproportionately hospital-based. However, the number of new nurses working in the hospital environment decreased from approximately 87% in 2005 to 76% in 2012 (Stempniak, 2016). Nevertheless, a plurality of nurses do work in hospitals. Nurses support hospitals not only through patient care but via research as well.

Salmond and Echevarria (2017) argue that the current healthcare environment is characterized by forces that require the use of transdisciplinary and/or interdisciplinary teams, and that nurses are critical components of such teams. Specifically, nurses are positioned to reduce excessive emergency department use, reduce hospitalization for conditions that are treatable on an outpatient basis, monitor the quality and quantity of diagnostics tests, review medical histories, decrease medication errors, and make other contributions that, when completed, will lead to fewer adverse outcomes via the disparity chain.

Premji and Hatfield (2016) argue that nurses can also increase the bidirectional flow of information between patients and the healthcare system by generating dialogue with patients that allows for a more refined way of delivering healthcare services. In addition, Smith (2007) introduced an interesting and humanistic argument regarding the roles that both hospital-based and nonhospital-based nurses can play in reducing disparities. This strategy is simply strengthening the mixture of caring for humankind in the medical care that is provided. Moreover, Smith proposed that this reintegration be provided to all patients, independent of subgroup characteristics. The American Hospital Association (2016) also makes an important observation, arguing that nurses, because they have access to the patients in hospitals on a continual basis, are positioned to identify the social determinants of health outcomes that may be shaping observed disparities. As a result, nurses can assist hospitals in referring and linking patients to the external services needed to reduce health disparities.

Determinants of health outcomes research estimates that health care only contributes 10% to 20% to health outcomes (McGovern, Miller & Hughes-Cromwick, 2014). Thus, the **accountable care health community model** seeks to link patients not only with physicians, hospitals, and other types of clinical care but with the broad range of community services that will allow these other health-related needs to be addressed (Shortell & Casalino, 2008). Nurses can serve as a liaison for hospitals and other healthcare systems as part of this model.

But couldn't healthcare disparities actually increase if the nurses are tribalistic in their orientation?

Yes, but we must remember that the conditions that generate excessive loyalty to one's subgroup, rather than the whole of humankind, can be changed as individuals participate in dialogue regarding the urgency of such a change!

Perceived threats to human survival are quite localized in a world in which communication and transportation are limited to smaller geographic areas. In the present, the capacity for global transportation or global communication allows an infrastructure for collective responses to threats by all persons on earth. Global transportation and communication systems permit persons, communities, regions, countries, and continents to act in unity against common threats whether they are localized food shortages, regional or global life-threatening changes in weather conditions, and/or the threat of a meteor moving along a pathway that will strike Earth. Accordingly, historical differences that have resulted in injuries to various groups and subgroups can no longer be the focus for they hinder the type of loyalty to humankind that is needed to support human survival. A narrative of change is needed that supports appreciation and love of one's subgroups but also embraces all of humankind.

It would be unreasonable for direct disparities in health care to *have not* occurred in a tribalistic world! Van Ryn and Fu (2003) introduced evidence regarding past provider behaviors that directly contributed to racial/ethnic disparities. Alexis, Vydelingum, and Robbins (2007) reported that in the National Health Services of England, nurses from Asia, Africa, and the Caribbean had no "voice" or occupational power to deliver services that were disparity-reducing in the healthcare system. However, Shavers et al. (2012) advance the argument that the magnitude of the operation of direct, interpersonal bias and systematic tribalism in hospitals and other healthcare settings has never been accurately measured because of the absence of appropriate instrumentation and methodological processes.

It is also important to remember that other research has revealed that disparities in hospital outcomes are oftentimes a result of the interaction of intersectoral forces. This was demonstrated via the earlier discussion of health disparities and hospitals. However, the continuing theme in this text is that such evidence, when available, must be used diagnostically and not in an accusatory fashion.

When historical facts and empirical research findings on disparities are used diagnostically, the focus is that of seeking to identify and treat remediable causes of such disparate outcomes so that those patterns do not repeat. Historical facts and empirical data that are used accusatorily deny opportunities for the harmonious merging of subgroups to support improvements in humankind. The past cannot be undone; it can only be used to inform change. Moreover, the accusatory use of past events oftentimes builds cases based upon oversimplification.

For example, Chakrabarti, Osborne, Rangnekar, and Mathur (2017) applied a multilevel hierarchical regression model to data from the American Hospital Association and the Nationwide Inpatient Sample (a longitudinal hospital inpatient, federal/private-sector database) in order to determine whether consumers receiving hospital-based services for cirrhosis had a higher rate of death while hospitalized by race/ethnicity. The answer was yes! However, the findings were highly instructive when the health disparity chain model was used in interpreting the results.

Based on their analysis, lower-resource hospitals operate in lower-resource neighborhoods and disproportionately serve lower-resource consumers, who tend to be disproportionately Latino Americans and African Americans. Lower-resource hospitals have, based upon this study, higher rates of mortality in general, as well as for specific illnesses and/or diseases. Thus, these circumstances created a chain reaction that led to significantly higher rates of deaths from cirrhosis among Latinos, African Americans, and Asian American subgroups (Chakrabarti et al., 2017).

However, when the data were disaggregated to account for differences in hospital resources and average mortality rates among patients with similar disease stage, education, and other characteristics, no racial/ethnic disparities were

revealed. The study by Chakrabarti et al. (2017) demonstrates the importance of healthcare administrators, public health professionals, and clinicians being able to enter into dialogue with statisticians so that observable disparities can be risk-adjusted. This study also documents the importance of examining the larger disparity chain of causation when analyzing hospital disparities. Hospitals receive patients whose status represents the end result of a lengthy group of factors that precede their hospital admissions and that may be nonremediable by the administrator of a particular hospital. However, as continually emphasized, all hospitals may wish to consider a comprehensive baseline disparity analysis that incorporates variables that exceed those most commonly used for quality measurement.

Are there areas of disparities that are directly sourced within the components of the health disparity chain that are remediable by the hospital administrators?

It was mentioned earlier that the services provided by nurses were causally related to identified health disparities. Some research suggests that subjective attitudes and behaviors of the hospital staff may differ across subgroups of consumers admitted to hospitals (Beckman, 2003; Manoach & Goldfrank, 2002). Johnstone and Kanitsaki (2008) reports similar behaviors in Australian hospitals which included language bias.

Do you mean the operation of contemporary tribalism?

Yes. *Homo sapiens* respond to individuals and groups at an affective level. By **affective level**, we refer to responses that occur at the level of emotions and/or feelings. Affective responses are a link in the health disparity chain because systems of social stratification generate affective responses to individuals and groups. Liu, Wen, Mohan, Bae, and Becker (2016) demonstrated the operation of the affective aspect of the health disparity chain in an extremely instructive article. By performing multivariate analyses with data from the Hospital

BOX 10.3 Development of Subtribal Bias Based on Affective Response

Affective Level 1

Individuals, whether through childhood conditioning or their own reasoning, develop an ontology that ranks subgroup differences based on non alterable characteristics such as racial/ethnic group, sex, etc., using a scale that ranges from inferiority to superiority. Individuals using such a framework also rate themselves as inferior and/or superior.

Affective Level 2

Individuals observe the learned behaviors and other norms of various subgroups and rank differences in learned behavior as inferior and/or superior. In this instance, subtribal differences in speech, dress, displays of affection, music and art preferences, public behaviors, etc., serve as the basis for different subgroups being assigned a rating of inferior or superior.

Affective Level 3

In some instances, disparities emerge in clinical care simply because the provider has an adverse response to the individual's personality.

Consumer Assessment of Healthcare Providers and Systems (HCAHPS) survey and from other sources, they determined that hospitals whose consumer base included certain thresholds of Latinos, Asians, and African Americans received lower overall patient satisfaction scores. These data indicate that interactions at the affective level are operative. The foundations of rudeness, curtness, and uncaring behaviors operate at the level of the emotional. Likewise, the study found that hospitals that served concentrated numbers of Medicaid patients also experienced lower patient satisfaction ratings. The data define a problem that has a simple solution—training that allows hospital staff to directly confront and reframe their responses to persons of different racial/ethnic groups and to persons of different socioeconomic subcultures. However, such an effort must exceed the use of mere cultural competency training in order to allow an authentic transformation in affective responses to occur.

How can change occur in affective responses if cultural competence training is insufficient?

Burgess, Fu, and Van Ryn (2004) advanced the theory that sometimes the pressures of

healthcare environments interact with unconscious bias and, in the process, generate subgroup bias. However, our team views the emergence of visible bias as being the result of the operation of an even more complex system comprising multiple levels of affective responses. **BOX 10.3** describes these levels. Our untested hypothesis is that when negative responses occur at any of these affective levels, the quality of the healthcare delivered may be affected.

▶ Other Correlates of Disparities in Hospital Care

Disparities in Ambulance Diversion

Another remediable area in which disparities in hospital care exist is in the area of ambulance diversion. **Ambulance diversion** is a process in which an emergency department at one hospital refers the patient to another hospital. Although ambulance diversion is most often capacity based, it also occurs for other reasons, such as a consumer's need for services outside of the hospital's area of expertise.

Pham, Patel, Millin, Kirsch, and Chanmugam (2006) reviewed the literature on ambulance diversion and highlighted a number of adverse outcomes. In addition, McCaughey, Erwin, and DelliFraine (2015) have argued that ambulance diversion leads to poorer quality care. However, Shen and Hsia (2016) analyzed data on Medicare patients from the records of ambulances across 26 California counties between 2001 and 2011. They demonstrated that ambulance diversion was a link in the disparity chain that creates severe asymmetries. Specifically, they found that hospitals that served large numbers of African Americans had a significantly greater rate of ambulance diversion than other hospitals. Moreover, such practices generated poorer health outcomes. Not only was access to state-of-the-art medical procedures bypassed, the 1-year mortality rates for hospital-diverted patients were 9.6% higher than for other consumers. While Massachusetts has literally made this practice illegal, every current or prospective hospital administrator may wish to research and implement alternative practices.

Disparities in Postsurgical Complications

It is important that current and future healthcare administrators know how to provide leadership to their respective institutions in analyzing their internal data to determine whether health disparities exist and the source of such disparities if they are discovered. Witt et al. (2016) examined disparities in in-hospital, postsurgical complications. This study demonstrated the role of social determinants of health in the chain that supports health disparities in hospitals. Specifically, persons with public insurance and/or who were uninsured were 30% to 50% more likely to have a postsurgical complication while in the hospital. Persons who reside in low-income communities had an almost 12% greater probability of an in-hospital postsurgical complication. However, status as a private insurance beneficiary, receipt of surgery in a not-for-profit hospital in a smaller or very small geographic area, and fewer patients for each nurse on duty corresponded with fewer in-hospital postsurgical problems. This study found no significant correlation between postsurgical complications by race/ethnicity once the disparity chain was followed to key sources.

Chapter Summary

This chapter began with an overview of the structure of the hospital industry and with a discussion of how the sector is changing. A statistical case study was introduced and completed that examined the relationship between lower quality hospitals in a state and the ethnic/racial and socioeconomic subgroups in each state. Readers were taught to use online statistical calculators to complete a health disparity analysis. A qualitative case study was used to demonstrate that hospitals play a highly critical role in the American healthcare system. Yet, because of the placement of hospitals within the health disparity chain, hospitals tend to treat consumers whose personal behaviors, socioeconomic status, environment, and other determinants of mortality and morbidity have fully or nearly fully matured into a state of severe illness. However, as this chapter also reveals, a number of disparities in both hospital and/or physician care are linked to differentials in access to care as a result of the presence or absence of health insurance. Most importantly, the chapter describes some approaches that hospitals can use to ensure that they do not produce disparate quality by subgroup and that they do not experience financial losses as a result of serving health disparity subgroups.

Review Questions and Problems

1. Summarize the current composition of the hospital sector in the U.S. healthcare

system, Then select a state or city and provide a summary of the hospital sector in that area. Census Bureau Quick Facts can be used to obtain demographic and socioeconomic data for the city or state that you select. Based on these data, what type of health disparities would you expect to exist among the hospitals in this city?

2. Note that most of the research cited in this chapter used primary sources of secondary data and some form of regression analysis. Choose one of the studies cited, and locate it online through your library. Examine the methods the authors used to complete their disparities study. Create a video in which you describe to a statistician the type of disparity study you would like them to complete for the hospital at which you are a healthcare administrator.

3. Reread the chapter and list any terms which are unclear to you. Go online and find definitions for these concepts.

4. Go to Hospital Compare and compare three hospitals in your area (e.g., Las Vegas) to determine which hospital would be best for a patient with heart attack symptoms.

Key Terms and Concepts

accountable care health community model Care model that seeks to link patients not only with physicians, hospitals, and other types of clinical care, but with the broad range of community services that will allow other health-related needs to be addressed.

affective level Responses that occur at the level of emotions and/or feelings.

ambulance diversion A process in which an emergency department at one hospital refers the patient to another hospital. Although most often capacity based, it also occurs for other reasons, such as a consumer's need for services outside of the hospital's area of expertise.

ANOVA (also known as analysis of variance) A statistical method used to test if there exists a significant degree of difference between two or more means (variables, observations, etc.). While the possible variances are being measured, the means are tested to identify significant differences.

community hospital Public institution that provides acute or short-term care. May provide general services and/or treatment for highly specialized illnesses and diseases.

degrees of freedom The abbreviation is "df" which tells us by how much a value can vary given the number of values that are fixed in a statistical calculation.

multicollinearity Defined as one or more significantly high correlations between two or more (independent) variables. When multicollinearity occurs it may indicate that there is too much correlation between variables to be able to support reliability of the regression.

prospective payment Payment system for healthcare services where services are first delivered and the provider is then reimbursed based on a predetermined, fixed amount.

registered hospital A hospital that has listed itself with the American Hospital Association (AHA), has met all accreditation standards of the Joint Commission on the Accreditation of Healthcare Organizations (JCAHO), and is certified under Titles 18 and 19 of the Social Security Act.

retrospective payment System in existence until 1983 whereby hospital services were not pre-priced. Hospitals delivered the service, decided on a price, and then billed Medicare after services were delivered.

standard error Based on statistics, the standard error measures spread between the observed data value and mean data values.

Variance Inflation Factor (VIF) A VIF is used in regression analysis to determine the existence of multicollinearity. The VIF, after being applied to all of the model's variables, will result in the R-square values.

References

Ailey, S. H., Johnson, T. J., Fogg, L., & Friese, T. R. (2015). Factors related to complications among adult patients with intellectual disabilities hospitalized at an academic medical center. *Intellectual and Developmental Disabilities, 53*(2), 114–119.

Akinyemiju, T., Jha, M., Moore, J. X., & Pisu, M. (2016). Disparities in the prevalence of comorbidities among U.S. adults by state Medicaid expansion status. *Preventive Medicine, 88*, 196–202.

Alexis, O., Vydelingum, V., & Robbins, I. (2007). Engaging with a new reality: Experiences of overseas minority ethnic nurses in the NHS. *Journal of Clinical Nursing, 16*(12), 2221–2228.

American Hospital Association. (2016). Ending health disparities: What can nurses do? *The Sentinel Watch*. Retrieved from https://americansentinel.edu

American Hospital Association. (2018). Fast facts on U.S. hospitals. Retrieved from https://www.aha.org/statistics/fast-facts-us-hospitals

Anderson, M. E., Glasheen, J. J., Anoff, D., Pierce, R., Capp, R., & Jones, C.D. (2015). Understanding predictors of prolonged hospitalizations among general medicine patients: A guide and preliminary analysis. *Journal of Hospital Medicine, 10*(9), 623–626. Doi: 10.1002/.jhm,2414

Armstrong, K., McMurphy, S. M., Ravenell, K., & Putt, M. (2007). Racial/ethnic differences in physician distrust in the United States. *American Journal of Public Health, 97*(7), 1283–1289. Doi: 10.2105/AJPH.2005.080762

Barish, R. A., Mcgauly, P. L., & Arnold, T. C., (2012). Emergency room crowding: A marker of hospital health. *Transactions of the American Clinical and Climatological Association, 123*, 304–311.

Barnett, J. C., & Berchick, E. R. Health Coverage in the U.S.: 2016. U.S. Bureau of the Census Report #P60-260. https://www.census.gov/library/publications/2017/demo/p60-260.html

Barnett, M. L., Hsu, J., & McWilliams, J. M. (2015). Patient characteristics and differences in hospital readmission rates. *JAMA Internal Medicine, 175*(11), 1803–1812. Doi:10.1001/jamainternmed.2015.4660

Beckman H. (2003). Difficult patients. In: M. D. Feldman & J. F. Christensen (Eds.), *Behavioral medicine in primary care: A practical guide* (pp. 23–32). New York: McGraw-Hill Medical.

Blair, I. V., Steiner, J. F., & Hanraner, E.P. (2011). Unconscious (implicit) bias and health disparities: Where do we go from here? *The Permanente Journal: Kaiser Permanente, 15*(2), 71–78.

Boulware, L. E., Cooper, L. A., & Ratner, L. E. (2003). Race and trust in the health care system. *Public Health Reports, 118*(4), 358–365.

Braveman, P. A., Heck, K., Egerth, S., Marchi, K. S., Dominguez, F. P., Cuffin C., Finger, K., . . . Curtis, M. (2015). The role of socioeconomic factors in black-white disparities in preterm birth. *American Journal of Public Health, 105*(4), 694–702.

Brooks-Carthon, J. M., Lasater, K. B., Rearden, J., Holland, S., & Sloane, D. M. (2016). Unmet nursing care linked to rehospitalizations among older black AMI patients: A cross-sectional study of US hospitals. *Medical Care, 54*(5), 457–465.

Burgess, D. J., Fu, S. S., & Van Ryn, M. (2004). Why do providers contribute to disparities and what can be done about it? *Journal of General Internal Medicine, 19*(11), 1154–1159.

Centers for Disease Control and Prevention (2018). *National Vital Statistics Reports, 67*(1), Births, Final Data for 2016. (Jan. 31).

Chakrabarti, A., Osborne, N. H., Rangnekar, A. S., & Mathur, A. K. (2017). The effect of hospital characteristics on racial/ethnic variation in cirrhosis mortality. *Journal of Racial and Ethnic Health Disparities, 4*(2), 243–251.

Chen, B. K., Cheng, X., Bennett, C., & Hibbert, J. (2015). Travel distances, socioeconomic characteristics, and health disparities in nonurgent and frequent use of Hospital Emergency Departments in South Carolina: A population based observational study. *BMC Health Services Research, 15*, 203.

Davis, J. L., Bynum, S. A., Katz, R. V., Buchanan, K., & Green, B. L. (2013). Sociodemographic differences in fears and mistrust contributing to unwillingness to participate in cancer screenings. *The Journal of Health Care for the Poor and Underserved, 23*(4 Suppl), 67–76. Doi: 10.1353/hpu.2012.0148.

Dickson, V. (2017). CMS says factoring patient socio-economic status into readmission penalties won't change much. Modern Health, www.modernhealthcare.com.

Englum, B. R., Hui, X., Zogg, C. K., Chaudhary, M. A., Villegas C, Bolorunduro, O. B., . . . Haider, A. H. (2016). Association between insurance status and hospital length of stay following trauma. *The American Surgeon, 82*(3), 281–288.

Fitzgerald, C. & Hurst, S. (2017). Implicit bias in healthcare professionals: A systematic review. *BMC Medical Ethics, 18*(19). doi: 10.1186/s12910-017-0179-8

Garfield, R., Damico, A., Stephens, J., & Rouhani, S. (2014). The coverage gap: Uninsured poor adults in states that do not expand Medicaid—an update. Kaiser Family Foundation.

Hasnain-Wynia, R., Baker, D. W., Nerenz, D., Feinglass, J., Beal, A. C., Landrum, C., Behal, R., & Weissman, J. S. (2007). Disparities in health care are driven by where minority patients seek care: Examination of the hospital quality alliance measures. *Archives of Internal Medicine, 167*(2), 1233–1239.

Havekes, E., Coenders, M., Dekker, K., & Van Der Lippe, T. (2014). The impact of ethnic concentration on prejudice: The role of cultural and socioeconomic differences among ethnic neighborhood residents. *Journal of Urban Affairs, 36*(5), 815–832. https://doi.org/10.1111/juaf.12091

Howell, E. A., Egorova, N. N., Balbierz, A., Zeitlin, J., & Hebert, P. L. (2016). Site of delivery contribution to black-white severe maternal morbidity disparity. *American Journal of Obstetrics and Gynecology, 215*(2), 143–52. doi: 10.1016/j.ajog.2016.05.007. Epub 2016 May 12.

Hu, J., Jordan, J., Rubinfeld, I., Schreiber, M., Waterman, B., & Nerenz, D. (2016). Correlations among hospital quality measures what "Hospital Compare" data tell us. *American Journal of Medical Quality, 32*(6), 605-610. https://doi.org/10.1177/1062860616684012.

Izugami, S., & Takase, K. (2016). Consumer perception of inpatient medical services. *PLoS One 11*(11). E0166117. Doi: 10.137/journal_pone_0166117.

Jha, A. K. (2016). The stars of hospital care: Useful or a distraction? *Journal of the American Medical Association*, 315(21), 2265–2266.

Johnstone, M., & Kanitsaki, O. (2008). Cultural racism, language prejudice and discrimination in hospital contexts: An Australian study. Diversity & Equality in Health and Care. Special Issue. http://diversityhealthcare.imedpub.com/cultural-racism-language-prejudice-and-discrimination-in-hospital-contexts-an-australian-study.php?aid=2186

Liu, S. S., Wen, Y. P., Mohan, S., Bae, J., & Becker, E. R. (2016). Addressing Medicaid expansion from the perspective of patient experience in hospitals. *Patient: Patient-Centered Outcomes Research*, 9(5), 445–455.

Manoach, S. M., & Goldfrank, L. R. (2002). Social bias and injustice in the current health care system. *Academic Emergency Medicine 9*(3), 241–247.

McCaughey, D., Erwin, C. O., & DelliFraine, J. L. (2015). Improving capacity management in the emergency department: A review of the literature, 2000–2012. *Journal of Healthcare Management*, 60(1), 63–75.

McGovern, L., Miller, G., & Hughes-Cromwick, P. (2014) The relative contribution of multiple determinants to health outcomes: Researchers continue to study the many interconnected factors that affect people's health. Health Policy Brief, August 21, 2014, Robert Wood Johnson Foundation, 4–5.

Merkow, R. P., Ju, M. H., Chung, J. W., Hall, B. L., Cohen, M. E., & Williams, M. V., . . . Bilimoria, K. Y. (2015). Underlying reasons associated with hospital readmission following surgery in the United States. *JAMA. 313*(5), 483–495.

National Center for Health Statistics. (2016). *Health, United States, 2015: With special feature on racial and ethnic health disparities*. Table 94. Hyattsville, MD.

Odd, D., Evans, D., & Emond, A. (2016). Preterm birth, age at school entry and long term educational achievement. *PLoS One 11*(5): e0155157. Doi:10.1371/journal.pone.0155157

Parikh, D. A., Chudasama, R., Agarwal, A., Rand, A., Qureshi, M. M., Ngo, T., & Hirsch, A. E. (2015). Race/ethnicity, primary language, and income are not demographic drivers of mortality in breast cancer patients at a diverse safety net academic medical center. *International Journal of Breast Cancer*. 2015. http://dx.doi.org/10.1155/2015/835074

Pham, J. C., Patel, R., Millin, M. G., Kirsch, T. D., & Chanmugam, A. (2006). The effects of ambulance diversion: A comprehensive review. *Academic Emergency Medicine*, 13(11), 1220–1227.

Phibbs, C. S., & Lorch, S. A. (2018). Choice of hospital as a source of racial/ethnic disparities in neonatal mortality and morbidity rates. JAMA Pediatrics. *172*(3), 221–223.

Premji, S. S., & Hatfield, J. (2016). Call to action for nurses/nursing. *Biomedical Research Journal*, 2016. doi: 10.1155/2016/3127543

Qualis Health. (2016). Qualis health communities for safer transitions of care (Washington). Retrieved from http://medicare.qualishealth.org/projects/care-transitions

Rangrass, G., Ghaferi, A. A., & Dimick, B. (2014). Explaining racial disparities in outcomes after cardiac surgery: The rule of hospital quality. *JAMA Surgery*, 149(3), 223–227.

Salmond, S. W., & Echevarria, M. (2017). Healthcare transformation and changing roles for nursing. *Orthopedic Nursing*, 36(1), 12–25.

Schindler, T., Koller-Smith, L., Lui, K., Bajuk, B., & Bolisetty, S. (2017). Causes of death in very preterm infants cared for in neonatal intensive care units: A population retrospective based cohort study. *BMC Pediatrics*, 17(1):59. doi:10.1186/s12887-017-0810-3

Sewell, A. A. (2015). Disaggregating ethnoracial disparities in physician trust. *Social Science Research 54*, 1–20. http://doi.org/10.1016/j.ssresearch.2015.06.020

Shavers, V. L., Fagan, P., Jones, D., Klein, W. M., Boyington, J., Moten, C., & Rorie, E. (2012). The state of research on racial/ethnic discrimination in the receipt of health care. *American Journal of Public Health*, 102(5), 953–966.

Shen, Y. C., & Hsia, R. Y. (2016). Do patients hospitalized in high-minority hospitals experience more diversion and poorer outcomes? A retrospective multivariate analysis of Medicare patients in California. *BMJ Open*, 6(3), e010263.

Shortell, S. M., & Casalino, L. P. (2008). Health care reform requires accountable care systems. *JAMA*, 300(1), 95–97.

Smith, J. K. (2007). Promoting self-awareness in nurses to improve nursing practice. *Nursing Standard, 21*(32), 47–52.

Steiner, C. A., Karaca, Z., Moore, B. J., Imshaug, M. C., & Pickens, G. (2017; Revised 2018). Surgeries in hospital-based ambulatory surgery and hospital inpatient settings, 2014: Statistical Brief #223. Healthcare Cost and Utilization Project (HCUP) Statistical Briefs (Internet). Rockville (MD): Agency for Healthcare Research and Quality (US).

Stempniak, M. (2016). Nurse watch: Nursing still the most trusted profession. Hospitals & Health Networks. Retrieved from https://www.hhnmag.com/articles/6834-nurse-watch-rns-still-the-most-trusted-profession-nurses-increasingly-move-to-community-based-settings

Tsugawa, Y., Jena, A. B., Figueroa, J. F., Blumenthal, D. M., & Jha, A. K. (2017). Comparison of hospital mortality and readmission rates for Medicare patient treated by male vs. female physicians. *JAMA Internal Medicine, 177*(2), 206–213.

U.S. Department of Health & Human Services. (2016). Office of the Assistant Secretary for Planning, Rural Hospital Participation and Performance in Value-Based Purchasing and Other Delivery System Reform Initiatives (Oct. 19). https://aspe.hhs.gov.

University of Warwick. (2016). Children born prematurely are disadvantaged at school and into adulthood but delaying school entry may not be the answer. (March 9).

Van Ryn, M., & Fu, S. S. (2003). Paved with good intentions: Do public health and human service providers contribute to racial/ethnic disparities in health? *American Journal of Public Health, 93*(2), 248–255.

Wang, H. X., Wang, J. J., Lawson, K. D., Wong, S. Y. S., Wong, M. C. S., . . . Mercer, S. W. (2015). Relationships of multimorbidity and income with hospital admission in three health care systems. *Annals of Family Medicine, 13*(2), 164–167.

Witt, W. P., Coffey, R. M., Lopez-Gonzalez, L., Barrett, M. L., Moore, B. J., Andrews, R. M., & Washington, R. E. (2016). Understanding racial and ethnic disparities in post-surgical complications occurring in U.S. hospitals. *Health Services Research, 52*(1), 220–243.

Worster, B., Bell, D. K., Roy, V., Cunningham, A., LaNoue, M., & Parks, S. (2018). Race as a predictor of palliative care referral time, hospice utilization, and hospital length of stay: A retrospective noncomparative analysis. *American Journal of Hospice and Palliative Medicine, 35*(1), 110–116.

Zhang, W., Lyman, S., Bouton-Foster, C., Parks M. L., Pan, T. J., Lan, A., & Ma, Y. (2016). Racial and ethnic disparities in utilization rate, hospital volume, and perioperative outcomes after total knee arthroplasty. *Journal of Bone & Joint Surgery, 98*(15), 1243–1252.

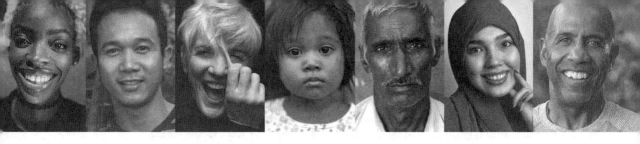

CHAPTER 11

Health Disparities in Health Insurance Markets

"He who has health, has hope; and he who has hope, has everything!"

—**Thomas Carlyle (1795–1881),** a Scottish philosopher

LEARNING OBJECTIVES

After completing this chapter, each learner will be able to:

- Summarize the structure of the health insurance market.
- Describe some of the trends that are currently taking place in the health insurance marketplace.
- Identify disparities in the health insurance market by type of insurance.
- Explain the implications of cancer as a pre existing condition for health insurance providers.
- Analyze how the operation of health insurance markets can impact healthcare disparities.

▶ Introduction

The passage of the **Affordable Care Act (ACA)** in 2010 had a number of impacts on the country's public and private health insurance markets. Perhaps most importantly, the ACA has served as a platform for reductions in health disparities by providing the uninsured with access to health care. Buchmueller, Levinson, Levy, and Wolfe (2016) confirmed that health insurance enrollment leads to decreases in healthcare disparities across all racial/ethnic subgroups. Over recent years, higher rates of health insurance coverage have coincided with the expansion of Medicaid that occurred in some states as part of the ACA (Antonisse, Garfield, Rudowitz, & Artiga, 2018). Case studies by Fletcher and Marriott (2014) of a unionized steel mill and a food processing plant suggest that although the presence of the ACA in health insurance markets may decrease healthcare disparities that are directly related to insured versus uninsured status, it may inadvertently create a new disparity issue that has been overlooked. Specifically, they suggest that to the degree that health insurance companies increase cost-sharing, currently insured workers may find themselves unable to access insurance despite their insured status. This would create a disparity in access to health care between lower and middle income workers and higher paid workers within the same organization.

Such a new disparity would conjoin currently operative differentials in the workplace. For example, Hammig, Henry, and Davis (2018) examined data from the 2010–2015 National Health Interview Survey (NHIS) and found that insurance coverage disparities between American-born workers and Mexican/Central American–born labor workers were extreme. The American-born workers were 100% more likely to have insurance coverage. The absence of health insurance coverage is a critical component of the disparity chain that can lead to severe disparities in mortality and morbidity among subgroups over time.

Hayes, Riley, Radley, and McCarthy (2015) examined data from the 2012–2013 Behavioral Risk Factor Surveillance System (BRFSS) to assess whether insurance status differences by income and racial/ethnic subgroup affected the presence of health disparities. They found that although insurance status did not have the power to completely eliminate disparities, it definitely reduced the size of disparities in the prevalence and incidence of selected illnesses and diseases.

Health insurance plays a unique role in ultimately determining health outcomes. Lee et al. (2016), in an examination of overall health outcomes of youth with below average educational outcomes, found that students without health insurance were more susceptible to depression and had lower self-ratings of wellness.

In this regard, this chapter examines the changes in health insurance markets that have occurred over recent years in order to explore their potential impact upon differential health and healthcare outcomes.

▶ Structure of the American Health Insurance System

It is often stated that the American healthcare system differs in its payment mechanisms relative to those of the American economy in general. Whereas the marketplace for clothing, automobiles, films, and other goods and services that we purchase on a day-to-day basis occurs through the interactions of only two parties—those who sell (suppliers) and those who buy (consumers)—this is not the case in the healthcare system. In order to buy most healthcare goods and services, and in order for health care providers to sell their goods and services, a third party is involved in the form of the healthcare insurance marketplace.

What exactly is health insurance?

Insurance of any type is a service that provides consumers with protection against risk. In this regard, **health insurance** can be defined as that component of the American healthcare system that assists Americans in purchasing the protection needed to prevent them from having to pay out-of-pocket costs for the full range of services and products needed in case of illness and disease treatment or illness and disease prevention.

The insurance marketplace in the United States consists of two separate marketplaces: a public insurance subsector and a private marketplace. **FIGURE 11.1** lists the components of the public insurance subsector.

As Figure 11.1 indicates, the public sector within the United States provides a wide range of healthcare insurance services. In 2014, approximately 36.5% of U.S. residents with health insurance received coverage through a public plan (National Center for Health

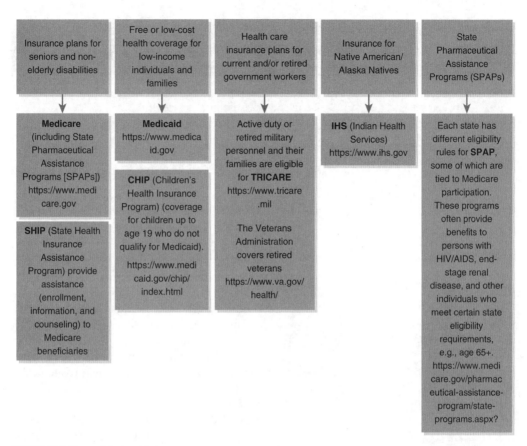

FIGURE 11.1 The public health insurance sector.

Statistics, 2016). The private insurance market provided risk protection to 66% of the healthcare marketplace (Smith and Medalia, 2015). The CDC's National Center for Health Statistics has identified a number of health insurance trends based on early release data from the 2016 National Health Interview Survey (2017) which covers data from 1997 to 2015 (**BOX 11.1**).

The data for the year 2016 presented thus far indicate that the American healthcare insurance market remains dominated by the private insurance sector. Approximately 69.2% of adults aged 18 to 64 received protection against insurance-related health disparities as a result of private insurance and 53.8% of children received such protection. Interestingly, only 20% of adults were reliant upon public-sector insurance for such protection. However, far more children (43%) were dependent upon the public sector to protect them against the type of healthcare disparities that may accrue when the individuals are uninsured.

FIGURE 11.2 provides a very loose overview of some types of private insurance. However, in many cases, each of these types of insurance may be provided by the same company.

Organizations That Provide Private Insurance

The private health insurance marketplace includes hundreds of insurers, but several

BOX 11.1 Overview of the American Health Insurance Market Based on Early Release Data from the 2016 National Health Interview Survey

- 12.3% of adults aged 18 to 64 years did not have health insurance.
- 5.0% of children younger than 18 years did not have health insurance.
- 69.0% of adults aged 18 to 64 years had access to health care via private insurance.
- 53.5% of children younger than 18 years had access to health care via private insurance.
- 20.3% of adults aged 18 to 64 had access to public health insurance.
- 43.4% of children younger than 18 years had access to public health insurance.

Date from: Tables 1.1a and 1.1b of the National Center for Health Statistics; Health Insurance Coverage, National Health Interview Survey Early Release Program 2016. Retrieved February 27, 2018, from https://www.cdc.gov/nchs/data/nhis/earlyrelease/earlyrelease201705.pdf

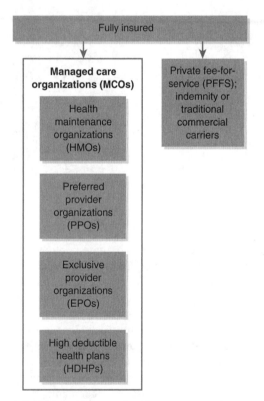

FIGURE 11.2 The private health insurance market.

companies dominate the market based upon size as measured by revenues and number of insureds. Private insurers in the United States disproportionately sell their services to employers who are providing healthcare benefits to their employees. The private health insurance market, although dominant in the United States, varies in market share by state. However, the Kaiser Family Foundation reports that in half of all states and the District of Columbia, private health insurance enrollees equaled 50% or more of all insured individuals. Yet, in the state of Utah, 60% of all insured persons were enrolled in private insurance (Kaiser Family Foundation, 2016). Interestingly, this source also reveals that three southern states had the lowest proportion of private health insurance enrollees per population at 42%. These states were Florida, Louisiana, and Mississippi.

However, America's Health Insurance Plans offers a listing of over 170 private insurance providers at https://www.ahip.org/about-us/. The National Association of Insurance Commissioners (2017) lists the top 10 health insurance companies by market share. **BOX 11.2** includes a listing of these companies.

In addition to the coverage provided by private insurance providers, a number of Americans receive healthcare insurance directly through their employer. These employers are considered as "self-insured or self-funded"

BOX 11.2 Major Private Health Insurance Providers

- UnitedHealth Group
- Kaiser Foundation
- Anthem
- Aetna
- Humana
- HCSC
- Centene
- Cigna
- Molina Healthcare
- Independence Health (Blue Cross)

Constructed by the authors with data found at The National Association of Insurance Commissioners (2017), 2016, Market Share Reports. Pg. 17. https://www.naic.org/prod_serv_alpha_listing .htm#market_share

providers. Because of the size of their workforce, the companies are able to assume the risks associated with healthcare insurance without using a private insurance company. These larger employers self-insure in order to address the healthcare needs of their employees. **BOX 11.3** lists a few of these companies.

The described listing is by no means exhaustive. There are literally thousands

of businesses and other organizations that self-insure in the country. However, insufficient data exist to determine whether disparities exist in the employer pool of companies who self-insure. Moreover, a search of the literature could not identify scholarly articles on differential health insurance outcomes between companies that self-insure and those that do not.

Panis & Brien (2017) report that self-insurance, employer-sponsored healthcare plans are a significant component in the healthcare insurance market. Utilizing data for the Form 5500 Annual Return/Report of Employee Benefit Plans, these researchers indicated that approximately 48% of the Forms 5500 filed reveal that the healthcare insurance provided was self-insurance and 7% of health care was provided as a combination of self-insurance and insurance benefits purchased from a private insurance company.

So, can smaller employers afford to self-insure?

These authors indicate that in 2014, 29% of the health insurance plans offered by companies with 100–199 employees were self-insured or mixed plan. In contrast, approximately 90% of companies with 5,000 or more employees

BOX 11.3 A Sample of Employers Who Provide Health Insurance Through Self-Funded Means

1. AT&T, Inc.	11. JC Penney Co	
2. Best Buy	12. Kraft Foods, Inc.	
3. Costco Wholesale Corporation	13. Kroger Co.	
4. David's Bridal	14. Macy's Inc.	
5. Direct TV Enterprises, LLC	15. Nestle Holdings	
6. FedEx Corporation	16. Pepsi Cola Bottling Co.	
7. General Foods, Corp.	17. Petsmart, Inc.	
8. Greyhound Bus Lines	18. Shell Energy North America, US	
9. Home Depot USA, Inc.	19. Tyson Foods	
10. Hyatt Hotels Corporation	20. UPS Freight Services	

were mixed-funded or self-insured. Diab (2018) introduces data confirming that self-insured, employer-owned health plans are becoming a dominant model in the United States healthcare insurance system. In the year 1999, an estimated 60% of employers with 200 employees or more provided healthcare insurance under the self-insured (or self-funded) model. In 2017, this number had increased to 79%—a growth rate of 31.6% (Diab, 2018).

What are the implications of this change for health disparities?

Miller (2016), using data from the Medical Expenditure Panel Survey (MEPS), revealed a decrease in the proportion of small employers who offer any type of healthcare insurance to their workers.

Can they do this legally?

Under the ACA, only employers with 50 or more full-time employees are mandated by law to provide healthcare insurance. Because small employers cannot afford to provide health insurance via self-insurance and cannot afford to purchase health insurance in the traditional private health insurance sector, this trend is accelerating. Such a trend can have adverse healthcare outcomes. Kugler et al. (2017) indicate that smaller businesses, particularly those in low-income communities, are more likely to employ low-income workers, females, and/or racial/ethnic minorities. Thus, this changing aspect of the structure of the health insurance market can potentially support health disparities.

Many healthcare administrators already work in the healthcare insurance marketplace, and a number of healthcare students will enter into this marketplace. Accordingly, it becomes appropriate to ask, "What other types of disparities exist in the health insurance sector?"

▶ Health Disparities and Health Insurance

Artiga, Young, Garfield, and Majeral (2015) identified a number of other patterns relative to disparities between public and private insurance beneficiaries. **BOX 11.4** summarizes some of these findings.

Despite disparities in the use of health insurance services, American are rejoicing because more individuals and families now have health insurance than at any other point in the country's history. For example, data from the CDC's 2016 National Health Interview Survey (NHIS) (which was published in 2017) indicate that the proportion of Americans in general who now participate in the health insurance marketplace has reached a 50-year high of 91%. As mentioned, this is the highest proportion of Americans who have ever been included in the healthcare marketplace since Medicare and Medicaid legislation was first implemented in 1965 amidst a plethora of criticism. Nevertheless, the available data must be closely examined in order to identify the types of disparities that may exist in this vital marketplace.

Disparities in Sources of Payment for Health Insurance

Disparities in the proportion of workers whose private health insurance is through employer self-insured have already been discussed. However, there are other disparities in the American health insurance marketplace. In 2016, whether through self-insured

> **Trend 1:** From 1987 to 2013, the proportion of White Americans who received their health insurance from public sources increased (**TABLE 11.1**).

BOX 11.4 General Disparities by Race/Ethnicity and by Public and Private Insurance Status

- In general, health disparities are less for racial/ethnic groups insured by Medicaid relative to private insurance. This suggests that private insurers may wish to consider adopting some of the access measures used by the Medicaid public insurance program. These strategies include case management services to assist in overcoming socioeconomic barriers to health care.
- For Medicaid enrollees, White Americans are most likely to postpone care despite having insurance. Thus, measures are needed to increase utilization rates for this group. Public health professionals may wish to take the lead in this effort.
- Interestingly, Latino Americans and African Americans who participate in the private insurance market are less likely to have a health home or a "usual source of care."
- Similarly, in the private insurance market, Latinos and African Americans are less likely to use those medical services that are covered by the insurance.
- Additionally, Hispanics/Latinos are less likely to receive preventive services. Thus, the private insurance submarket may wish to design culture-specific services to support greater participation in preventive services.
- For groups and subgroups who do not participate in the public or private insurance marketplace, White Americans are "worse off," because they are more likely to completely forego or to delay health care. Thus, special outreach is also needed for this group.

TABLE 11.1 Percentage Change from 1987 to 2013 of Americans Receiving Insurance Through Public Sources by Race/Ethnicity

Race/Ethnicity	1987	2013	% Change
White, non-Hispanic Americans	15.9%	21.3%	+33.96
African American, non-Hispanic Americans	47.2%	46.4%	−1.69
Latino/Hispanic	35.8%	42.4%	+18.43
Asian Americans	—	17.9%	—
American Indian, Alaska Native, Native Hawaiian, and Other	—	42.8%	—

Calculated from data in Health, 2016, Table 98, pg. 328.

or fully-insured, 63.7% of the population received insurance through private sources. However, data from *Health, United States, 2016 (2017)* revealed a number of other interesting trends. Specifically, an increase occurred in the percent of nearly all American subgroups who were insured through public insurance. This trend can potentially increase the public sector's financial burden thereby creating instabilities in the very health insurance marketplace which serves health disparity populations. Moreover, the data reveal that some interesting trends are a part of this shift.

As Table 11.1 indicates, disparities existed relative to the proportion of Americans who participated in insurance markets via public sources in both 1987 and 2013. Despite having the lowest percentage participation rates in the public insurance market, in 1987, White Americans had the greatest growth in participation over the period, with a 33.96% increase. In contrast, the proportion of African Americans receiving insurance coverage through the public health market decreased by 1.7%.

TABLE 11.2 describes disparities by sex. In 1987, males (23.9%) were less likely to receive health insurance through public sources than were their female counterparts (19.2%). In 2013, approximately 25.7% of females and 29.7% of males were reliant on the public sector for coverage of their healthcare costs. Moreover, the increase in participation over the 1987 to 2013 time periods was 24.27% for males but only 33.85% for females.

> **Trend 2:** Females became significantly more dependent upon public sources for health care from 1987 to 2013.

TABLE 11.2 Changes in Participation in Public Health Insurance by Sex, 1987 and 2013

Sex	1987	2013	% Change
Male	23.9%	29.7%	+24.27
Female	19.2%	25.7%	+33.85

Calculated from data in Health, 2016, Table 98, pg. 328.

In 1987, 28.6% of all Americans had no health insurance of any kind. By 2016, this percentage had dropped to 8.6% (Barnett and Berchick, 2017). Because much of the increase in the insured occurred under the 2010 ACA, the role of the public sector in paying for care increased. Today, Americans must now decide whether the improvements in life expectancy and decreased death rates that correlate with the increases in insurance coverage are consistent with their personal and collective values. **TABLE 11.3** in the following section demonstrates this point by aligning death rate disparities by state next to the % uninsured by state for persons age 18 to 64 years.

Okay, so are death rates higher in the states that report a greater percentage of uninsured persons?

Correlation or regression analyses were applied to the data in Table 11.3 to determine if death rates are higher in states with a greater percentage of uninsured persons. Thus, a correlation coefficient calculator was used to answer this question (the results are displayed at the bottom of the table). Interestingly, the correlation coefficient reveals a positive but weak association between the % of the population who are uninsured in a state and the death rates for those states ($r = 0.2510$). The weak association simply informs us that multiple variables are associated with this outcome. Moreover, the correlation is only marginally significant ($p < .0756$).

However, we also ask a different question of the data, "Is there a stronger correlation between uninsurance status and death rates in the states that selected to not expand their Medicaid insurance requirements under the ACA?" We therefore calculated the correlation between uninsured status and death rates for the 19 highlighted states. As mentioned, these are the states that did not expand Medicaid coverage under the ACA. The results

TABLE 11.3 Percentage of Uninsured, Death Rates, and Medicaid Expansion Status by State (2016)

Civilians non-institutionalized population	Percentage Uninsured (2016)[a] Independent Variable (*x*)	Death Rate per 100,000 (2016) (age-adjusted)[b] Dependent Variable (*y*)	Expanded Medicaid[c] (Yes/No) (states that did not expand Medicaid are bolded)
United States	8.6%	728.8	
Alabama	**9.1%**	**920.4**	**No**
Alaska	14.0%	745.6	Yes
Arizona	10.0%	675.8	Yes
Arkansas	7.9%	893.2	Yes
California	7.3%	619.9	Yes
Colorado	7.5%	669.5	Yes
Connecticut	4.9%	654.0	Yes
Delaware	5.7%	746.2	Yes
District of Columbia	3.9%	766.0	Yes
Florida	**12.5%**	**666.6**	**No**
Georgia	**12.9%**	**800.4**	**No**
Hawaii	3.5%	572.0	Yes
Idaho	**10.1%**	**725.0**	**No**
Illinois	6.5%	724.3	Yes
Indiana	8.1%	835.0	Yes

(continues)

	Percentage Uninsured (2016)[a]	Death Rate per 100,000 (2016) (age-adjusted)[b]	Expanded Medicaid[c] (Yes/No) (states that did not expand Medicaid are bolded)
Civilians non-institutionalized population	Independent Variable (x)	Dependent Variable (y)	
Iowa	4.3%	721.1	Yes
Kansas	**8.7%**	**756.8**	**No**
Kentucky	5.1%	938.4	Yes
Louisiana	10.3%	870.5	Yes
Maine	**8.0%**	**759.0**	**No**
Maryland	6.1%	717.6	Yes
Massachusetts	2.5%	669.0	Yes
Michigan	5.4%	785.4	Yes
Minnesota	4.1%	648.1	Yes
Mississippi	**11.8%**	**948.9**	**No**
Missouri	**8.9%**	**808.2**	**No**
Montana	8.1%	743.2	Yes
Nebraska	**8.6%**	**707.0**	**No**
Nevada	11.4%	762.6	Yes
New Hampshire	5.9%	721.5	Yes
New Jersey	8.0%	668.5	Yes
New Mexico	9.2%	753.4	Yes
New York	6.1%	640.7	Yes

TABLE 11.3 Percentage of Uninsured, Death Rates, and Medicaid Expansion Status by State (2016) *(continued)*

North Carolina	**10.4%**	**782.4**	**No**
North Dakota	7.0%	688.4	Yes
Ohio	5.6%	832.3	Yes
Oklahoma	**13.8%**	**888.4**	**No**
Oregon	6.2%	705.9	Yes
Pennsylvania	5.6%	770.1	Yes
Rhode Island	4.3%	690.1	Yes
South Carolina	**10.0%**	**829.8**	**No**
South Dakota	**8.7%**	**719.5**	**No**
Tennessee	**9.0%**	**886.3**	**No**
Texas	**16.6%**	**730.6**	**No**
Utah	**8.8%**	**714.7**	**No**
Vermont	3.7%	712.8	Yes
Virginia	**8.7%**	**715.5**	**No**
Washington	6.0%	672.0	Yes
West Virginia	5.3%	943.3	Yes
Wisconsin	**5.3%**	**717.9**	**No**
Wyoming	**11.5%**	**720.9**	**No**

r (correlation coefficient) = 0.2510

p-value = .0756

N (number) = 51

[a] Barnett, Jessica C. and Edward R. Berchick, Current Population Reports, P60-260, *Health Insurance Coverage in the United States: 2016*, pg. 19. U.S. Government Printing Office, Washington, DC, 2017.

[b] Centers for Disease Control and Prevention, National Center for Health Statistics. CDC WONDER Online Database. Underlying Cause of Death 1999–2016. Retrieved from https://wonder.cdc.gov/ on June 8, 2018.

[c1] Advisory Board (2018). Where the states stand on Medicaid expansion: 33 states, D.C. have expanded Medicaid. Retrieved from https://www.advisory.com/daily-briefing/resources/primers/medicaidmap

[c2] Kaiser Family Foundation (2018). Status of State Action on the Medicaid Expansion Decision. Retrieved from https://www.kff.org/health-reform/state-indicator/state-activity-around-expanding-medicaid-under-the-affordable-care-act/?currentTimeframe=0&sortModel=%7B%22colId%22:%22Location%22,%22sort%22:%22asc%22%7D

are quite interesting. Specifically, the second Pearson correlation coefficient was even lower ($r = 0.1031$) and the p-value was $p < .6745$. Again, this suggests that any association between uninsured status and death rates would exist as a "lagged" association.

What do you mean by "lagged"?

A **lag variable** is used when the relationship between the independent and dependent variables did not occur within the same time period.

So, why did you include this exercise?

This exercise was included because it demonstrates the iterative progress that healthcare professionals must use in seeking to formulate and test hypotheses. But, let's for a moment, return to a discussion of the shift from private to public insurance. As a part of this discussion, let's not merely examine the data by race/ethnicity and sex but by as many subgroups as can be identified.

▶ The Decline of the Private Health Market: Additional Observations

From 1984 to 2015, the national effort to improve life expectancy and reduce death rates across all groups in America co-occurred with decreases in the purchase of private insurance by *every single group and/or subgroup in America* except for Asian Americans. Indeed, these subgroups in the country have acted in their own self-interest by decreasing their participation in the private insurance market. As **TABLE 11.4** reveals, not a single subgroup in America increased their participation in the private health insurance marketplace between 1984 and 2015, other than Asian Americans.

BOX 11.5 summarizes the many subgroups in the United States who reduced their

TABLE 11.4 Changes in the Percentage of the Population with Private Insurance: 1984 and 2015			
	1984	**2015**	**% Change**
Total number (in millions)	157.5	176.6	+12.13
Total percentage of population	76.8	65.5	−14.58
Age			
Younger than 19 years	72.6	55.0	−24.24
Younger than 6 years	68.1	51.0	−25.11
6–18 years	74.8	56.7	−24.20
Younger than 18 years	72.6	54.6	−24.79
6–17 years	74.9	56.2	−24.97

18–64 years	78.6	69.7	−11.32
18–44 years	76.5	66.8	−12.68
18–24 years	67.4	64.8	−3.86
19–25 years	67.4	65.5	−2.82
25–34 years	77.4	65.1	−15.89
35–44 years	83.9	70.0	−16.57
45–64 years	83.3	73.6	−11.64
45–54 years	83.3	74.1	−11.04
55–64 years	83.3	73.1	−12.24

Sex

Male	77.3	65.4	−15.39
Female	76.2	65.6	−13.91

Sex and Marital Status

Male			
Married	85.0	78.3	−7.88
Divorced, separated, widowed	65.5	56.6	−13.59
Never married	71.3	60.6	−15.01
Female			
Married	83.8	78.0	−6.92
Divorced, separated, widowed	63.1	58.1	−7.92
Never married	72.2	60.4	−16.34

Race/Ethnicity

White only	79.9	68.2	−14.64
Black or African American only	58.1	50.6	−12.91
American Indian or Alaska Native only	49.1	41.1	−16.29
Asian only	69.9	73.8	+5.58
Native Hawaiian or other Pacific Islander only	—	—	
Two or more races	—	55.3	
Hispanic origin			
Hispanic or Latino	55.7	43.8	−21.36
Mexican	53.3	40.9	−23.26
Puerto Rican	48.4	48.0	−.83
Cuban	72.5	61.7	−14.90
Other Hispanic or Latino	61.6	47.8	−22.40
Not Hispanic or Latino	78.7	70.7	−10.17
White only	82.4	75.2	−8.74
Black of African American only	58.2	51.2	−12.03

(continues)

TABLE 11.4 Changes in the Percent of the Population with Private Insurance: 1984 and 2015 *(continued)*

	1984	2015	% Change
Age and Percent of Poverty Level			
Younger than 65 years			
Below 100	32.2	18.6	−42.24
100-199	70.3	39.8	−43.39
100-133	59.4	30.6	−48.48
134-199	75.2	45.1	−40.03
200-399	89.3	73.4	−17.81
400 or more	95.4	91.9	−3.67
Younger than 19 years			
Below 100	29.6	10.6	−64.19
100-199	73.6	30.3	−58.83
100-133	63.8	22.3	−65.04
134-199	78.4	35.5	−54.72
200-399	91.1	71.1	−21.95
400 or more	96.2	92.7	−3.64
Younger than 18 years			
Below 100	28.5	9.3	−67.37
100-199	73.9	30.1	−59.26
100-133	63.9	21.9	−65.73
134-199	78.6	35.3	−55.09
200-399	91.3	71.1	−22.12
400 or more	96.1	92.7	−3.54
18-64 years			
Below 100	35.0	24.3	−30.57
100-199	68.3	44.6	−34.70
100-133	56.6	35.4	−37.46
134-199	73.3	49.8	−32.06
200-399	88.3	74.3	−15.86
400 or more	95.2	91.8	−3.57
Geographic Region			
Northeast	80.5	70.2	−13.94
Midwest	80.6	70.1	−13.93
South	74.3	62.5	−15.88
West	71.9	62.6	−12.93
Location of Residence			
Within MSA	77.5	66.7	−13.94
Outside MSA	75.2	57.8	−23.14

Calculated based on data from National Center for Health Statistics. (2017). *Health, United States, 2016: With Chartbook on Long-term Trends in Health.* Hyattsville, MD. Table 102, p 334–335.

BOX 11.5 Subgroups That Have Decreased Their Participation in the Private Insurance Market

- All Americans in general
- Americans in every single age category
- Americans who were male
- Americans who were female
- Married, divorced, separated, widowed, and never married males
- Married, divorced, separated, widowed, and never married females
- Whites only and whites, non-Hispanic
- African Americans
- Alaska Natives
- Mexican Americans
- Puerto Rican Americans
- Cuban Americans
- Other Latinos
- Persons with incomes 400% or more above poverty
- Persons with income 200%–399% above poverty
- Persons with incomes 134%–199% above poverty
- Persons with incomes 100%–133% above poverty
- Persons with incomes below 100% of poverty
- Persons who live in the Northeast
- Persons who live in the Midwest
- Persons who live in the South
- Persons who live in the West
- Persons living outside metropolitan areas
- Persons living inside metropolitan areas

participation in the private insurance marketplace over recent years.

Given this shift away from private insurance to that provided by state and federal governments, why do so many Americans still favor repealing the ACA?

This question can only be answered by the readers.

Are you saying that the data reveal that most Americans are now on Medicaid?

No, not at all. In 2016, only 21.92% of Americans were covered through Medicaid.

Were they getting Medicare?

No, only 17.65% of Americans were receiving Medicare as of 2016 (source: https://www.ncpssm.org/our-issues/medicare/medicare-fast-facts/). However, the Health Exchanges that

were established under the ACA provided subsidies to persons with incomes up to 400% of the poverty level. In addition, all other sources of public insurance as a collective listed allowed this major shift in the health insurance market to occur.

▶ Healthcare Disparities in the Public Insurance Marketplace

Health disparities research focuses on avoidable disparities in healthcare outcomes as measured by differences in mortality and morbidity. Healthcare disparities reference differences in the healthcare treatment and services between groups and subgroups. Thus, it becomes important to ask, "What type of healthcare disparities exist in public health insurance markets?"

Medicare and Healthcare Disparities

Schneider, Zaslavsky, and Epstein (2002) examined data from the 1998 Health Plan Employer Data and Information Set (HEDIS) to determine whether racial disparities existed in terms of quality of care for those with Medicare as their insurance plan. They found that African American and White American Medicare recipients received differential treatment in terms of the following areas: (1) breast cancer screening, (2) eye examinations for persons diagnosed with and in treatment for diabetes, (3) the use of beta blockers after myocardial infarction, and (4) posthospitalization follow-up. Trivedi, Zaslavsky, and Schneider (2016) applied a multilevel regression model to a dataset consisting of 431,573 persons from 151 Medicare health plans. They identified disparities in control of blood pressure, diabetes, and cholesterol by race/ethnicity. Additionally, these Medicare plans exhibited tremendous variations on a plan-by-plan basis. Braun et al. (2015) found disparities with regard to cancer mortality rates across various demographic subgroups, but determined that the use of patient navigators could reduce these disparities in Asian and Pacific Islander Medicare beneficiaries.

Similarly, Lopez, Bailey, and Rupnow (2015) found interesting disparities in treatment outcomes of Medicare beneficiaries with type 2 diabetes. First, disparities existed in the prevalence of diabetes in Medicare beneficiaries for Latino Americans and African Americans relative to their American counterparts of European descent. In addition, treatment outcomes were not equivalent. Specifically, hypertension and diabetic retinopathy were also more common in Latino American and African American Medicare beneficiaries.

In contrast, disparate outcomes relative to **lipid metabolism** disorders or differences in the process by which fats in the body were converted to energy, and **atrial fibrillation**, or irregularities in the heart rates that affect the flow of blood in the body were more common in White Americans. Other disparities also exist among beneficiaries who are insured through Medicare. For example, 2015 data collected by the CMS, Office of Minority Health and the Rand Corporation (2017) revealed that White American women were less likely than their Hispanic American counterparts to undergo colorectal cancer screenings. Additionally, it was found that White American women were less likely than their Asian/Pacific Islander and Hispanic American counterparts to have lower HbA1c levels. Other disparities discussed in the report were also surprising. For example, disparities were found in the incidence of high-risk medication prescriptions given to elderly males. Specifically, a lower number of Asian/Pacific Islander and Hispanic American males were prescribed high-risk medications than were their African American and White American counterparts. Conversely, when data were collected for the prescriptions of high-risk medications to Medicare-covered senior women, it was found that White American women were prescribed these medications at a higher rate than their non-White counterparts.

▶ Medicaid Insurance and Healthcare Disparities

Disparities also exist in the outcomes among Medicaid healthcare beneficiaries. Indeed, an abundance of research has documented disparities in healthcare services among persons insured by Medicaid. Brunner et al. (2006) in a study of 295 children with rheumatoid arthritis obtained interesting results. They found that the Medicaid-insured children had significantly ($p < .05$) poorer outcomes than children insured by private health insurance.

Couldn't these disparities reflect differences in the progression of the disease?

Although it is true that such disparities could have reflected different baseline clinical conditions, this was not the case. The disparities persisted even when statistical techniques were applied to ensure that the study was not comparing "apples and oranges." Thus, the outcomes among the Medicaid population were "worse" than for children with private insurance. Likewise, Knight, Xie, and Mandell (2016) conducted a study of youth aged 10 to 18 years with **systemic lupus erythematosus (SLE)** and identified treatment disparities. Systemic lupus erythematosus (SLE) is a chronic disease of the immune system that involves circumstances where the body of an individual misreads healthy tissue as being infected and begins attacking itself.

Mental health disorders are relatively common among children and adults. Knight, Xie, and Mandell (2016) in an examination of data from this federal primary source of secondary data called the Medicaid Analytic eXtract database also found that there was a high correlation between children with SLE and mental health conditions. The **Medicaid Analytic eXtract (MAX)** is a set of person-level data files on Medicaid eligibility, service utilization, and payments. The MAX data are created to support research and policy analysis.

How valid are the data?

Each state's Medicaid Office serves as a central repository for data from the Medicaid and CHIP programs. The data are then standardized across states and electronically submitted to a Centers for Medicare and Medicaid Services (CMS) database that captures this data with an emphasis upon chronic illnesses. The data used in the study was for 2006–2007. Logistic regression revealed that African American youth within the population

of Medicaid insurers were less likely to be screened, diagnosed, and/or treated for mental illness. Additional examples could be cited due to the large numbers of published articles on this issue. However, the broader portrait demonstrates that health disparities within the Medicaid population are not as great as those between public and private insurance markets.

Does Medicaid show any healthcare disparities by sex?

Differences do exist by sex. Sabik, Tarazi, and Bradley (2015) discovered that geographic differences exist in breast and cervical cancer screening for women based upon whether they live in states that expanded Medicaid as requested under the ACA. Using data from the CDC 2012 Behavioral Risk Factor Surveillance System (BRFSS), logistic regression was used to determine if there were differences in cervical and breast cancer screening rates across states. The null hypothesis was rejected and the study revealed that these important medical services were accessed more often in states that did expand Medicaid than those that did not as part of the ACA.

The above example was based more on geography than sex. Are there any other examples?

There are many examples. However, as mentioned, overall, the research reveals that health disparities are generally less severe among Medicaid recipients. In 1973, the National Cancer Institute recognized that data were needed to track and analyze the nature of various types of cancers and established the Surveillance, Epidemiology and End Results (SEER). In 1992, the National Program of Cancer Registry Amendment Act was passed to collect and manage data on cancer nationwide in order to develop a **cancer registry**. Felder et al. (2016) used data from the South Carolina Central Cancer Registry to assess racial differences in access to one of the major treatments offered to women with cancer, **adjuvant hormonal therapy**, a treatment that specifically targets the hormones that are associated with the growth of breast tumors in order to reduce their levels. South Carolina is a state in which contemporary tribalism may be operative. Yet, the female Medicaid participants in this study, based upon both bivariate and multivariate analysis, did not experience any differences in use of this therapy by race/ethnicity.

▶ Healthcare Disparities in the Private Insurance Market

Researchers have compared healthcare outcomes of uninsured and Medicaid participants with those who have been treated for the same diseases through private insurance providers. Such studies indirectly address disparities. Because the race/ethnicity, income, age, and sex of these two groups of insurance beneficiaries differ, outcome comparisons between the two groups suggest disparities. However, in general, findings from such studies reveal better outcomes for those persons covered by private insurance (Dayaratna, 2012; Bisgaier and Rhodes, 2011). Gupta, Sonis, Schneider, and Villa (2018) reported that patients with head and neck cancer who had private insurance have much better outcomes than those with Medicaid, Medicare, or no insurance. Ellis et al. (2018) reported higher mortality rates for all lung cancer except for publicly insured versus privately insured patients.

Despite the shift from private to public health insurance that has occurred since the passage of the Affordable Care Act, research continues to confirm that the source of health insurance is associated with differential outcomes. Niedzwiecki, Hsia, and Shen (2018) argue that while Medicaid-insured and/or uninsured patients who had heart attacks did experience better access to some healthcare services, persons with private insurance had lower death rates and hospital readmission rates. Other research could be cited. However,

the overall finding in the research appears to support the conclusion that persons who are insured by the private sector have better health care than those who are publicly insured. Thus, the documented shift in the insurance marketplace away from private insurance may be aligned with worse healthcare and health outcomes in the future.

This is not to say that disparities do not exist in private insurance markets. Gonzales and Ortiz (2015), based on data from the American Community Survey, found disparate rates of participation in the employer-based private insurance market for same-sex couples relative to White American, opposite-sex couples. However, the study also found that White American same-sex couples had higher rates of private insurance participation than non-White same-sex couples. Shires and Jaffee (2013) reported general discrimination in insurance markets against female-to-male transgendered people.

Spencer, Roberts, and Gaskin (2015) identified another disparity across insurance types. When data were compared for Medicare, Medicaid, and privately insured hospitalized consumers, the use of multivariate regression indicated that privately insured patients had fewer adverse safety accidents.

Moreover, Siddiqui, Heney, McDougal, and Feldman (2016) completed a study of the relationship between mortality from urothelial carcinoma and type of insurance. The researchers ensured that they were not comparing "apples to oranges" by stratifying the data to reflect persons with similar genders, ages, stage of cancer, etc. They found that 1-year and 5-year mortality rates were lower for those higher socioeconomic groups who selected to use private insurance compared to lower-income groups with public insurance. In this case, the disparity chain is so complex that it is difficult to sort out the exact causes of such circumstances.

Why did several of the examples used focus on cancer when the issue at hand is health disparities and insurance?

These examples were selected simply because various types of cancers are the first or the second major causes of death for all racial/ethnic groups (Heron, 2017). Both pharmacologic and innovative surgical modalities have emerged that have reduced the progression of various carcinogenic tumors. As a result, 5-year survival rates for most cancers are considerably higher than in the past. However, health insurance markets intermediate access to these treatments.

▶ Key Facts About Cancer and Health Disparities That All Administrators in Public and Private Insurance Organizations Should Know: A Case Study

It is highly critical that healthcare administrators in the insurance sector be knowledgeable regarding cancer as a disease in general and the various disparities that can arise with regard to diagnosis and treatment. Under the ACA, insurers cannot deny coverage to persons based on preexisting conditions. This policy change places health insurance providers at greater risk of enlarged health disparities with regard to all diseases, but to cancer in particular. While actuaries include disease-specific risk data in their analyses, health insurance administrators can also benefit by remaining updated on areas in which health disparities can occur among those whom they insure. While cancer was selected as the case study for this exercise, similar research must be conducted in other disease areas. Thus, this section is designed to provide some steps that healthcare administrators in the insurance sector can take to minimize cancer-related disparities.

Recommendation 1: Know How Cancer Disparities Are Distributed Across Various Healthcare Populations

Due to the continuous efforts of the Centers for Disease Control and Prevention (CDC), the trends and patterns that characterize cancer are now well known. For example, the CDC's U.S. Cancer Statistics, contrary to popular belief, show that the incidence of cancer is greatest among White Americans and African Americans (CDC, 2014). Moreover, entities such as The National Cancer Institute, collect information and data regarding cancer-related health disparities. For example, the NCI's SEER states that the incidence of thyroid cancer per 100,000 females increased in non-Hispanic White American from 16.7617 in 2005 to 23.0033 in 2015. Moreover, their data show that there was a slight uptick for the same time frame in the incidence of myeloma among American males of Asian/Pacific Islander lineage (from 4.7567 to 4.8350). Thus, as an insurance provider enrolls an increased proportion of these two populations, the risk of disparities increases. However, African Americans experience new cancers at a rate that is *not* statistically higher than White Americans. In contrast, although cancer is the primary cause of death for Asian/Pacific Islanders, they actually have the lowest incidence of cancer of any demographic subpopulation.

However, as more health disparity populations are enrolled in public and private insurance, it is important for healthcare administrators to know that those new African American enrollees are currently more likely to *die* from cancer than their White American counterparts. The healthcare administrator should also know that both White and African American new insurance enrollees are far more likely to die from cancer than the other racial/ethnic populations served by the health insurer. For example, both White

Americans and African Americans die from cancer more often than do Native Americans/Alaskan Natives. These two groups die from cancer more often than Asian Americans. White and African American new enrollees also have a greater risk of dying from cancer than Latinos.

Isn't the probability of survival intimately linked with the type of cancer these newly insured health disparity populations have?

Healthcare managers in a State Medicaid program should know that African Americans are more likely to experience colorectal cancers. African American women experience colon and rectal cancer more often than their majority counterparts (Howlader et al., 2013). The lowest-risk female groups for colon and rectal cancer are Native Americans, Latinos, and Asian/Pacific Islanders. White females are also significantly more likely to acquire colon and/or rectal cancer than are Native American, Latina, or Asian/Pacific Islander women. The inclusion of coverage for cancer screenings and tracking of participation rates in screening can ultimately reduce insurance costs.

African American and White American women have similar lung cancer rates. The rates of lung cancer are much lower for women who are of Asian/Pacific Islander, Hispanic/Latino, and/or Native American/Alaskan Native ancestry.

White American women experience the highest rates of breast cancer. However, although White women are diagnosed with breast cancer more often than African American women, African American women *die* of breast cancer more often than White women. Similarly, although Asian American women are diagnosed with breast cancer more often than American women who are classified as Latinas, Latinas die from breast cancer more often than Asian American women. Insurance companies can ultimately lower their insurance costs by having a greater understanding of how and why these trends occur.

African American men experience prostate cancer more often than White American males and are more likely to die from this condition compared to white males. However, white males experience prostate cancer more often than Asian/Pacific Islander males. Additionally, white males die from prostate cancer more often than Asian Pacific Islander males.

If, as a healthcare administrator, your geographic area serves more Latinos, expect cervical/uterine cancers to decrease. Latinas have lower rates of cervical/uterine cancer than do African American women. Moreover, African American women die from cervical/uterine cancer more often than Latinas, whites, or other ethnicities of women.

Healthcare administrators who work in insurance programs that enroll Asian/Pacific Islanders may see increases in liver cancer. This group experiences liver cancer more often than whites and African Americans. Asian Americans also experience gastric carcinoma more often than do whites and African Americans. Indeed, Asian American males die from liver cancer and stomach cancer more often than white males. However, overall, Asian/Pacific Islanders have the lowest death rates from all cancers than any other racial/ethnic group.

Simply being familiar with these trends will allow a healthcare administrator in a health insurance program to better prepare to address health disparities in their organizations.

Recommendation 2: Healthcare Administrators in the Insurance Industry Need to Have Knowledge Regarding the Nature of the Diseases of New Enrollees with Preexisting Conditions

Despite access to some of the country's most skilled actuaries and statisticians, healthcare administrators in the insurance industry need to have a greater degree of knowledge regarding the nature of the diseases of those new enrollees with preexisting conditions. Again, the case study of cancer can be continued. Through the sponsorships of the National Cancer Institute, the CDC's U.S. Cancer Statistics, the American Cancer Society, and/or other public and private agencies, an abundance of research now exists that provides a much more detailed portrait of health disparities in the area of cancer. For example, one factor that leads to the continuation of health disparities across ethnic groups in the area of cancer is the underrepresentation of ethnic/racial groups in clinical trials.

Health administrators in insurance companies are perfectly positioned to serve as a source of referral of advanced stage cancer beneficiaries to clinical trials. One group that was quite successful in the recruitment of both Latinos and African Americans through community-based strategies was the San Francisco Bay Lung Cancer Study (Cabral et al. 2003). Researchers have found that minority groups are less likely to see themselves as at risk of cancer (Orom, Kiviniemi, Underwood, Ross, & Shavers, 2010) and may be less likely to be aware of the evidence-based risk factors that are associated with the development of cancer. Healthcare administrators in insurance companies can address this aspect of the disparity chain through an institutional program that simultaneously educates their beneficiaries on risk prevention and self-management in all diseases/illnesses. The higher death rates for certain subgroups are not only associated with later diagnosis but also with limited medical care after the cancer is in remission. Thus, ensuring the inclusion of transition services after hospitalization is also an important option.

All insurance companies seek to prevent late diagnosis through screening services. However, interventions are needed to increase the *use* of mammograms and other screening services by low-income groups and minorities.

Additionally, some low-income and/or minority females who have stage I, II, or III breast cancer are less likely to psychologically confront the true threat embodied in their disease. Rather, they seek to "find the good in their illness" For example, they may feel it is fate to have the disease and/or their Creator's will (Tomich & Helgeson, 2004). Self-management supports are needed because African Americans are less likely to maintain the recommended level of surveillance. These trends lead, of course, to higher death rates.

In particular, healthcare administrators in insurance programs must understand that health disparities in outcomes of any disease or illness will not only reflect patient-generated factors. They must ensure that quality of care differences do not exist. Healthcare administrators in insurance companies also can reduce disparities by choosing to provide supports for people with disabilities. For example, a healthcare administrator would want to ensure that deaf women know that mammogram and Pap smear services are available.

Although the insurance company will seek an enrollee's medical history, ethnic minorities may be less likely to participate in information-seeking regarding whether a genetic basis for cancer or other diseases exist in the family (Hann et al., 2017; Saulsberry and Terry, 2013). Insurance companies can lower their costs by providing much needed prevention and information.

Some studies have suggested the existence of pain management disparities among racial and ethnic minorities (Hoffman, Trawalter, Axt, & Oliver, 2016; Shah et al., 2015; Mossey, 2011). Moreover, these disparities may be related to factors involving the patient and/or healthcare provider as well as the healthcare system. Thus, minorities with cancer and other illnesses may experience greater pain. Policies to ensure equality in this area could be incorporated into quality control measures.

Chapter Summary

This chapter began with an overview of the American insurance market. In particular, it introduced data to confirm increases in the proportion of Americans with health insurance. Americans across all groups and subgroups are extremely grateful for increased access to public and private health insurance as a key component of the American healthcare system. Whether the health problem involved is a severe chronic illness such as cancer or a more acute and less threatening problem such as a sprained ankle, the expansion of health insurance market participation to the country's millions of previously excluded residents has already stimulated a new chain of causation that will result in greater life expectancy.

Nevertheless, it is important that all healthcare administrators understand current trends in the insurance marketplace. Four approaches have been used in this chapter. First, data on past and current insurance marketplace participation rates were introduced and disparities in these rates discussed. Second, the importance of inclusion in the health insurance marketplace was hypothesized by presenting data on disparities in death and insurance market nonparticipation rates by state. Third, research on health disparities in the operation of Medicaid, Medicare, and private insurance markets was briefly described. Finally, cancer disparities were used as a case study in order to make recommendations that healthcare administrators may wish to consider as they seek to address disparities in this one area of morbidity and/or in others as well.

Review Questions and Problems

1. Summarize the structure and organization of the health insurance market within the United States (250 to 350 words).
2. Based on the discussion in the chapter, apply difference analysis and identify how much each subgroup has decreased their participation in the private insurance market. Complete some research, and write a blog entry regarding this trend.
3. Supplement the data in this chapter by performing additional research and constructing a fact sheet on 10 disparities in the public and private insurance marketplaces.
4. Reviewing the materials on cancer as a case study, which of the proposed disparity-reducing strategies would you support as a current or future healthcare administrator in the health insurance sector?
5. Did any of the cancer disparity trends mentioned surprise you? If so, which ones?
6. Did learning about datasets and regression help you to understand scholarly articles on health disparities?

Key Terms and Concepts

adjuvant hormonal therapy Breast cancer treatment that specifically targets the hormones that are associated with the growth of breast tumors in order to decrease their size.

Affordable Care Act (ACA) Nicknamed "Obamacare," this statute was signed into law by Barack Obama in 2010. It was the first major overhaul of the U.S. healthcare system and expansion of coverage since the passage of Medicare and Medicaid in 1965. Among its many goals, it seeks to reduce the number of uninsured Americans.

atrial fibrillation Condition whereby irregularities in heart rate distort the flow of blood in the body.

cancer registry Registry established in 1992 as part of the National Program of Cancer Registry Amendment Act to collect and manage data on cancer nationwide.

health insurance Component of the American healthcare system that assists Americans in purchasing the protection needed to prevent them from having to pay out-of-pocket costs for the full range of services and products needed in case of illness and disease treatment or illness and disease prevention.

lag variable A lag variable is used when the relationship between the independent and dependent variables did not occur within the same time period.

lipid metabolism The process by which fats in the body are converted into energy.

Medicaid Analytic eXtract (MAX) A set of person-level data files on Medicaid eligibility, service utilization, and payments. The MAX data are created to support research and policy analysis.

systemic lupus erythematosus (SLE) Chronic disease of the immune system where the body misreads healthy tissue as being infected and begins attacking itself.

References

Antonisse, L., Garfield, R., Rudowitz, R., & Artiga, S. (2018). The effects of Medicaid expansion under the ACA: Updated findings from a literature review. Issue brief. Kaiser Family Foundation. Retrieved from https://www.kff.org/medicaid/issue-brief/the-effects-of-medicaid-expansion-under-the-aca-updated-findings-from-a-literature-review-march-2018/

Artiga, S., Young, K., Garfield, R., & Majeral M. (2015). Racial and ethnic disparities in access to and utilization of care among insured adults, Kaiser Commission on Medicaid and the Uninsured. Issue brief. Retrieved from https://www.kff.org/disparities-policy/issue-brief/racial-and-ethnic-disparities-in-access-to-and-utilization-of-care-among-insured-adults/

Bisgaier, J., & Rhodes, K. V. (2011). Auditing access to specialty care for children with public insurance. *New England Journal of Medicine, 364*, 2324–2333. DOI: 10.1056/NEJMsa1013285

Braun, K. L., Thomas, W. L., Domingo, J. L., Ponce, A., Haunani, K. P., Brazzel, S. S., . . . Tsark, J. U. (2015). Reducing cancer screening disparities in Medicare beneficiaries through cancer patient navigation. *Journal of the American Geriatrics Society, 63*(2), 365–370.

Brunner, H. I., Taylor, J., Britto, M. T., Corcoran, M. S., Kramer, S. L., Melson, P. G., Kotagal U. R., . . . Passo, M. H. (2006). Differences in disease outcomes between Medicaid and privately insured children: Possible health disparities in juvenile rheumatoid arthritis. *Arthritis Care & Research, 55*(3), 378–384.

Buchmueller, T. C., Levinson, Z. M., Levy, H. G., & Wolfe, B. L. (2016). Effect of Affordable Care Act on racial and ethnic disparities in health insurance coverage. *American Journal of Public Health, 106*(8), 1416–1421.

Cabral, D. N., Napoles-Singer, A. M., Mike, R., McMillon, A., Sisow, J. D., Wensch, M. R., . . . Wiencke, J. K. (2003). Population and community-based recruitment of African Americans and Latinos: The San Francisco Bay Area Lung Cancer Study. *American Journal of Epidemiology, 158*(3), 272–279.

Centers for Disease Control and Prevention. (2012). Behavioral Risk Factor Surveillance System (BRFSS) Prevalence and Trends Data, 2012 by state. Retrieved from https://www.cdc.gov/brfss/brfssprevalence/index.html

Centers for Disease Control and Prevention. (2018) Cancer Prevention and Control, Cancer Data and Statistics. Retrieved from https://www.cdc.gov/cancer/dcpc/data/index.htm

CMS Office of Minority Health and RAND Corporation. Racial and Ethnic Disparities by Gender in Health Care in Medicare Advantage (2017). 12, 25. Baltimore, MD.

Clarke, T. C., Norris, T., & Schiller, J. S. (2017). Early release of selected estimates based on data from 2016 National Health Interview Survey. National Center for Health Statistics. Retrieved from https://www.cdc.gov/nchs/data/nhis/earlyrelease/earlyrelease201705.pdf

Dayaratna, K. D. (2012) Studies Show: Medicaid Patients Have Worse Access and Outcomes than the Privately Insured. Heritage Foundation Backgrounder. No. 2740. Retrieved from http://thf_media.s3.amazonaws.com/2012/pdf/bg2740.pdf

Diab, A. (2018). American employers are in the healthcare business. Collective Health, https://blog.collectivehelath.com

Ellis, C., Canchola, A. J., Spiegel, D., Ladabaum, U., Haile, R. & Gomez, L. (2018). Trends in cancer survival by health insurance status in California from 1997 to 2014, *JAMA Oncology* 4(3), 317–323. doi: 10.1001/jamaoncol.2017.3846.

Felder, T. M., Do, D. P., Lu, Z. K., Lal, L. S., Heiney, S. P., & Bennett, C. L. (2016). Racial differences in receipt of adjuvant hormonal therapy among Medicaid enrollees in South Carolina diagnosed with breast cancer. *Breast Cancer Research and Treatment, 157*(1), 193–200.

Fletcher, J., & Marriott, J. (2014). Beyond the market: The role of constitutions in health care system convergence in the United States of America and the United Kingdom. Symposium: The buying and selling of health care. *Journal of Law, Medicine, & Ethics, 42*(4), 455–474.

Gonzales, G., & Ortiz, K. (2015). Health insurance disparities among racial/ethnic minorities in same-sex relationships: An intersectional approach. *American Journal of Public Health, 105*(6), 1106–1113.

Gupta, A., Sonis, S. T., Schneider, E. B., & Villa, A. (2018). Impact of the insurance type of head and neck patients on their hospitalization utilization patterns. *Cancer, 124*(4), 760–768. doi: 10.1002/cncr.31095

Hammig, B., Henry, J., & Davis, D. (2018). Disparities in health care coverage among U.S. born and Mexican/Central American born labor workers in the U.S. *Journal of Immigrant and Minority Health.* https://doi .org/10.1007/s10903-018-0697-6

Hann, K. E. J., Freeman, M., Fraser, L., Waller, J., Sanderson, S. C., Rahman, B., . . . Lanceley, A. (2017). Awareness, knowledge, perceptions, and attitudes towards genetic testing for cancer risk among ethnic minority groups: A systematic review. *BMC Public Health, 17*(1), 503. doi: 10.1186/s12889-017-4375-8.

Hayes, S. L., Riley, A., Radley, D. C., & McCarthy, D. (2015). Closing the gap: Past performance of health insurance in reducing racial and ethnic disparities in access to care could be an indication of future results. Issue brief. Commonwealth Fund, pub. 1805, *5.*

Heron, M. Deaths: Leading causes for 2015. National Vital Statistics Reports; vol 66 no 5. Table 1, 24–61. Hyattsville, MD: National Center for Health Statistics. 2017.

Hoffman, K. M., Trawalter, S., Axt, J. R., & Oliver, M. N. (2016). Racial bias in pain assessment and treatment recommendations, and false beliefs about biological differences between blacks and whites. *PNAS,* DOI: 10.1073/pnas.1516047113

Howlader, N., Noone, A. M., Krapcho, M., Garshell, J., Neyman, N., Altekruse, S., . . . Tatalovich, Z. (2013). SEER Cancer Statistics Review, 1975–2010. [Based on the November 2012 SEER data submission, posted to the SEER website, April 2013.]. Bethesda, MD: National Cancer Institute.

Kaiser Family Foundation (2016). Health Insurance Coverage of the Total Population. All states. https:// www.kff.org/other/state-indicator/total-population/? currentTimeframe=0&sortModel=%7B%22colId%22 :%22Location%22,%22sort%22:%22asc%22%7D

Knight, A. M., Xie, M., & Mandell, D. S. (2016). Disparities in psychiatric diagnosis and treatment for youth with systemic lupus erythematosus: Analysis of a national U.S. Medicaid sample. *Journal of Rheumatology, 43*(7), 1427–1433.

Kugler, M., Michaelides, M., Nanda, N., & Agbanyani, C. (2017). Entrepreneurship in low-income areas. IMPAQ International LLC for the Office of Advocacy, U.S. Small Business Administration under contract number SBAHQ-15-M-0150. Sept. No. 437.

Lee, J. O., Kosterman, R., Jones, T. M., Herrenkohl, T. I., Rhew, I. C., Catalano, R. F., & Hawkins, J. D. (2016).

Mechanisms linking high school graduation to health disparities in young adulthood: A longitudinal analysis in the rate of health behaviors, psychosocial stressors, and health insurance. *Public Health, 13,* 61–69.

Lopez, J. M. S., Bailey, R. A., & Rupnow, M. F. T. (2015). Demographic disparities among Medicare beneficiaries with Type 2 diabetes mellitus in 2011: Diabetes prevalence, comorbidity and hypoglycemic events. *Population Health Management, 18*(4), 283–289.

Miller, S. (2016). Small businesses are dropping health coverage: Large employers hold steady. Society for Human Resource Management, Aug. 4. https://www .shrm.org.

Mossey, J. M. Defining racial and ethnic disparities in pain management. (2011). *Clinical Orthopaedics and Related Research. 469*(7), 1859–70. doi: 10.1007 /s11999-0111770-9.

National Association of Insurance Commissioners. (2017). 2015 Market Share Reports for the Top 125 Accident and Health Insurance Groups and Companies by State and Countrywide. Retrieved from http://www.naic .org/prod_serv/MSR-HB-16.pdf

National Cancer Institute. Examples of Cancer Disparities. Cancer health disparities: Did you Know? Retrieved from https://www.cancer.gov/about-cancer/understanding /disparities#ui-id-2).

National Center for Health Statistics. (2016). *Health, United States, 2015: With special feature on racial and ethnic health disparities.* Hyattsville, MD.

National Committee to Preserve Social Security & Medicare. (2018, April). Medicare Fast Facts. Retrieved June 25, 2018, from https://www.ncpssm.org/our -issues/medicare/medicare-fast-facts/.

National Institutes of Health, National Cancer Institute. Surveillance, Epidemiology, and End Results Program. https://seer.cancer.gov/ Fast Stats. Interactive Tool using 2000-2015 (SEER 18). Accessed June 9, 2018.

Niedzwiecki, M. J., Hsia, R. Y., & Shen, Y. C. (2018). Not all insurance is equal: Differential treatment and health outcomes by insurance coverage among nonelderly adult patients with heart attack. *Journal of the American Heart Association, 7*(11). doi: 10.1161 /jaha.117.008152.

Orom, H., Kiviniemi, M. T., Underwood, W., Ross, L., & Shavers, V. L. (2010). Perceived cancer risk: Why is it lower among non-whites than whites? *Cancer Epidemiology, Biomarkers and Prevention, 19*(3), 746–754.

Panis, C. W. A., & Brien, M. J. (2017). Self-Insured Health Benefit Plans 2017: Based on Filings through Statistical Year 2014. Advanced Analytical Consulting Group, 1–39. Retrieved from https://www.dol.gov/sites/default /files/ebsa/researchers/statistics/retirement-bulletins /annual-report-on-self-insured-group-health-plans -2017-appendix-b.pdf

Sabik, L. M., Tarazi, W. W., & Bradley, C. J. (2015). State Medicaid expansion decisions and disparities in women's cancer screening. *American Journal of Preventive Medicine*, *48*(1), 98–103.

Saulsberry, K., & Terry, S. F. The need to build trust: a perspective on disparities in genetic testing. *Genetic Testing and Molecular Biomarkers*, *17*(9), 647–648. doi: 10.1089/gtmb.2013.1548

Schneider, E. C., Zaslavsky, A. M., & Epstein, A. M. (2002). Racial disparities in the quality of care for enrollees in Medicare managed care. *JAMA*, *287*(10), 1288–1294.

Shah, A. A., Zogg, C. K., Zafar, S. N., Schneider, E. B., Cooper, L. A., Chapital, A. B., . . . & Castillo, R. C. (2015). Analgesic access for acute abdominal pain in the emergency department among racial/ethnic minority patients: A nationwide examination. *Medical care*, *53*(12), 1000–1009.

Shires, D. A., & Jaffee, K. (2015). Factors associated with health care discrimination experiences among a national sample of female-to-male transgender individuals. *Health & Social Work*, *40*(2), 134–141.

Siddiqui, M. M., Heney, N. M., McDougal, W. S., & Feldman, A. S. (2015). Disparities in overall and urothelial carcinoma specific mortality associated with healthcare insurance status. *Bladder*, *2*(1), e10.

Smith, J. C., & Medalia, C. (2015). *U.S. Census Bureau, Current Population Reports, P60–253, Health Insurance Coverage in the United States: 2014*. Washington, DC: U.S. Government Printing Office.

Spencer, C. S., Roberts, E. T., & Gaskin, D. J. (2015). Differences in the rates of patient safety events by payer: Implications for providers and policymakers. *Medical Care*, *53*(6), 524–529.

Tomich, P. L., & Helgeson, V. S. (2004). Is finding something good in the bad always good? Benefit finding among women with breast cancer. *Health Psychology*, *23*(1), 16–23.

Trivedi, A. N., Zaslavsky, A. M., Schneider, E. C., & Ayanian, J. Z. (2006). Relationship between quality of care and racial disparities in Medicare health plans. *Journal of the American Medical Association*, *296*(16), 1998–2004.

U.S. Cancer Statistics Working Group. *United States Cancer Statistics: 1999-2014 Incidence and Mortality Web-based Report*. Atlanta: U.S. Department of Health and Human Services, Centers for Disease Control and Prevention and National Cancer Institute; 2017. Retrieved from http://www.cdc.gov/uscs

U.S. Census Bureau. (n.d.). 1-Year American Community Survey. Retrieved from https://factfinder.census.gov/faces/nav/jsf/pages/searchresults.xhtml?refresh=t

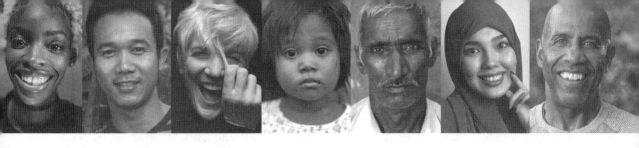

CHAPTER 12

Healthcare Disparities in Long-Term Care Institutions

"Count your age by friends, not years. Count your life by smiles, not tears."

—**John Lennon**, an English singer, songwriter, and a co-founder of the Beatles

▶ Introduction

Since the nineteenth century, a plethora of medical advances have expanded knowledge of disease and illness and exponentially increased the number and nature of life-prolonging treatment modalities. Relatively simple technologies such as the electron microscope, as well as more complex processes such as the development of techniques for the successful transplantation of organs and tissues, have conjoined to extend longevity and, consequently, to create magnified growth in the elderly population. Although the medical advances of the nineteenth and twentieth centuries have successfully expanded the life span of the American population, neither the most refined surgical techniques nor the most exciting oncological and/or virological advances have been sufficient to eliminate the full impact of aging.

Whether the aging process occurs through interval cell damage as a consequence of free radicals and/or radiation (Amarya, Singh, & Sabharwal, 2015; Harman, 1956) and/or in the event systematic immunological changes occur (Wang & Casolaro, 2014), it is clear that aging creates physical and psychological conditions that are both medically and surgically irreversible (Faragher, 2015; Schneider & Reid, 1996). Of importance to our discussion is that aging brings an increased need for both medical and nonmedical services.

Because more than 80% of elderly persons suffer from at least one chronic illness (Ward, Schiller, & Goodman, 2014) and, consequently, require substantially more healthcare services than their nonelderly counterparts, both researchers and policy makers have primarily focused on health issues that are specific to the aging process. Such a focus, however, has obscured the fact that the aging process limits the ability of the elderly to execute activities associated with daily living (Collerton et al., 2012; Hayflick, 1993). Yet, significant numbers of elderly persons are limited in their ability to carry out activities associated with daily living (Quick-Stats, 2016). A study by Harris-Kojetin, et al. (2016) reported that in 2014, 41% of elderly people who were receiving long-term care of some kind required help with a minimum of one daily living activity. Heart conditions, diabetes mellitus, asthma, and arthritis lead the list of diseases and illnesses that may affect the ability of the elderly to perform daily living activities (Mielenz et al., 2013; Woods et al., 2016). More recently, Alzheimer's, as well as other forms of dementia, have been added to this listing of problems (Yu, Mathaison, & Lin, 2016; Hoffman, et al., 2014).

The long-term care system has developed over time as the infrastructure for the delivery of health-related services to those who have age-related and/or other disabilities. Over the next few decades, as the U.S. population continues to age, the populations requiring long-term care will increase. Additionally, the elderly and disabled population is diverse. It serves various subgroups including African Americans, Asians, and other races/ethnicities; sexual minorities; religious minorities; various socioeconomic groups; and so on. Females, in particular, are disproportionately served by the long-term care industry (Harris-Kojetin et al., 2016). Moreover, the U.S. Bureau of the Census (March 13, 2018) reveals that based upon projected population trends, the older population will exceed the number of children in the United States within twelve or fewer years. Older women will be over-represented in this growth pattern. As the U.S. population continues to become more diverse, so will the population served by the long-term care industry.

The projected demographic changes in the composition of the elderly and/or disabled population complicate the service needs of those who are in need of long-term care services. Martinovich (2017) highlights trends on the type of inequalities in health, income, employment, and/or other areas that characterize key subgroup populations in the United States, including the elderly. First, most non-majority subgroups are, independent of age, significantly poorer than their majority counterparts (Semega, Fontenot, & Kollar, 2017). Second, some subgroups have higher rates of mortality and morbidity than majority subgroups (Xu, 2017). Indeed, as a consequence of subgroup differences in access to health care, lifestyle, and other factors, significant differences in mortality rates exist among subgroups. When racial/ethnic subgroup status is compounded by low socioeconomic status, the probability of disease, illness, or death is exponentially increased thereby disproportionately affecting the representation of these groups among those Americans who seek long-term care services (Williams, Mohammed, Leavell, & Collins, 2010; Hayward, Crimmins, Miles & Yu, 2000). Moreover, data from the Congressional Budget Office (2016) indicate that in 2015, approximately 6 million persons age 65 and over were Medicaid as well as Medicare enrollees as a result of their low-income status.

More recently, a number of questions have emerged with regard to health care associated with age and aging. For example, to what degree "should" the healthcare community engage in research activities designed to expand the length and quality of human life? Does an ontological framework that is built upon improving the human condition support healthcare research that is designed to radically extend the years of human life? And, if such expansions of the life span occur, would disparities exist in access to the medical technology and/or yet-to-be-derived pharmaceutical products that will successfully achieve cellular immortality?

The field of health and healthcare disparities is currently insulated from addressing such futuristic notions. Rather, the question becomes, "What are the processes, institutions, and care networks available to the aging and/or the disabled in the present and near future, and do these systems and their personnel deliver differential health care to those who utilize such services?" Thus, queries such as those listed in **BOX 12.1** become relevant.

This chapter does *not* answer each of the questions presented in Box 12.1. The questions are provided to show how important it is for a current or future healthcare administrator, public health professional, or clinician to be able to formulate key disparity questions.

▶ Overview of the Long-Term Care Industry

Long-term care refers to medical and non-medical services that are provided in order to help people with age-related limitations and/or disabilities to maximize their physical, social, mental, psychological, and spiritual outcomes despite the irreversibility and progression of their disabling physical and/or cognitive status.

The long-term care industry in the United States has a number of components. Harris-Kojetin et al. (2016) in a National Centers for Health Statistics 2016 report provide descriptive data on the long-term care industry for 2013–2014. **TABLE 12.1** provides an overview of key components of the long-term care industry for that data collection period.

BOX 12.1 Key Questions on Healthcare Disparities in Long-Term Care

Do unfavorable disparities exist in terms of:

- Access to long-term care for persons age 60 or older and/or to other fragile groups or subgroups?
- The impact of the caregiving activities upon the mental, physical, and financial health of various subgroups?
- The relative role of formal versus informal caregiving among key subgroups?
- The rates of utilization of available long-term services by selected subgroups?
- The mean length of time for the elderly persons from subgroups to transition from informal to formalized caregiving?
- The causes and correlates of the transition process by subgroup?
- The degree of congruence between the level of services provided and the needs of the served populations by subgroup?
- Long-term care trends and patterns by subgroup?
- The probability that a frail elderly person and/or other disabled individual has access to appropriate services by subgroup?
- The probability of elder abuse?

TABLE 12.1 Structure of the Long-Term Care Industry, 2013–2014

Service or Setting	Number of People Served Per Year[a]	Number of Providers[b]
Community-based providers	Hospices serve 1,340,700 patients per year.	4,000
	Adult day services serve approximately 282,200 participants per year.	4,800
	Home health agencies serve approximately 4,934,600 patients per year.	12,400
Quasi-institutional providers	Assisted living and other residential care facilities serve approximately 835,200 residents per year.	30,200
Institutional providers	Nursing homes serve an estimated 1,369,700 residents per year.	15,600

[a] Harris-Kojetin, L., Sengupta, M., Park-Lee, E., Valverde, R., Caffrey, C., Rome, V., & Lendon, J. (2016). Long-term care providers and services users in the United States: Data from the National Study of Long-Term Care Providers, 2013–2014. *Vital Health Statistics, 3*(38), 34.

[b] Harris-Kojetin, L., Sengupta, M., Park-Lee, E., Valverde, R., Caffrey, C., Rome, V., & Lendon, J. (2016). Long-term care providers and services users in the United States: Data from the National Study of Long-Term Care Providers, 2013–2014. *Vital Health Statistics, 3*(38), 102.

▶ Informal Caregiving: An Overview

Data from a joint report of the National Alliance for Caregiving (NAC) and the American Association of Retired Persons (AARP) indicate that in 2015 approximately 43.5 million Americans were family and/or informal caregivers (AARP Public Policy Institute & National Alliance for Caregiving, 2015). Moreover, according to the report, 34.2 million of these individuals cared for an individual age 50 years or older including the frail elderly or disabled and/or those with dementia or cognitive problems. Although caregiving by its very nature tends to be burdensome, it may be particularly stressful for caregivers who are also employed full or part-time. Given the hours devoted to paid work and caregiving, few waking hours are left to attend to other activities of life. Additionally, because only

a few caregivers live with their frail relative or friend, the commuting process further marginalizes the individual's remaining time. Although some caregivers manage to maintain this strenuous schedule for decades, the AARP/NAC report indicates that the mean length of time of informal caregiving is approximately 4 years.

The costs to caregivers can be enormous. Another report by the AARP states that various subgroups spend 9% to 44% of their annual income on caregiving (Rainville, Skufca, & Mehegan, 2016). Wages, Social Security benefits foregone, and other workplace-related losses were as high as $659,139 per person over the lifetime for caregivers (MetLife Mature Market Institute, 1999). More recent estimates place this amount even higher (Kaufman, Lee, Vaughon, Unuigbe, & Gallo, 2018).

Additionally, when queried regarding their own health status, nearly a quarter of caretakers for the aged assessed their health as below average in the AARP/NAC report. In some respects, the impact of caretaking on a person's mental health far exceeds the physical health costs. Caretakers are more apt to be diagnosed as depressed (Gallagher, Rose, Rivera, Lovett, & Thompson, 1989; Kaufman et al., 2018). Consequently, this unique population segment may become reliant on psychotropic drugs to treat their depression.

In spite of these high personal costs, relatively few support services are available to caregivers. Many primary caregivers access no external support services. Of those who do receive support services, only a small percentage solicit formalized caretaker services. As the U.S. population ages, the entire caregiver system will require numerous supports in order for this informal caretaking system to be strengthened (Schulz & Tompkins, 2010).

Because of the increase in informal caretaking, customized supports may be needed for persons who care for seniors with various impairments. Financial supports may also be required to offset some of the financial losses that are associated with caregiving. Public health programs may be needed that specifically address the disproportionate impact of caregiving upon women. Indeed, social workers may need to customize referrals and other available supports to reflect the differential impact of caregiving upon spouses versus adult children. And, for all caregivers, programs are needed to ameliorate the adverse impact of extended caregiving on their health.

▶ Disparities in Caretaking Among Subgroup Populations

National data on the elderly are inclusive of some data on caretaking among various subgroups. Data from the report, Caregiving in the U.S. 2015 by the National Alliance for Caregiving and AARP Public Policy Institute

(2015), reveal some interesting differences by race/ethnicity, as summarized in **TABLE 12.2**.

There are also age characteristics of adult caregivers to consider as provided in **TABLE 12.3**.

The data in Table 12.2 confirm that informal caretaking is more prevalent among certain racial/ethnic subgroups. For example, 16.9% of White Americans were caregivers, but 20.3% of African Americans were involved in various levels of informal caregiving. Thus, African Americans were 20.11% more likely to be involved in informal caretaking than were their white counterparts. The rate for Latino Americans was even higher at 21%. Approximately 19.7% of Asian Americans were involved in informal caretaking. Therefore, Asian Americans were 16.5% more likely to provide informal care than were White Americans.

Table 12.2 also reveals differences in the percentage of time devoted to caretaking. Approximately 57% of African American caregivers spent 30 hours per week performing various caretaking duties (percentage difference 71.7%). In contrast, 45% of Latino Americans provided high-intensity informal care (percentage difference 36.36%). For White Americans, 33% spent approximately 20 hours per week in informal caregiving. Finally, an estimated 30% of Asian Americans spent 16 hours per week providing informal caregiving.

Disparities in caregiving also exist by sex. Approximately 75% of persons who place their own health at risk through informal caregiving are female (AARP and NAC, 2015). Moreover, even when males serve as informal caretakers, they devote up to 50% less time in caretaking activities than do females. Additionally, the same dataset reveals that males are more likely to perform tasks associated with instrumental activities of daily living such as assistance with home repairs, finance, transportation, etc. In contrast, females assume the caretaking tasks associated with fragilities in the activities of daily living, such as toileting needs, bathing, etc.

Gender minorities play a critical role in informal long-term care. The 2010 MetLife

TABLE 12.2 Informal Caregiving Differences by Race/Ethnicity, 2015

	Percentage Providing Long-Term Care	Mean Age of Caregivers	Difference in Mean Hours Per Week Spent on High-Burden Caregiving
Whites (Reference Group)	16.9%	52.5 years	33% spend a mean of 20 hours per week
African Americans	20.3%	44.2 years	57% spend a mean of 30 hours per week
Percentage Difference from Reference Group	20.11%	15.8 years	72.72% higher than reference group
Latino/Hispanics	21%	42.7 years	45% spend a mean of 30 hours per week
Percentage Difference from Reference Group	24.26%	18.66 years	36.36% higher than reference group
Asian Americans	19.7%	46.6 years	30.0% spend a mean of 16 hours per week
Percentage Difference from Reference Group	16.56%	11.23 years	9.09% lower than reference group

Calculated by Authors from data found at National Alliance for Caregiving and AARP (2015) Caregivers in the U.S. https://www.aarp.org/content/dam /aarp/ppi/2015/caregiving-in-the-united-states-2015-report-revised.pdf

TABLE 12.3 Informal Caregiving by Age

Age Characteristics	
Mean age of caregivers (years):	49.2
Age groups (%)	
18–49 years	48%
65 years and older	34%

publication, "Still Out, Still Aging: Study of Lesbian, Gay, Bisexual, and Transgender Baby Boomers," found that LGBT males provided approximately 41.38% more hours of care per week than did males with traditional sexual identities. However, Frederickson-Goldsen et al. (2011) determined that this group of Americans have greater concerns regarding accessing care as the aging process occurs.

Are there disparities in informal caretakers who commit elder abuse?

The National Council of Aging (2018) estimates that approximately 10% of Americans age 60 years and older have been victims of elder abuse or neglect and that in 60% of these cases the abuser is a family member. Moreover, in approximately 66.66% of the cases, the abusers are not merely family members, but are either the spouse or the child of the person who has been or is being abused. Although white females have a higher rate of abuse than other groups, the actual magnitude of elder abuse disparities has not been fully characterized because of underreporting and faulty measurement in data collection systems.

How can caregiving be better supported?

Not only are new and qualitatively different programs needed to support informal caregivers, outreach and education interventions may be needed to encourage caregivers to more fully utilize current and prospective programs. The evidence is quite clear: Caregivers who access support services experience lower levels of depression and fewer adverse effects in general (Sibalija, 2017; Potter, 2017). Indeed, one study found that even access to information about caregiver support services through telephonic means alone had a positive impact upon depression of participating caregivers (Tremont et al., 2014). **Respite care** can also reduce adverse outcomes among caregivers. However, respite care is underutilized. But, when caregivers do utilize support services, the institutionalization of the elderly is less likely. Adult day care is correlated with similar outcomes (Klein et al., 2016).

Although the use of respite care is highly correlated with positive impacts on both caregivers and the frail elderly, interventions as straightforward as counseling can also provide measurable benefits (Lopez-Hartmann, Wens, Verhoeven, & Remmen, 2012). Likewise, group counseling through caregiver support groups is also associated with positive outcomes (Senanarong et al., 2004). Thus, outreach by public health professionals or outreach through other mechanisms is needed to increase the use of caretaker support systems in various communities. Additionally, healthcare providers can

inform families of such options. In order to develop such systems, however, more information is needed regarding the dynamics of caregiving at the community level.

▶ Nursing Homes

Despite the criticality of informal care, community-based care options, and quasi-institutional care, nursing homes are, in some respects, the very foundation of the long-term care industry. Accordingly, the country's nursing home industry is disproportionately financed through public funding. Moreover, given the high level of vulnerability of the clients, the nursing home industry is also highly regulated. Boccuti, Casillas, and Neuman (2015) reported that as of 2015 more than 15,500 nursing homes were in operation in the United States. These healthcare facilities are licensed at the state level and most are also certified to deliver care via the Centers for Medicare and Medicaid Services (CMS). In addition to being one of the most highly regulated components of the healthcare system, nursing homes also differ in another important aspect. Although the healthcare industry includes a disproportionate number of nonprofit healthcare institutions, this is not the case with nursing homes. The more than 1.3 million residents of nursing homes are served by an industry in which 70% or providers operate as for-profit organizations.

A plurality of nursing homes (52%) are moderate in size, containing 60 to 120 beds. Approximately 29% of nursing homes exceed this range in bed size, and 19% have fewer than 60 beds (Boccuti, et al., 2015).

Quality of Care

Similar to hospitals, hospices, and other healthcare institutions, the quality of care provided by certified nursing homes is regularly assessed and made publicly available through Nursing Home Compare. Nursing

Home Compare (https://www.medicare.gov/nursinghomecompare/) is a CMS database that includes data collected as part of its certification process. The CMS requires all nursing homes that it certifies to meet a comprehensive set of standards that are designed to ensure that the best quality of care is provided to each patient. It uses a 5-star rating system, with five stars being the highest rating possible. In order to assess whether these standards are being met, a team of health inspectors makes unannounced visits to nursing homes. The health inspectors are assigned at the state level. This is because CMS contracts with state agencies for nursing home oversight.

Research by Boccuti et al. (2015) determined that in 2015 nearly 40% of nursing home residents lived in facilities that had combined ratings of only one or two stars and approximately 41% resided in nursing homes that had ratings of four or five stars.

Couldn't the lower ratings simply indicate that some residents were merely "sicker"?

Not really, the rating system takes the patient mix into consideration. **Patient mix** refers to the characteristics of the patients served by a healthcare facility, including the severity of the patients' health needs. Patient mix identifiers may also include patient demographics and socioeconomic characteristics.

▶ Healthcare Disparities in Long-Term Care: The Case of Nursing Homes

With an American population that is projected to consist of 20% seniors by 2050, the imperative to strengthen the range of services that comprise long-term care is a critical one. Whether the objective of the intervention is the informal care system, the community-based service system, and/or the quasi-institutional care system, it becomes important to determine whether conditions that adversely affect patients/clients in any of these systems are operative across subgroups.

An abundance of data reveal that, in some respects, consumers of long-term care services may be at a higher risk of remediable differences in care because of the multiple intersectionalities that characterize the aged and/or those with disabilities. Harley and Teaster (2018), for example, describe some of the healthcare barriers impacting females, older adults, LGTB populations, and persons in rural communities. These access and quality issues are enlarged when a single individual is included in each of these groupings. Moreover, disparities can occur at many points in long-term care. For example, Haines et al. (2018) in an analysis of data for 2,966,444 patients found that statistically significant differences existed for the transfer of Asian Americans, African Americans, and Latino Americans to hospice care relative to their White American counterparts even when the data were adjusted to reflect the differences in initial circumstances.

It is interesting, however, that providers may, in an effort to prevent disparities, always interpret decreases in disparities as a positive sign. However, this may not always be the case. For example, disparities do exist in the treatment of hypertension (Ferdinand et al., 2017). Thus, a nursing home administrator may be anxious to ensure that such differences do not continue in their facility. However, Goodwin (2018) notes that if blood pressure measures decrease among the elderly without the use of a medical intervention, it is a sign of impending death. Yet, a healthcare administrator in a long-term care facility will, without consultation with a clinician, view such reductions in blood pressure control as indicative of the narrowing of healthcare disparities.

As one reviews subgroup disparities in health care in the United States, it is again important to recognize that subgroup differences in long-term care also extend worldwide. For example, Dahlberg, Berndt, Lennartsson, and Schon (2017) reported on differences in home-based, long-term care services by gender, socioeconomic status, parental status, and living status in Sweden. Specifically, the study revealed that the women participants relied less on informal care and more on formal care than did males.

Disparities research in the United States is oftentimes so focused on racial/ethnic and gender subgroup differences that the statistical data are not analyzed to include other differentials in care that are also operative. For example, disparities in falls occur between those with sight impairments and those without (Brundle et al., 2015). Long-term care disparities are not only characterized by racial/ethnic, gender, and/or socioeconomic subgroups. Some disparities, for example, occur between the aged and the nonaged. One area in which age-based remediable disparities have been documented is in the area of oral health. Kohli et al. (2017) summarize research regarding documented differences in oral health care by age. They then propose a public health training program for long-term care administrators, clinicians, and informal caregivers to reduce such differentials.

Does CMS report healthcare disparities in nursing homes on Nursing Home Compare?

No, healthcare disparities are not routinely reported by Nursing Home Compare. However, a large body of research does describe some of the types of disparities that researchers have identified as characteristic of the nursing home market (Konetzka & Werner, 2009).

How accurate are these studies?

Like all research, studies on healthcare disparities in nursing homes vary in quality. For example, Grabowski and McGuire (2009) argued that although a large body of research published over 2003–2008 identified disparities by race/ethnicity in nursing home outcomes, these studies failed to distinguish two sets of confounding variables.

What do you mean by "confounding variables"?

Confounding variables are unforeseen "extraneous" variables that affect the dependent and independent variables. Thus, a confounding variable distorts or renders the study inaccurate by its presence.

Could you provide an example?

Disparities can occur because a patient's family selects a nursing home that has a lower rating because of organizational characteristics that correlate with poorer care. Health disparities can also exist in nursing homes because formal caregivers deliver lower quality care to some individuals versus other individuals.

What did Grabowski and McGuire (2009) find when they looked at both of these approaches to disparities?

Grabowski and McGuire (2009) found that multiple variables were operative. Some families were selecting the lowest-cost nursing homes. These nursing homes had fewer resources and, as a result, delivered poorer care in general. However, within the nursing homes, individual African Americans were more likely to be subjected to physician restraints, more likely to be sedated, and more likely to be fed using feeding tubes.

Could these "differences" be explained by differences in needs?

Almost all of the differences did reflect higher levels of need when adjustments were made for health status and for socioeconomic variables. The only outcome that was not explained was the disproportionate use of feeding tubes. Further analysis of the data revealed that the observed differences in care were related to differences in need and not to maltreatment based upon the subjective responses of the nursing home staff.

Other research also demonstrates that some demographic differences in nursing home care outcomes reflect the fact that selected racial/ethnic subgroups disproportionately enter into nursing homes with low-quality ratings (Campbell, Cai, Gao, & Li, 2016).

What other factors are operative?

Travers, Schroeder, Blaylock, and Stone (2017) indicate that partnerships are needed between nursing home residents and their families and nursing home staff in order to reduce disparities. Specifically, these researchers determined that White residents of nursing homes were significantly ($p < .05$) more likely to have had an influenza and/or pneumococcal vaccination than their counterparts of other races/ethnicities. Two factors interacted to produce this outcome: (1) some subgroups were less likely to be offered the vaccination, and (2) African Americans were more likely to refuse the vaccination even when it was offered.

Are there studies that reveal disparities by factors other than race/ethnicity?

Yes. Yang, Meng, and Miller (2011) utilized data from the 2004 National Nursing Home Survey and multilevel regression to determine whether nursing home residents in rural areas had "worse" outcomes than their urban counterparts. They used the method **multilevel regression**, which allows multiple clusters of associated variables (that are grouped into individual categories) to be simultaneously examined as sources of causation. In the analysis of nursing home outcomes, a number of patient- and facility-level variables interacted to affect resident outcomes.

Yang et al. (2011) found that even when all other variables were held constant, residents in rural nursing homes were hospitalized 50% more often and experienced moderate to severe pain 68% more frequently. Additionally, the facilities that served them were more likely to have foregone the chore of seeking accreditation for purposes of quality measurement.

Analyzing Disparities in Long-Term Care

The factors associated with disparities in long-term care are, like healthcare disparities in general, **nonlinear**. By *nonlinear*, we mean that there is not a straight-line causal relationship between age, racial/ethnic, gender, sexual preference, etc., and disparate outcomes. For example, Konetzka and Werner (2009) suggest

that disparities associated with formal care have actually decreased. However, disparities in the quality of care as measured by incidence of pressure ulcers and other variables continue to exist. Baumgarten et al. (2004) also identified other differences in care according to race/ethnicity. Campbell et al. (2016) analyzed more recent data regarding nursing home quality of life and found similar trends in the incidence of pressure ulcers. Bliss et al. (2015) found that African Americans developed pressure ulcers earlier in nursing homes than those in other subgroups. However, they found no differences in treatment for this condition. Thus, rather than inequalities in care occurring as the outcome of direct prejudice and/or discrimination by caregivers, it appears that they may reflect two sets of factors. At the first level, healthcare quality differences appear to occur because the long-term care facilities that serve lower socioeconomic groups and minorities have fewer resources with which to provide care to their residents. Second, they reflect public policies that seek to allow market forces to serve as the primary mechanism for the management of long-term care markets.

I'm not quite sure what you mean by that statement.

Recall that the long-term care industry, unlike hospitals and other healthcare institutions, is disproportionately dominated by for-profit providers. Moreover, a review of the history of long-term care reveals that, to a large degree, public policies have helped shape this outcome.

Why is this the case?

When the Social Security Act of 1935 was passed, an Old Age Assistance component was included. Title 1 of this legislation allocated matching grants to states so that elderly persons who lived in private facilities could receive payments to pay for services. Thus, seniors contracted with private citizens to provide their housing and other needed services. In 1950, still another amendment to the

Social Security Act allowed dollars allocated for long-term care to be paid directly to nursing homes. Policies such as these have supported the development of nursing homes as market-driven facilities. These market-driven forces, despite the presence of an abundance of regulations, could be associated with disparities in nursing home quality. This statement is based on the fact that an analysis of data in Nursing Home Compare reveals that for-profit nursing homes have lower star ratings than their nonprofit counterparts.

Is there additional evidence that disparities in nursing home quality may be related more to socioeconomic variables rather than tribalist tendencies?

Let's quickly analyze some data to see if this is indeed the case. First, let's give this exercise a title. Let's call it, "Assessing the Relationship Between Nursing Home Quality and Socioeconomic Variables: A Macro-Level Analysis."

What do you mean by "macro-level" analysis?

Macro-level refers to the larger forces that impact individual nursing homes. *Micro-level* approaches to nursing homes focus on the operations and characteristics of each nursing home. Nursing home quality varies based upon micro-level variables. Data from the Centers for Medicare and Medicaid Nursing Home Compare site (Medicare.gov, 2018) reveal that in 2015 only 19% of the nation's 15,505 nursing homes who participated in Nursing Home Compare achieved a score of five stars. Approximately 23% were awarded a score of four stars; 22% achieved three stars. Approximately 20% received a score of two stars; 16% were designated as receiving one star. Thus, collectively, 36% of all reporting nursing homes received a score of only one or two stars in 2015.

Research reveals that multiple variables impact nursing home performance. Zhang, Lu, Xu, Rodriguez-Monguio, and Gurwitz (2016), in a study that focused on the adoption of health information technologies, found that, although not the focus of the research, micro- and macro-level variables interacted in the nursing home marketplace. Using data from the Online Survey Certification and Reporting (OSCAR) system, in combination with findings from the Healthcare Information and Management Systems Society (HIMSS) database, the researchers found that factors internal to the nursing home and socioeconomic factors impacted nursing home quality. Specifically, investigators found that nursing homes that were resource-rich in terms of personnel and other resources were more likely to use health information technology that could benefit patient care. Likewise, they discovered that nursing homes that serve patients of higher socioeconomic status as reflected by a lower ratio of Medicaid patients were also more likely to have engaged in the purchase of a health management information system (HMIS).

Based on the dependent variable, utilization of health information technology systems, the study by Zhang et al. (2016) suggests that nursing home outcomes are not merely a function of the skills and operational aspects of the organization itself. Rather, nursing home quality outcomes are potentially influenced by the socioeconomic parameters that provide the larger context in which nursing homes operate. *Stated differently, macro-level variables and not merely variables specific to each nursing home determine overall quality of care.*

The study by Zhang et al. (2016) differs from the more standard approaches used in evaluations of nursing home quality by its examination of macro-level variables. The importance of macro-level variables was also demonstrated by Estabrooks, Knopp-Sihota, Cummings, and Norton (2016) in their examination of data generated as part of the Translating Research in Elder Care (TREC) initiative in Canada. They determined that macro-level variables outside of the direct organization impacted quality of care as measured by rates of urinary tract infections, catheter use, overall commitment, use of best practices, and other outcomes. Similarly, Lutfiyya, Gessert, and Lipsky (2013), based on the 15,177 nursing homes that reported to Nursing Home Compare, confirmed the importance of a macro-level variable, rural/urban geographic site, as a predictor of a four star or higher rating. Utilizing t-tests to assess significance, they found that nursing homes located in rural areas, a macro-level variable, were less likely to have a rating of four stars than their urban counterparts.

As mentioned, such studies contrast sharply with research on nursing home quality that tends to focus on micro-level measures of quality that are implicit to each nursing home. The nature and number of nursing home staff are key micro-level variables that impact nursing home quality, according to Harrington, Schnelle, McGregore, and Simmons (2016). Trinkoff et al. (2015) in a study of 16,628 nursing homes throughout the United States discovered that nursing homes that had nursing home administrators and directors of nursing with higher levels of education and certifications were associated with a higher nursing home quality as measured by significantly better pain management outcomes ($p < .05$). Other studies have also focused upon staffing mixes and patterns of other facility-specific characteristics.

Cognizant of the complexity of the task of introducing macro-level determinants into the quality measurement equation, some analysts have sought to integrate such variables into their analyses of micro-level forces. Lee, Blegen, and Harrington (2014) analyzed the impact of a micro-level variable, registered nurse staffing hours, on three key quality measures—pressure ulcers, urinary tract infections, and weight loss—while controlling for macro-level independent variables such as geographic location, comparability of patient case mix, and organizational parameters. These researchers found that the increase in RN hours was positively associated with fewer incidences of patient pressure ulcers.

Both micro- and macro-level analyses are important to healthcare administrators, public health professionals, and clinicians as they seek to elevate the quality of care received by nursing home residents. However, a preliminary analysis suggests that inquiries into the sources of nursing home quality are disproportionately aligned with an investigation of variables that are controllable within the nursing home context. In this regard, we will now perform an exercise to answer the question, "What is the relationship between the percentage of 1- and 2-star nursing homes in each state and the District of Columbia as a function of demographics (i.e., percentage of the population older than 65 years and the percentage of the population who are minority in each state)?" We will introduce key socioeconomic determinants of health into our model as measured by (1) the percentage of the population with incomes at and/or below poverty level and (2) the percentage of persons in each state with 4 or more years of college. Before describing the methods that we will use to assess the impact of these macro-level variables upon nursing home quality, let's briefly review the literature that rationalizes the selection of these variables for inclusion in the analysis.

Measuring Nursing Home Quality

Nursing home quality is, as are other aspects of health care, highly patient focused. This focus is driven by the Institute of Medicine's directives that emphasize individuals and populations as the subject of healthcare delivery systems in general, including nursing homes and other long-term care facilities (IOM, 2001). Castle and Ferguson (2010) reported that in the years from 2005 to 2010, 57% of the 3,950 articles published on nursing home quality used indicators based on the well-known model by Donabedian (1985).

What is Donabedian's model, and why is it important?

Avedis Donabedian (1985) created a model that asserted that healthcare quality is a function of three interrelated components. First, a *structure* must exist that supports the delivery of high-quality health care. Second, processes must be identified that address every aspect of the steps needed to support the diagnosis and treatment of the illness or disease. Through the combination of a high-quality structure and the use of *processes* that adhere to current evidence on how to complete processes for the diagnosis and treatment of the illness or disease, the patient's *outcome* (as measured by mortality, treatment complications, and related measures) will be maximized.

This model is important to long-term care because it is the basis of Nursing Home Compare. The *structural, process,* and *outcome* quality indicators identified by Donabedian's model currently guide which data are collected, analyzed, and reported in Nursing Home Compare. Donabedian's model of quality necessarily focuses on the micro-level variables that characterize each healthcare delivery setting. Although numerous criticisms have been levied against currently established nursing home quality indicators, these criticisms primarily address the ability of these micro-level variables to encompass the most relevant measures of the structure, process, and outcomes associated with each individual nursing home. Less attention has been paid to the demographic and socioeconomic context in which a healthcare organization delivers service. Yet, it is critical that healthcare administrators, public health professionals, and clinicians analyze their quality outcomes within such a framework.

Can you provide examples of researchers who have been critical of Nursing Home Compare?

Williams, Straker, and Applebaum (2016) argue that the current model used as the basis for Nursing Home Compare does not consider the level of satisfaction of nursing home residents and their families. Werner, Konetzka, and Kim (2013) imply that the linkages between the care processes used in measuring quality and nursing do not necessarily lead to improved outcomes. They analyzed changes in

a number of facility-level processes in 16,623 nursing homes over the period 2000 to 2009. These researchers determined that improvements occurred in only one of five outcome measures used in the analysis. Thus, the authors concluded that the process measures used to assess quality in nursing homes are disconnected from the outcomes.

However, the current critiques of the micro-level quality indicators do not, for the most part, include the need to integrate macro-level parameters that may affect nursing homes' ability to deliver quality as measured by the selected structural, process, and outcome indicators currently used.

Why is this important?

The failure to integrate macro-level influences into measurements of quality is not benign. Werner, Konetzka, and Polsky (2016) found that despite limitations in the use of quality data by consumers, the introduction of Nursing Home Compare's easier-to-read star ratings led to an 8% loss in market share by 1-star facilities and a 6% gain in market share for 5-star nursing homes. However, if macro-level variables are also operative, then ratings that do not address such interactions will lead consumers to make decisions based on compromised data. For example, a patient mix that includes a disproportionate number of frail and/or prefrail patients will affect nursing home outcomes (Kojima, 2015). The disproportionate alignment of frailty and/or prefrailty data with macro-level social determinants of health such as the number of residents from impoverished neighborhoods and/or communities with lower-educated residents introduces greater risk of poor quality at the micro-level. Such a statement is consistent with findings from a study by Gohil et al. (2015). In this study, the authors recalculated hospital performance ratings based on the impact of infection-based readmission rates. When these readmission rates were recalculated by accounting for poverty, education, and other socioeconomic variables; ethnicity as a demographic variable;

as well as initial differences in health status as measured by number of coexisting diseases and illnesses, nearly one-third of the 322 hospitals in the analysis changed rankings based on alterations in quality as measured by infection-based readmission rates. Gilstrap and Joynt (2014), in a systematic review of literature, also critiqued the use of only micro-level variables in the analysis of heart failure readmission rates as a measure of quality of care in hospitals.

You've convinced me that we need to do this analysis to see if we can find new information about the factors associated with quality disparities in nursing home ratings. Where do we begin? What are our variables?

The first step is to identify a reliable data source. We have used data from Medicare's Nursing Home Compare that identify the percentage of nursing homes in each state by their star rating for 2015. For each state and the District of Columbia, the percentage of nursing homes with a rating of one or two stars were added together and used as the dependent variable, for a total of 51 observations. The first independent variable selected for inclusion in the analysis was the population per nursing home. Data for this variable, the population per nursing home, were calculated by dividing the total population of each state by the number of total nursing homes in each state. The total number of persons was not limited to those older than age 65 years, because some nursing home residents are younger than age 65. The other independent variables used were the percentage of the population age 65 and over; the percentage of the population who were minority in each state; the percentage of the state's population who were impoverished; and the percentage of each state's population with 4 or more years of college.

How do we prepare the data for analysis?

Because the purpose of this exercise is to support readers in learning the importance of using data to gain new insights into the causes and correlates of disparities, the data have already been included. Nevertheless, read up

on how the data were collected so that you understand their limitations. First, look at the headings in the table located in the appendix. Starting with each state, read across the rows. You are now engaging in a process that we call **data validation and verification**, whereby anytime data are copied, typed, or otherwise imported from the source of origin the data must be carefully checked to ensure that they are accurate and consistent.

The first step of data verification is that of reviewing every line in Table 12.4 to ensure that there are no missing values. If the verification process reveals missing values, one must return to the original data source and then find and insert the missing values.

The data also must be reviewed to determine which values will be used in the actual analysis. An examination of the table in the appendix shows that data on Guam and Puerto Rico, two U.S. territories, are not included. When Nursing Home Compare is checked, the data verification process reveals that incomplete values are available for these territories. Thus, because of the missing values, we have excluded these territories from the analysis that we are about to complete.

Given that our research question focuses on states, why do we include the District of Columbia?

Article 1, Section 8, Clause 17 of the U.S. Constitution does not allow any area that serves as the host site for the U.S. government to have statehood. However, in order to protect the residents of the District of Columbia (which has served as the capital since 1790) researchers usually include this area in their analyses.

What else do we review in data verification other than missing data?

As part of the data validation and verification process we will next perform a range check. A **range check** is a check to make sure that the data all fall within numerical intervals that are consistent with that variable. Numerical data for all measurable phenomenon generally have upper and lower limits in which they will fall.

For example, human age falls between 1 and 120 years. Although the mean height of an adult male differs by country, state, income, profession, and other variables, a value of 16 feet for height may suggest a data error in a survey. Similarly, if in Table 12.4, a listing appeared that indicated that the state of Delaware had 4,500 nursing homes, this would obviously be a mistake since Delaware is a small state, and the total number of nursing homes nationwide is only 15,000. Similarly, if in Table 12.5, you found an entry that recorded 41% as the percentage of the population who are impoverished, this would also be an obvious mistake. Additionally, if the data indicated that the 73% of the population in one state were 65+ years and older, that would be a mistake since most states have under 20% of the population in that age group.

Can missing values and range checks be completed electronically rather than manually using statistics software?

Yes, these initial steps can be performed by statistical software packages. However, every data point listed in the table should be checked against the original source by someone other than the individual who initially constructed the table. Thus, as part of this exercise, you may want to form a group with whom to work so that all data provided to you for this simple analysis can be checked against the listed source.

Researchers should never use "dirty" data. Although this is true of all research areas, it is particularly true in the area of health care because lives are oftentimes at stake. In the area of health disparity research, false findings from the use of poorly "cleansed" data can aggravate subgroup tensions. Now, please validate and verify the data in the table found in the chapter appendix and Table 12.4.

Why is there so much emphasis in this text on data and original analyses?

The field of health and healthcare disparities relies on data and statistics. Thus, current and future healthcare administrators, public health professionals, and clinicians must be able to convert data into information and information into knowledge.

What Is the Difference Between Data, Information, and Knowledge?

When we examine the Nursing Home Compare dataset and "count" the number of nursing homes with 1- or 2-star ratings, we are using data. When we review the data to determine which states have a higher percent of 1- or 2-star ratings, we are converting the data into information. When we conduct a literature search, review studies on nursing homes, reflect on current data and patterns that exist, and draw conclusions, we are "manufacturing" knowledge. When we ask new questions and use statistical processes to answer those questions, we are producing new knowledge. When healthcare professionals use new knowledge to improve health outcomes, we are advancing the human condition.

Statistical analysis, data science, transdisciplinary inquiry, etc., are tools needed in each step of this process. However, Cresswell, Bates, and Sherkh (2017) argue that whereas banking, retailing, and other industries have integrated data science into their organizations, the healthcare industry has lagged in this area. Yet, the benefits that can accrue from the incorporation of even data science approaches alone can support healthcare administrators in making quality improvements. But, data science approaches can also improve "learning health systems" that can support public health professionals by improving predictability. Data science can also advance the growth of "prevention medicine" by clinicians. Accordingly, this exercise seeks to demonstrate the benefits of even simple forays into the use of secondary data for uncovering new knowledge.

The following table (**TABLE 12.4**) contains the data that we will be using for our exercise.

TABLE 12.4 Assessing the Relationship Between the % of Nursing Homes with 1- or 2-Star Ratings and Key Demographics and Socioeconomic Characteristics in Each State

	Dependent Variable (y)	Independent Variables (x)				
		x_1	x_2	x_3	x_4	x_5
State	Percentage of Nursing Homes with Nursing Home Compare Ratings of One or Two Stars[a]	Percentage of Minorities[b]	Percentage of the Population Who Are Impoverished[b]	Percentage of the Population with 4 or More Years of College[b]	Population per Nursing Home[c]	Percentage of the Population Age 65 and Older[b]
Alabama	31.86%	33.7%	18.8%	23.5%	21,374	14.890%
Alaska	27.78%	37.6%	10.2%	28.0%	40,743	8.959%
Arizona	29.37%	43.5%	18.2%	27.5%	46,447	15.358%
Arkansas	30.40%	26.4%	19.3%	21.1%	13,032	15.345%
California	26.66%	61.3%	16.3%	28.8%	31,806	12.496%
Colorado	28.17%	30.9%	12.7%	38.1%	24,783	12.215%
Connecticut	29.69%	30.8%	10.5%	37.6%	15,691	15.091%
Delaware	24.44%	36.1%	12.0%	30.0%	20,579	15.889%
D.C. (District of Columbia)	21.05%	64.4%	18.0%	54.6%	34,078	11.320%
Florida	30.81%	43.9%	16.5%	27.3%	28,555	18.584%
Georgia	37.18%	45.4%	18.4%	28.8%	28,188	11.896%
Hawaii	21.74%	77.1%	11.2%	30.8%	30,572	15.619%

Idaho	21.79%	16.9%	15.5%	25.9%	18,029	13.283%
Illinois	37.47%	37.5%	14.3%	32.3%	2,133	13.500%
Indiana	31.81%	19.5%	15.4%	24.1%	24,521	13.901%
Iowa	28.93%	12.6%	12.5%	31.0%	14,963	15.508%
Kansas	33.04%	23.0%	13.6%	20.0%	9,125	13.975%
Kentucky	42.11%	14.4%	18.9%	22.3%	10,151	14.394%
Louisiana	46.95%	40.5%	19.8%	22.5%	15,761	13.246%
Maine	18.45%	6.1%	13.9%	29.0%	44,905	17.614%
Maryland	32.74%	47.0%	10.0%	37.9%	5,881	13.340%
Massachusetts	29.54%	25.7%	11.6%	40.5%	14,360	14.695%
Michigan	31.32%	24.1%	16.7%	26.9%	15,582	14.977%
Minnesota	25.00%	18.3%	11.3%	33.7%	26,614	13.904%
Mississippi	36.63%	42.6%	22.5%	20.7%	26,828	13.882%
Missouri	35.42%	19.8%	15.6%	27.1%	5,848	14.963%
Montana	30.00%	13.0%	15.2%	29.5%	75,568	16.190%
Nebraska	33.65%	19.2%	12.7%	29.3%	4,809	14.125%
Nevada	32.08%	48.0%	15.5%	23.0%	35,271	13.603%

(continues)

TABLE 12.4 Assessing the Relationship Between the % of Nursing Homes with 1- or 2-Star Ratings and Key Demographics and Socioeconomic Characteristics in Each State *(continued)*

| State | Dependent Variable (y) | Independent Variables (x) | | | | |
	Percentage of Nursing Homes with Nursing Home Compare Ratings of One or Two Stars[a]	x_1 Percentage of Minorities[b]	x_2 Percentage of the Population Who Are Impoverished[b]	x_3 Percentage of the Population with 4 or More Years of College[b]	x_4 Population per Nursing Home[c]	x_5 Percentage of the Population Age 65 and Older[b]
New Hampshire	30.26%	8.6%	8.9%	34.9%	36,824	15.251%
New Jersey	26.10%	42.8%	10.8%	36.8%	3,638	14.366%
New Mexico	37.14%	60.8%	21.0%	26.3%	127,206	14.705%
New York	39.52%	43.2%	15.7%	34.2%	3,335	14.336%
North Carolina	39.76%	35.8%	17.4%	28.4%	46,841	14.232%
North Dakota	26.25%	13.0%	11.5%	27.7%	123,067	14.223%
Ohio	41.00%	19.7%	15.8%	26.1%	764	15.094%
Oklahoma	43.42%	32.7%	16.7%	24.1%	38,079	14.213%
Oregon	29.63%	22.8%	16.5%	30.8%	28,517	15.405%
Pennsylvania	39.89%	21.9%	13.5%	28.6%	5,652	16.310%
Rhode Island	22.62%	25.5%	14.2%	31.9%	152,138	15.402%

South Carolina	34.76%	36.1%	17.9%	25.8%	5,635	15.212%
South Dakota	26.13%	16.8%	14.1%	27.0%	43,041	14.897%
Tennessee	36.91%	25.3%	17.6%	24.9%	2,660	14.621%
Texas	47.92%	56.2%	17.3%	27.6%	5,407	11.184%
Utah	28.87%	20.5%	12.3%	31.1%	273,594	9.740%
Vermont	27.03%	6.4%	11.5%	36.0%	78,470	16.322%
Virginia	38.03%	36.6%	11.5%	36.3%	2,206	13.342%
Washington	27.40%	29.2%	13.3%	32.9%	37,702	13.575%
West Virginia	45.24%	7.5%	18.0%	19.2%	55,440	17.246%
Wisconsin	27.79%	17.6%	13.0%	27.8%	4,809	14.771%
Wyoming	27.78%	15.5%	11.5%	25.7%	159,503	13.455%

a   Compiled by authors from data found in the archived datasets of Centers for Medicare & Medicaid Services. (2015). Nursing Home Compare Database. 2015 Annual Files. ProviderInfo_2015.zip. https://data.medicare.gov/data/archives/nursing-home-compare

b   Census Bureau. (2015). American Fact Finder. American Community Survey. ACS Demographic and Housing Estimates. 2012–2016 American Community Survey 5-Year Estimates.

c   Calculated by authors with data found from Census Bureau. (2015). American Fact Finder. American Community Survey. ACS Demographic and Housing Estimates. 2012–2016 American Community Survey 5-Year Estimates. Population by State. https://factfinder.census.gov/faces/nav/jsf/pages/community_facts.xhtml# and Centers for Medicare & Medicaid Services. Data.Medicare.gov. Nursing Home Compare Database. 2015 Annual Files. ProviderInfo_2015.zip. https://data.medicare.gov/data/archives/nursing-home-compare

What Is the First Step?

Please validate and verify the data to ensure that they are clean data by using the steps already described.

Now, we summarize the data in the table.

How do we summarize the data in the table?

We can summarize the data by simply initiating a conversation with the data. This is accomplished by asking a series of questions of the data such as those provided in **BOX 12.2**.

Does having the fewest 1- or 2-star ratings mean the same as having the best nursing homes?

As you can see from Table 12.4, these measures may be quite different. Because the focus of this exercise is on states with the "lowest overall quality" in terms of nursing homes, we focused on the sum of the 1- and 2-star quality nursing homes in this initial set of questions. Each reader can expand his or her information regarding the nursing home industry by "conversing" with the data based on the question, "Which states had the best nursing home quality as measured by the percentage of nursing homes in each state that received a 5-star rating?" But, in order to begin transforming the information into knowledge, we can ask different questions.

What factors explain the tremendous differences in the percentage of 1- or 2-star nursing homes in each state?

One strategy to exploring this question would be to take a micro-level approach. As discussed earlier, Nursing Home Compare data are compiled based upon three sets of aggregate data that are necessarily specific to each nursing home in each state. The first set of data includes key measures that have been collected based upon state health inspection reports. These items include nursing home–specific data on variables such as differences in food storage, healthcare quality as measured by the number and severity of pressure ulcers, etc. By using these variables, our analysis would tell us whether nursing homes in West Virginia had more of these quality issues than those in Washington, D.C., for example.

Other micro-level variations could exist in terms of staffing measures, such as number of nursing hours per resident day. Likewise, the differentials by states could be related to direct patient care "quality measures" from the CMS's Minimum Data Set (MDS).

For example, because nursing homes in Texas and other states have a larger percentage of 1- or 2-star ratings, a micro-level analysis would allow us to determine whether the low

---

BOX 12.2 Transforming the Data in Table 12.4 into Knowledge

Question: On average, what percentage of U.S. nursing homes were low performing in 2015, as measured by having an overall rating of one or two stars?
Answer: 34.64%
Question: Which state had the absolute "worst" nursing home ratings as measured by the highest percentage of nursing homes with one or two stars?
Answer: Texas (47.92%)
Question: What were the next four states with the worst ratings?
Answer: Louisiana (46.95%), West Virginia (45.24%), Oklahoma (43.42%), and Kentucky (42.11%).
Question: Which state had the absolute best overall nursing home quality in 2015, as measured by the lowest percentage of nursing homes with one or two stars?
Answer: Maine (18.45%)
Question: What were the next four "top" states in terms of the lowest percentage of nursing homes with one or two stars?
Answer: District of Columbia (21.05%), Hawaii (21.74%), Idaho (21.79%), and Rhode Island (22.62%)

ratings were related to nursing home–specific factors. These factors would include whether they had patients who had more falls and/or had more residents with poorly managed pain, etc. The inclusion of these types of variables in the estimation of a regression analysis would allow us to understand which sets of nursing home–specific variables were most "deficient" in these states.

That seems valuable. So why aren't we using this type of analysis as an exercise?

As mentioned earlier, considerable attention has been paid to nursing home–specific variables. This exercise seeks to answer the question, "To what degree is the percentage of nursing homes with 1- or 2-star ratings related to the overall demographics and socioeconomic composition of all residents in that state?"

As can be seen, the table also presents the total population per nursing home, the percentage of the population who had 4 or more years of college, the percentage of the population age 65 and older, the percentage of the population that is minority, and the percentage of the population that was impoverished in 2015. Here, too, we can ask questions of the data.

This is a lot of data! What do we do with it?

As mentioned, first, review it. Second, validate and verify it. Third, you may want to look for patterns in it. For example, you could check to see if Texas ranks higher in the percentage of residents living in poverty or in the percentage of persons age 65 or over or if it ranks lower in the percentage of persons with a 4-year college degree or higher. Look for any patterns that suggest that there may be a relationship between the dependent and independent variables.

Are there tools we may use?

Yes, you could construct a scatterplot. As you can see in Table 12.4, it includes the % of persons age 65 and older. We calculated the percentage of population age 65 and older in each state since this will be a variable for our analysis. We also used Census Bureau data in order to populate the columns for the percentage minority and percentage poverty for each state.

So, do we recheck the data entry sheet for more errors?

Yes. After rechecking the data entry sheet, use the multiple regression calculator in Excel and see what you can discover regarding the macro-level variables.

Why don't we just use a multiple regression calculator?

We do not use a multiple regression calculator because we have five independent variables. Few online multiple regression calculators can accommodate more than three independent variables.

How do we use Excel to run a multiple regression?

Multiple regression is a statistical tool to study the relationship between a dependent (outcome) variable and two or more independent (predictor) variables. With regards to our question, we want to know whether the percentage of nursing homes with one or two stars can be predicted based on the five independent variables.

However, before starting a multiple regression analysis, one must check that the data meet several assumptions that are necessary in order for multiple regression to be used as the analytical tool. These assumptions should be assessed before moving forward. Please note that it is not uncommon when analyzing data that one or more assumptions will not be met. However, in the event that certain assumptions are not met, a statistician can often find solutions for the issues.

- **Assumption 1:** The dependent variable is measured on a continuous scale (i.e., interval or ratio).
- **Assumption 2:** The model has two or more independent variables. They can be either continuous or categorical (i.e., ordinal or nominal).
- **Assumption 3:** The independent variables cannot be highly correlated (no multicollinearity).

- **Assumption 4:** The residuals must have a normal distribution.
- **Assumption 5:** Little variability exists across the error terms (homoscedasticity).
- **Assumption 6:** The relationship between the dependent and independent variables clusters around a straight line (linearity).

Now let's run the regression.

BOX 12.3 outlines how to run a multiple regression in Excel (version 16.9). **TABLE 12.5**

provides a summary of the output of the regression statistics. **TABLE 12.6** provides summary statistics for each variable.

Now, let's look at the output. But, first, ask yourself what you think our analysis will find. That is, do you think there is or is not a relationship between our hypothesized variables and the percent of 1- and 2-star rated nursing homes in each state? Are you anxious to view the results? Is our heart beating more rapidly?

BOX 12.3   How to Use Excel to Perform a Multiple Regression

Step 1: Identify the Variables

For this exercise, the *y* value, or dependent variable, is the percentage of nursing homes with 1- or 2-star nursing home ratings in each state as of 2015.

The five independent variables that were used for these calculations are:

1. The percentage of the population in each state with 4 years or more of college
2. The percentage of the population in each state who are impoverished
3. The percentage of the population in each state who are minorities
4. The percentage of the population who are age 65 and older
5. The mean population per nursing home in each state

Step 2: Set Up Excel to Analyze the Data

1. Open Excel, and enter all the data on one sheet in separate columns.
2. Check to see if the Data Analysis ToolPak is activated. If it is, you should see Data Analysis under the Data tab. If it has not been activated, click Tools, then Excel Add-ins. In the Add-ins window, check Analysis ToolPak and then OK.

Step 3: Prepare the Data File

Open the data file and export the data or enter the data by yourself. When entering the data, they must be in adjacent columns and rows, as any empty cells will be treated as missing data. As can be seen when you open the Excel window, all labels (i.e., variable names) should be in the first row. In this example, our dependent variable is the percentage of nursing homes with 1- or 2-star nursing home ratings; the independent variables are percentage minorities, percentage impoverished, percentage with 4 or more years of higher education, per capita population per nursing home, and percentage of the population age 65 and older.

Step 4: Select the Tool for the Analysis

Under the Data tab, click Data Analysis, Scroll, and then select Regression. Click OK.

Step 5: Input the Data Range and Select the Output Options

1. **Input the dependent variable.** In the Regression dialog window, place your cursor in the [Input Y Range] and then highlight the column of data in the spreadsheet. In this case, you should highlight the data for the dependent variable (i.e., percentage of nursing homes with 1- or 2-star ratings).

2. **Input the independent variables.** Do the same by placing your cursor in the "Input X Range" then highlighting multiple columns of the independent variables; that is, highlight the data including all five independent variables in the spreadsheet.
3. **Select the desired options for checking assumptions.** Select "Options" in the Residuals and Normal Probability categories. These are the options to check the key assumptions that must be met in order to perform a multiple regression that we mentioned earlier.

Step 6: Run the Analysis

Click OK to generate the results. You will find the following information.

TABLE 12.5 Summary Output: Regression Statistics

Multiple *R*	0.57931637	The multiple R tells us the correlation coefficient between the dependent variable and the five independent variables as a collective.
R Square	0.33560746	A measure of the degree to which the changes in the five independent variables predict a unit change in the dependent variables.
Adjusted *R* Square	0.26178606	A measure of the impact of adding and/or deleting variables.
Standard Error	0.05877867	The average measure of variation or dispersion in the data.
Observations	51	The number of states and the District of Columbia.

TABLE 12.6 Summary Output: Variables

Variables	β Value	*p*-Value
Percentage minorities	−0.0257	0.6837
Percentage of the population who are impoverished	0.7522	0.0278**
Percentage of the population who hold a 4-year degree or higher	−0.0031	0.0680*
Per capita population per nursing home	−3.1E-07	0.0832*
Percentage of the population who are 65 years and older	−0.7728	0.1490

$N = 51$ (all states and the District of Columbia); dependent variable, percentage of nursing homes in each state with Nursing Home Compare ratings of one or two stars (poor quality); Adjusted $R^2 = 0.2618$; level of significance at $*p < 0.1$; $**p < .05$; B, regression coefficient; CI, confidence interval. The β value is the coefficients of the variables. It tells us how much dependent variable changes when each independent variable changes. The sign of the coefficient tells us whether the change is direct or inverse. The *p*-value is a measure of whether an association is likely to be based on chance alone or is greater than chance alone.

Please review the above data and concepts, and ensure that they are clear. Complete Internet research if more in-depth information is required. Now, let's continue.

How can we interpret these findings?

Three variables were significant based on the p values of $p < .1$ and $p < .05$. Overall, states with a higher percentage of impoverished residents had a higher percentage of nursing homes with one or two stars. With regards to the steps in Box 12.3, the following information is needed to interpret the multiple regression results.

Multiple Correlation Coefficient (Multiple R)

The multiple R, ranging from -1 to $+1$, indicates the correlation between the dependent and independent variables ("+" is a positive correlation; "−" is a negative correlation). The p-values indicate that a number of the results are significant. For example, a positive and significant ($p < .02$) relationship exists between the percentage of the population who are impoverished and nursing home ratings (0.02783987). This suggests that if a nursing home is located in a high-poverty state, there is a greater chance that it will have a higher percentage of lower-quality nursing homes. In contrast, a negative and marginally significant relationship exists between the percentage of persons with 4 or more years of college and nursing home ratings (0.06799783). Stated differently, because higher education is associated with better health outcomes, it is not surprising that a higher percentage of persons in a state who are college educated is part of a trajectory that is associated in fewer low-quality nursing homes.

Interestingly, the results also indicate a negative relationship between the percentage of different subgroups comprising a state's population and nursing home quality. On average, as the number of minorities as a percent of the total population increases, nursing home quality decreases. However, the magnitude is such that the degree of change is not even mildly significant ($p < .68372399$). Similarly, a negative relationship exists between the percentage of population that is age 65 and older and nursing home quality; that is, as the percentage of the population that is age 65 and older increases, nursing home quality decreases slightly but not significantly ($p < .14902076$). A marginally significant negative relationship exists between the size of the per capita population per nursing home and nursing home quality ($p < .08322592$). In other words, if the per capita population per nursing home in a state is too high, it may have a mild impact on the percent of 1- and 2-star nursing homes.

Are you saying that the data indicate that as the size of the per capita population per nursing home increases, other factors come into play that reduce nursing home quality?

Yes, that is the case.

Coefficient of Determination (R Square)

The R^2, which ranges from 0 to +1, is used to determine the proportion of the variance in the dependent variable that can be predicted from the independent variable. In this case, 33.56% of the change in the percentage of nursing homes with one or two stars is associated with the changes in: (1) percentage minorities, (2) percentage impoverished, (3) percentage with 4 years or more of higher education, and (4) percentage of the population 65 years and older. This suggests that it may be worthwhile for nursing home administrators to know that the demographic and socioeconomic status of the overall state will indirectly affect their measured quality outcomes.

Adjusted R Square

We usually do not interpret this statistic because it is just a modified version of R^2 based on the number of predictors in the model.

Standard Error

The standard error of the regression is 0.05877867 (or 5.87%). This number is an estimate of the variation of the observed percentage of nursing homes with one or two stars along the regression line.

Analysis of Variance (ANOVA)

The ANOVA table in **TABLE 12.7** includes four components:

- sum of squares (SS): a measure that is used to calculate the all of the observations with regard to the distance from the mean. The difference from the mean of each observation is squared and then the sum of all the resulting measurements is added.
- degrees of freedom (df): represent the number of values or parameters which may be independently varied in a calculation.
- mean squares (MS): used to estimate variances across values, variables and/or, other groups of data.
- F statistic (F): created when running a regression analysis or ANOVA. This value identifies whether there is a significant difference between two variables.

What does this all mean?

Three independent variables were found to be statistically significant when looking at the variation in the percentage of nursing homes with 1- or 2-star nursing home ratings: percentage of the population who are impoverished, percentage of the population with 4 or more years of higher education, and the population per nursing home.

In today's world of big data and a healthcare environment that has shifted to an emphasis on quality, every single healthcare administrator, public health professional, and clinician should have the basic skills required to analyze disparities data and test their own theories regarding the possible causes of disparities in their health care institution. This exercise demonstrates this point by using long-term care.

Why did you select long-term care for this exercise?

Long-term care organizations are highly regulated and frequently assessed. Moreover, the assessment tools to measure quality are micro-level. However, a long-term care administrator can use a simple analysis such as this one to supplement findings obtained from the Conditions of Participation data. This analysis clearly reveals that nursing homes that operate in high-poverty states are at greater risk of lower quality. However, a continuing theme throughout the text has also been the intimate relationship between health and health care disparities and original hypotheses that can be tested via data.

TABLE 12.7 ANOVA Table					
ANOVA	df	SS	MS	F	Significance F
Regression	5	0.07853422	0.01570684	4.54620861	0.00193498
Residual	45	0.15547197	0.00345493		
Total	50	0.23400619			

These types of findings signal a need for nursing home administrators and other healthcare professionals to identify similar data in order to study and eventually implement processes that can mitigate the existing causes of such disparities in nursing home patients and the lower threshold of nursing home care that they receive.

Chapter Summary

This chapter began by providing an overview of the long-term care industry. It then utilized a brief review of selected literature on health care disparities in nursing home care. This review demonstrated that, for the most part, quality issues in general (and healthcare disparities are a quality issue) in long-term care are most often viewed as institutional rather than as both systemic and institutional. A brief case study was completed in order to re-emphasize the importance of healthcare professionals seeking new insights into healthcare outcomes and disparities in their institution. Disparities can be identified in virtually all healthcare institutions, and particularly in long-term care settings. An accurate understanding of the variables associated with disparate outcomes is necessary in order for remediable disparities to be identified and reduced. This chapter trains readers to ask and answer new questions regarding the healthcare disparities.

Review Questions and Problems

1. Write a 1,000-word summary regarding Alabama's population characteristics. Identify which health disparities are likely to exist in this state using data found in the tables in this chapter and your own research.
2. Compare and contrast two states and their nursing home star rating data. Discuss which state you would choose for yourself or a family member if a nursing home environment was required.
3. Redo the entirety of the analysis based on the following variables: (a) percentage of the total population that is female, (b) percentage of the population that is married, (c) per capita income, and (d) percentage of the population who are college graduates. Now write a public health paper regarding your findings.

Key Terms and Concepts

confounding variables Unforeseen "extraneous" variables that affect the dependent and independent variables. Thus, a confounding variable distorts or renders the study inaccurate by its presence.

data validation and verification The process of carefully checking that data that have been copied, typed, or otherwise imported are accurate and consistent.

long-term care Medical and nonmedical services that are provided in order to help people with age-related limitations and/or disabilities to maximize their physical, social, mental, psychological, and spiritual outcomes despite the irreversibility and progression of their disabling physical and/or cognitive status.

multilevel regression Also known as a hierarchical linear model or multilevel model, this statistical model may have variances at one or more levels.

multiple regression A statistical regression that is used to identify relationships between two or more independent variables and one dependent variable.

nonlinear The absence of a straight-line causal relationship between two variables.

patient mix The characteristics of the patients served by a healthcare facility including the severity of the patients' health needs. May also incorporate patient demographics and socioeconomic characteristics.

range check A check to make sure that the data all fall within a certain range.

respite care Short-term, temporary caregiving for an elderly, ill, incapacitated or handicapped person provided by a secondary caregiver. Primary caregivers are given time away from their duties for a brief period in order to rest. Respite care is provided in a variety of settings, including homes and institutionally based sites.

References

AARP Public Policy Institute & National Alliance for Caregiving. (2015). Caregiving in the U.S. 2015 report. Retrieved from https://www.aarp.org/content/dam/aarp/ppi/2015/caregiving-in-the-united-states-2015-report-revised.pdf

Amarya, D., Singh, K., & Sabharwal, M. (2015). Changes during aging and their association with malnutrition. *Journal of Clinical Gerontology and Geriatrics, 6*(3), 78–84.

Baumgarten, M., Margolis, D., van Doorn, C., Gruber-Baldini, A. L., Hebel, J. R., Zimmerman, S., & Magaziner, J. (2004). Black/white differences in pressure ulcer incidence in nursing home residents. *Journal of the American Geriatrics Society, 52*(8), 1293–1298.

Bliss, D. A., Gurvich, O., Savid, K., Eberly, L. E., Harms, S., Mueller, C., . . . Virnig, B. (2015). Are there racial/ethnic disparities in types of pressure ulcer development and pressure ulcer treatment in older adults of after nursing home admission. *Journal of Aging and Health, 27*(4), 571–593.

Boccuti, C., Casillas, G., & Neuman, T. (2015). Reading the stars: Nursing home quality star ratings, nationally and by states. Kaiser Family Foundation. Retrieved from https://www.KFF.org/medicare/issue-breifing/reading-the-stars=nursing-home-quality-star-ratings-nationally-and-by-state

Brundle, C., Waterman, H.A., Ballinger, C., Olleveant, N., Skelton, D.A., Stanford, P. and Todd, C. (2015). The causes of falls: Views of older people with visual impairment, *Health Expectations, 18*(6), 2021–2031. Doi: 10.1111/hex.12355

Campbell, L. J., Cai, X., Gao, S., & Li, Y. (2016). Racial/ethnic disparities in nursing home quality of life deficiencies, 2001 to 2011. *Gerontology and Geriatric Medicine, 2*, 1–9. doi: 10.1177/2333721416653561

Castle, N. G., & Ferguson, J. C. (2010). What is nursing home quality and how is it measured? *Gerontologist, 50*(4), 426–442.

Centers for Disease Control and Prevention (Jan. 15, 2016). QuickStats: Percentage of adults with activity limitations, by age group and type of limitation – National Health Interview Survey, United States, 2014: *MMWR Morbidity and Mortality Weekly Report* 2016; 65:14. DOI: http://dx.doi.org/10.15585/mmwr.mm6501a6.

Collerton, J., Kingston, A., Bond, J., Davies, K., Eccles, M. P., Jagger, C., Kirkwood, T. B., & Newton, J. L. (2012). The personal and health service impact of falls in 85 year olds: Cross-sectional findings from the Newcastle 85+ cohort study. *PLoS One, 7*(3), e33078. doi:10.1371/journal.pone.0033078

Congressional Budget Office (2016). Enrollment and spending in Medicaid estimates for FY 2015, Office of Management and Budget. https://www.cbo.gov. March.

Cresswell, K. M., Bates, D. W., & Sheikh, A. (2017). Why every health care organization needs a data science strategy. *NEJM Catalyst.* Retrieved from https://catalyst.nejm.org/healthcare-needs-data-science-strategy/

Dahlberg, L., Berndt, H., Lennartsson, C., & Schon, P. (2017). Receipt of formal and informal help with specific care tasks among older people living in their own home. National trends over two decades. *Social Policy & Administration, 52*(1), 91–110.

Donabedian, A. (1985). Twenty years of research on the quality of medical care: 1964–1984. *Evaluation & Health Professions, 8*(3), 243–265.

Estabrooks, C. A., Knopp-Sihota, J. A., Cummings, G. G., & Norton, P. G. (2016). Making research results relevant and useable: Presenting complex organizational context data to nonresearch stakeholders in the nursing home setting. *Worldviews on Evidence-Based Nursing, 13*(4), 270–276.

Faragher, R. G. A. (2015). Should we treat aging as a disease? The consequences and dangers of miscategorization. *Frontiers in Genetics, 6*, 171.

Ferdinand, K. C., Yadav, K., Nasser, S. A., Clayton-Jeter, H. D., Lewin, J., Cryer, D. R., & Senatore, F. F. (2017). Disparities in hypertension and cardiovascular disease in blacks: The critical role of medication adherence. *Journal of Clinical Hypertension, 19*(10) 1015–1024. Doi: 10.111/jch.13089.

Fredriksen-Goldsen, K. I., Kim, H.-J., Emlet, C. A., Muraco, A., Erosheva, E. A., Hoy-Ellis, C. P., Goldsen, J., & Petry, H. (2011). *The Aging and Health Report: Disparities and resilience among lesbian, gay, bisexual, and transgender older adults.* Seattle: Institute for Multigenerational Health.

Gallagher, D., Rose, J., Rivera, P., Lovett, S., & Thompson, L. (1989). Prevalence of depression in family caregivers. *The Gerontologist, 29*(4), 444–456.

Gilstrap, L. G., & Joynt, K. E. (2014). Understanding the relationship between readmission and quality of hospital care in heart failure. *Current Heart Failure Reports, 11*(4), 347–353.

Gohil, S. K., Datta, R., Cao, C., Phelan, M. J., Ngyen, V., Rowther, A. A., & Huang, S. S. (2015). Impact of hospital population case-mix, including poverty, on hospital all-cause and infection-related 30-day readmission rates. *Clinical Infectious Diseases, 61*(8), 1235–1243.

Goodwin, J. S. (2018). Decreasing blood pressure in older patients. *JAMA Internal Medicine, 178*(1), 100–101.

Grabowski, D. C., & McGuire, T. G. (2009). Black-white disparities in care in nursing homes. *Atlantic Economic Journal, 37*(3), 299–234.

Haines, K. L., Jung, H. S., Zens, T., Turner, S., Warner-Hillard, C., & Agarwal, S. (2018). Barriers to hospice care in trauma patients: The disparities in end-of-life care. *American Journal of Hospice and Palliative Medicine.* https://doi.org/10.1177/1049909117753377

Harley, D. A., & Teaster, P. B. (2018). Women, older adult, and LGBTQ populations with disabilities in rural, frontier, and territory communities. In D. Harley, N. Ysasi, M. Bishop, & A. Fleming (Eds.), *Disability and vocational rehabilitation in rural settings*. New York: Springer.

Harman, B. (1956). Aging: A theory based on free radical and radiation chemistry. *Journal of Gerontology*, 11280–11360.

Harrington, C., Schnelle, J. F., McGregore, M., & Simmons, S. F. (2016). The need for higher minimum staffing standards in U.S. nursing homes. *Health Services Insights, 9*, 13–19.

Harris-Kojetin, L., Sengupta, M., Park-Lee, E., Valverde, R., Caffrey, C., Rome, V., & Lendon, J. (2016). Long-term care providers and services users in the United States: Data from the National Study of Long-Term Care Providers, 2013-2014. *Vital Health Statistics, 3*(38), x–xii, 1–105.

Hayflick, L. (1993). Biology of human aging. *American Medicine and Science, 285*, 432–468.

Hayward M. D., Crimmins E. M., Miles T. P., & Yu Y. The significance of socioeconomic status in explaining the racial gap in chronic health conditions. *American Sociological Review. 2000;65*, 910–930.

Hoffman, K., Frederiksen, K. S., Sobol, N. A., Beyer, N., Vogel, A., Andersen, B. B., . . . Hasselbach, S. G. (2014). Impact of physical activity and cognition on activities on daily living in home-dwelling patients with mild to moderate Alzheimer's disease, *Journal of Alzheimer's Disease, 10*(4), Suppl. S761-762. https://aanddjournal .net/article/S1552-5260(14)02098-6/fulltext

Institute on Aging. (n.d.). Read how IOA views aging in America. Retrieved from https://www.ioaging.org /aging-in-america

Institute of Medicine. (2001). Improving the quality of long-term care. Washington, D.C.: National Academies Press.

Kaufman, J. E., Lee, Y., Vaughon, W., Unuigbe, A., & Gallo, W. T. (2018). Depression associated with transitions into and out of spousal caregiving. *International Journal of Aging and Human Development.* https://doi .org/10.1177/0091415018754310

Klein, L. C., Kim, K., Almeida, D. M., Femia, E. E., Rovine, M. J., & Zarit, S. H. (2016). Anticipating an easier day: Effects of adult day services on daily cortisol and stress. *The Gerontologist, 56*(2), 303–312. https://doi .org/10.1093/geront/gnu060

Kohli, R., Nelson, S., Ulrich, S., Finch, T., Hall, K., & Schwarz, E. (2017). Dental care practices and oral health training for professional caregivers in long-term care facilities: An interdisciplinary approach to address oral health disparities. *Geriatric Nursing, 38*(4), 296–301.

Kojima, G. (2015). Prevalence of frailty in nursing homes: A systematic review and meta-analysis. *Journal of the American Medical Directors Association, 16*(11), 940–945.

Konetzka, R. T., & Werner, R. M. (2009). Disparities in long-term care, building equity in market-based reforms. *Medical Care Review and Research, 66*(5), 491–521.

Lee, H. Y., Blegen, M. A., & Harrington, C. (2014). The effects of RN staffing hours on nursing home quality: A two-stage model. *International Journal of Nursing Studies, 51*(3), 409–417.

Lopez-Hartmann, M., Wens, J., Verhoeven, V., & Remmen, R. (2012). The effect of caregiver support interventions for informal caregivers of community-dwelling frail elderly: A systematic review. *International Journal of Integrated Care, 12*, e3133.

Lutfiyya, M. N., Gessert, C. E., & Lipsky, M. S. (2013). Nursing home quality: A comparative analysis using CMS Nursing Home Compare data to examine differences between rural and nonrural facilities. *Journal of the American Medical Directors Association, 14*(8), 593–598.

Martinovich, M. (2017). Significant racial and ethnic disparities still exist, according to Stanford Report, Stanford News, https://news.stanford.edu. June 16.

Medicare.gov. (n.d.). Nursing Home Compare. Retrieved from https://www.medicare.gov/NursingHomeCompare /About/howcannhchelp.html

MetLife Mature Market Institute. (2010). Still out, still aging: The MetLife study of lesbian, gay, bisexual, and transgender baby boomers. https://www.giaging.org /documents/mmi-still-out-still-aging.pdf

MetLife Mature Market Institute. (1999, November). The MetLife Juggling Act Study: Balancing caregiving with work and the costs involved. Metropolitan Life Insurance Company. Retrieved from http://www .caregiving.org/data/jugglingstudy.pdf

Mielenz, T.J., Kubiak-Rizzone, K.I., Alvarez, K.J., Hlavacek, P.R., Freburger, J.K., Giulani, C., Mercer, V.S. & Callahan, L.F. (2013) Association of self-efficacy and outcome expectations with physical activity in adults with arthritis. *Arthritis, 2013, Article 621396.* Doi: 10.1155/2013/621396.

National Council of Aging. (2018). Elder abuse facts. Retrieved from https://www.ncoa.org/public-policy-action/elder -justice/elder-abuse-facts/

National Council of Aging. (2015). Senior Centers. Fact Sheet. https://www.ncoa.org/wp-content/uploads/FactSheet _SeniorCenters.pdf

Potter, A. J, (2017). Factors associated with caregiver's use of support services and caregivers' nonuse of services sought. *Journal of Aging & Social Policy, 30*(2), 155–172, doi:10.1080/08959420.2017.1414539.

QuickStats: Percentage of Adults with Activity Limitations, by Age Group and Type of Limitation — National Health Interview Survey,† United States, 2014. MMWR Morb Mortal Wkly Rep 2016;65:14. DOI: http://dx.doi.org/10.15585/mmwr.mm6501a6

Rainville, C., Skufca, L., & Mehegan, L. (2016). Family Caregivers Cost Survey: What they spend and what they sacrifice. Family caregiving and out-of-pocket costs: 2016 report. AARP Research. Retrieved from https://www.aarp.org/research/topics/care/info-2016/family-caregivers-cost-survey.html

Schneider, E. J., & Reed, J. D. (1996). Life extension. *New England Journal of Medicine. 312*(18), 1158–1197.

Schulz, R., & Tompkins, C. A. (2010). Informal caregivers in the United States: Prevalence, caregiver characteristics, and ability to provide care. In: The Role of Human Factors in Home Health Care: Workshop Summary. National Academies Press: Wash. D.C.

Semega, J. L., Fontenot, K. R., & Kollar, M. A. U.S. Census Bureau, Current Population Reports, P60–259, *Income and Poverty in the United States: 2016*,U.S. Government Printing Office, Washington, DC, 2017.

Senanarong, V, Jamjumras, P., Harmphadungkit. K., Klubwongs, M., Udomphanthurak, S., Poungvarin, N., . . . Cummings J. L. (2004). A counseling intervention for caregivers: effect on neuropsychiatric symptoms. International *Journal of Geriatric Psychiatry, 19*(8), 781–788.

Sibalija, J., (2017). Social Support, Social Participation, and Depression among Caregivers and Non-Caregivers in Canada: A Population Health Perspective (2017). Electronic Thesis and Dissertation Repository. 4638. https://ir.lib.uwo.ca/etd/4638

Travers, J. L., Schroeder, K. L., Blaylock, T. E., & Stone, P. W. (2017). Racial/ethnic disparities in influenza and pneumococcal vaccination among nursing home residents: A systematic review. *The Gerontologist.* doi: 10.1093/geront/gnw193

Tremont, G., Davis, J. D., Papandonatos, G. D., Ott, B. F., Fortinsky, R. H. Gozalo, O., Yue, M. S., . . . Bishop, D.S. Psychosocial telephone intervention for dementia caregivers: A randomized, controlled trial. *Alzheimer's & Dementia*, 2014; DOI: 10.1016/j.jalz.2014.05.1752

Trinkoff, A. M., Lerner, N. B., Storr, C. L., Han, K., Johantgen, M. E., & Gartrell, K. (2015). Leadership education, certification and resident outcomes in US nursing homes: Cross-sectional secondary data analysis. *International Journal of Nursing Studies, 52*(1), 334–344.

U.S. Bureau of the Census (March 13, 2018). Older people projected to outnumber children for first time in

U.S. history, Release Number: CB18–41 https://www.census.gov. Accessed June 15, 2018.

U.S. Department of Agriculture. (2018). USDA support for older Americans. Release no. 0202.15. Retrieved from https://www.fns.usda.gov/pressrelease/2015/020215

Wang, G. C., & Casolaro, V. (2014). Immunologic changes in frail older adults. *Translational Medicine, UniSa, 9*, 1–6.

Ward, B. W., Schiller, J. S., & Goodman, R. A. Multiple chronic conditions among U.S. Adults: A 2012 update. *Preventing Chronic Disease*, 11, E62.

Werner, R. M., Konetzka, R. T., & Kim, M. M. (2013). Quality improvement under nursing home compare: The association between changes in process and outcome measures. *Medical Care, 51*(7), 582–588.

Werner, R. M., Konetzka, R. T., & Polsky, D. (2016). Changes in consumer demand following public reporting of summary quality ratings: An evaluation in nursing homes. *Health Services Research*, 51(Suppl 2), 1291–1309.

Williams, A., Straker, J. K., & Applebaum, R. (2016). The nursing home five star rating: How does it compare to resident and family views of care. *The Gerontologist, 56*(2), 234–242.

Williams, D. R., Mohammed, S. A., Leavell, J., & Collins, C. (2010). Race, socioeconomic status and health: Complexities, ongoing challenges and research opportunities. *Annals of the New York Academy of Sciences*, 1186, 69–101. doi: 10.1111/j.1749-6632.2009.05339.x

Woods, E.C., O'Conor, R., Martynenko, M., Wolf, M.S., Wisnivesky, J.P., & Federman, A.D. (2016). Associations of asthma control and airway obstruction with performance of activities of daily living among older asthmatics. *Journal of American Geriatrics Society, 64*(5), 1046-1053. Doi: 10.1111.jgs.14108

Xu, J. (2017). QuickStats: Age-Adjusted Death Rates, by Race/Ethnicity — National Vital Statistics System, United States, 2014–2015. *MMWR Morb Mortal Wkly Rep 2017;66:375.* DOI: http://dx.doi.org/10.15585/mmwr.mm6613a6

Yang, Y., Meng, H., & Miller, N. A. (2011). Rurality and nursing home quality: Evidence from the 2004 National Nursing Home Study. *The Gerontologist, 51*(6), 761–773.

Yu, F., Mathaison, M. A., & Lin, F. (2016) Interactive effects of cognitive and physical predictors of ADL in Alzeimer's disease. *The Journal of the Alzheimer's Association, 12*(7), Suppl. https://www.alzheimersanddementia.com/article/S1552-5260(16)30872-X/abstract?code=jalz-site

Zhang, N., Lu, S. F., Xu, B., Rodriguez-Monguio, R., & Gurwitz, J. (2016). Health information technologies: Which nursing homes adopted them? *Journal of the American Medical Directors Association, 17*(5), 441–447.

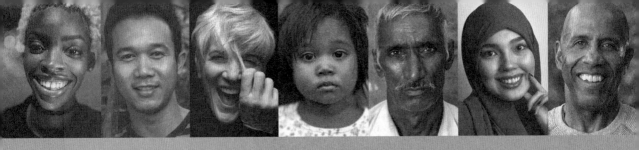

Appendix

State	Number of Nursing Homes	Nursing Home Star Ratings					Number Facilities with 1 or 2 Stars	Percentage of Facilities with 1 or 2 Stars
		5 Stars	4 Stars	3 Stars	2 Stars	1 Star		
Alabama	226	46	66	42	57	15	72	31.86%
Alaska	18	5	2	6	5	0	5	27.78%
Arizona	143	45	28	28	27	15	42	29.37%
Arkansas	227	60	54	44	45	24	69	30.40%
California	1,208	407	281	198	238	84	322	26.66%
Colorado	213	53	67	33	37	23	60	28.17%
Connecticut	229	63	62	36	47	21	68	29.69%
Delaware	45	19	7	8	10	1	11	24.44%
District of Columbia	19	10	3	2	3	1	4	21.05%
Florida	688	162	172	142	136	76	212	30.81%
Georgia	355	71	82	70	53	79	132	37.18%
Hawaii	46	18	12	6	8	2	10	21.74%

Nursing Home Compare Star Ratings for Each State

Nursing Home Star Ratings

Idaho	78	25	16	20	12	5	17	21.79%
Illinois	758	172	177	125	159	125	284	37.47%
Indiana	525	134	127	97	94	73	167	31.81%
Iowa	439	113	122	77	80	47	127	28.93%
Kansas	339	76	86	65	61	51	112	33.04%
Kentucky	285	37	66	62	50	70	120	42.11%
Louisiana	279	31	56	61	64	67	131	46.95%
Maine	103	33	29	22	16	3	19	18.45%
Maryland	226	61	57	34	47	27	74	32.74%
Massachusetts	413	109	107	75	78	44	122	29.54%
Michigan	431	125	99	72	84	51	135	31.32%
Minnesota	372	111	97	71	58	35	93	25.00%
Mississippi	202	37	52	39	36	38	74	36.63%
Missouri	511	111	117	102	102	79	181	35.42%
Montana	80	18	15	23	15	9	24	30.00%
Nebraska	211	46	47	47	51	20	71	33.65%
Nevada	53	15	11	10	8	9	17	32.08%
New Hampshire	76	20	23	10	17	6	23	30.26%
New Jersey	364	110	91	68	73	22	95	26.10%
New Mexico	70	9	21	14	15	11	26	37.14%
New York	625	136	125	117	126	121	247	39.52%
North Carolina	420	82	92	79	71	96	167	39.76%
North Dakota	80	21	24	14	16	5	21	26.25%

(continues)

Nursing Home Compare Star Ratings for Each State								
		Nursing Home Star Ratings						
State	**Number of Nursing Homes**	**5 Stars**	**4 Stars**	**3 Stars**	**2 Stars**	**1 Star**	**Number Facilities with 1 or 2 Stars**	**Percentage of Facilities with 1 or 2 Stars**
Ohio	944	173	216	168	204	183	387	41.00%
Oklahoma	304	33	72	67	59	73	132	43.42%
Oregon	135	32	38	25	26	14	40	29.63%
Pennsylvania	697	144	146	129	149	129	278	39.89%
Rhode Island	84	23	18	24	14	5	19	22.62%
South Carolina	187	40	42	40	32	33	65	34.76%
South Dakota	111	25	31	26	13	16	29	26.13%
Tennessee	317	59	75	66	53	64	117	36.91%
Texas	1,202	147	227	252	286	290	576	47.92%
Utah	97	32	20	17	17	11	28	28.87%
Vermont	37	11	7	9	7	3	10	27.03%
Virginia	284	51	66	59	60	48	108	38.03%
Washington	219	59	62	38	44	16	60	27.40%
West Virginia	126	18	28	23	27	30	57	45.24%
Wisconsin	385	115	100	63	69	38	107	27.79%
Wyoming	36	8	9	9	5	5	10	27.78%
Total	**15,522**	**3,561**	**3,650**	**2,934**	**3,064**	**2,313**	**5,377**	
Percentage of Nursing Homes with 1- and 2-Star Ratings								**34.64%**

Source: Compiled by Authors from data found in the archived datasets of Centers for Medicare and Medicaid Services (2015). Nursing Home Compare Database. 2015 Annual Files. ProviderInfo_2015.zip. https://data.medicare.gov/data/archives/nursing-home-compare

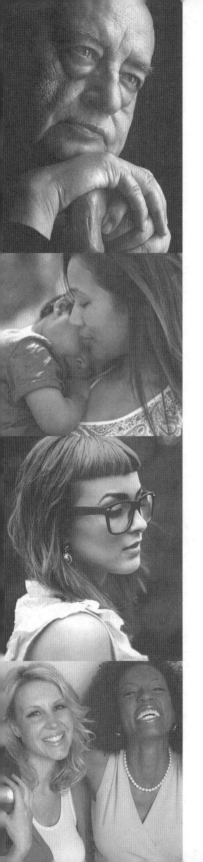

PART IV

Reanalyzing Health Disparities: Two Case Studies

"The aim is to get the students actively involved in seeking this evidence: their role is not simply to do tasks as decided by teachers, but to actively manage and understand their learning gains."

—**John Hattie**, the author wrote in his book - Visible Learning for Teachers: Maximizing Impact on Learning (2012)

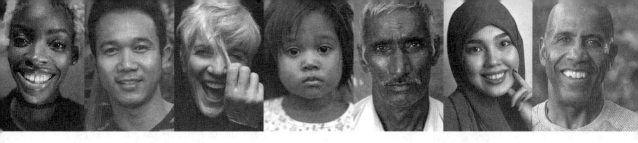

CHAPTER 13

"They Protect Eagles, Don't They?": Using Health Disparity Research to Tell New Stories

"There is often a big disparity between the way in which we perceive things and the way things really are."

— **The 14th Dalai Lama**

▶ Introduction

Health outcomes are generally based on two variables: (1) mortality as measured by life expectancy and death rates, and (2) morbidity as measured by the prevalence and incidence of disease and illness. Such topics are normally relegated to the domain of public health students and personnel rather than discussed in the arena of healthcare administration and/or clinical courses. However, knowledge of the public health and the clinical side of health care is necessary because it is those with illnesses and diseases who are served by the various components of the healthcare system, and by those who serve as the administrators of those systems. This case study focuses on a description of disparities in life expectancy and death rates by race/ethnicity, sex, and age. In doing so, it demonstrates how a narrow definition of health disparities can allow key health disparity issues to remain inadequately addressed.

The linkages between health disparities and healthcare disparities are linear. In this text, the concept of health disparities has been defined as any remediable differences in health characteristics and *health* outcomes across *any* identifiable subgroup in human society. This definition suggests that it is critical for current and future healthcare administrators, public health professionals, clinicians, healthcare researchers, policy makers, communities, and individuals and their families to engage in a data mining process so that remediable causes and correlates of current and emerging differentials can be identified and addressed.

▶ The Ultimate Health Outcome: Life Expectancy

Consider the following definitions of life expectancy from some of the more popular English dictionaries:

- "The average number of years that a person or animal can expect to live" (*Merriam Webster's Learner's Dictionary*, n.d.)
- "The probable number of years remaining in the life of an individual or class of persons as determined statistically, and as affected by factors such as heredity, physical condition, nutrition, and occupation" (Dictionary.com, n.d.)
- "The statistically determined average number of years of life remaining after a specified age for a given group of individuals" (*Collins Dictionary*, n.d.)

Despite the existence of a multiplicity of definitions of **life expectancy**, the one most commonly used is the number of years that an individual can expect to live at birth.

In the United States, life expectancy differs not only by race/ethnicity and sex but also by geography. **TABLE 13.1** presents life expectancy by state in 2014 without regard to race/ethnicity or sex. (Note, however, that life expectancy has, on average, fallen for both males and females over the last few years for which data are available.) Kochanek, Murphy, Xu, and Arias (2017) found that life expectancy at birth in the United States decreased from 78.7 years for the population as a whole in 2014 to 78.6 in 2016. However, life expectancy also decreased from 2014 to 2015. But even before this trend began, another rather alarming health disparity also existed. So, let's go backwards for a moment to 2014, the last year for which life expectancy was increasing and uncover some trends that were masked at that time.

As Table 13.1 demonstrates, although there are small observable differences in life expectancy among most states, a number of states have much lower life expectancy than others. For example, using Hawaii, the state with the highest life expectancy, as the reference point (81.15 years), some states have disparities of 5 or more years less in life expectancy than Hawaii. While this might seem to be a dramatic difference, if the geographic comparisons are based upon U.S. counties, the disparities sometimes exceed 20 years!

	TABLE 13.1 Life Expectancy and Disparities by U.S. State, 2014				
Rank	**States with Life Expectancies Above Mean Years at Birth**	**Life Expectancy (years)**	**Rank**	**States with Life Expectancies Below Mean Years at Birth**	**Life Expectancy (years)**
1	Hawaii	81.15	26	Montana	78.93
2	Minnesota	80.90	27	Pennsylvania	78.76
3	California	80.82	28	Kansas	78.74
4	Connecticut	80.56	29	Delaware	78.72
5	Massachusetts	80.41	30	Wyoming	78.62
6	New York	80.36	31	Texas	78.54
7	Vermont	80.24	32	Alaska	78.41
8	Colorado	80.21	33	New Mexico	78.35
9	New Hampshire	80.15	34	Michigan	78.26
10	New Jersey	80.04	35	Nevada	78.11
11	Washington	79.99	36	Ohio	77.91
12	North Dakota	79.95	37	North Carolina	77.86
13	Utah	79.91	38	Missouri	77.73
14	Wisconsin	79.79	39	Indiana	77.69
15	Rhode Island	79.76	40	Georgia	77.38
16	Iowa	79.73	41	District of Columbia	76.86
17*	Arizona	79.58	42	South Carolina	76.89
17*	Nebraska	79.58	43	Tennessee	76.33
18	South Dakota	79.57	44	Kentucky	76.26

(continues)

TABLE 13.1 Life Expectancy and Disparities by U.S. State: 2014 *(continued)*

Rank	States with Life Expectancies Above Mean Years at Birth	Life Expectancy (years)	Rank	States with Life Expectancies Below Mean Years at Birth	Life Expectancy (years)
19	Idaho	79.49	45	Arkansas	76.18
20	Florida	79.48	46	Oklahoma	76.09
21	Oregon	79.44	47	West Virginia	76.03
22	Maine	79.32	48	Louisiana	75.82
23	Virginia	79.18	49	Alabama	75.65
24	Maryland	79.16	50	Mississippi	74.91
25	Illinois	79.02		**All states**	**79.1**

* indicates duplicate ranking

Institute for Health Metrics and Evaluation Life expectancy at birth, both sexes, 2014 figures. Seattle, WA: IHME, University of Washington, 2014. www.healthdata.org/us-health.

In a seminal study, Dwyer-Lindgren and colleagues (2017) introduced the argument that research insufficiencies characterize data on life expectancy by state. This is because numerous differentials within and between states can be identified when the data are disaggregated into smaller geographic units such as counties. To examine their hypothesis, the authors analyzed data on America's 3,142 counties. The analysis revealed a life expectancy disparity that exceeded 20 years between the county with the highest life expectancy, Summit County, Colorado, an area with an overall life expectancy at birth of 86.83 years, and Oglala Lakota County of South Dakota, a community with a life expectancy of a mere 66.81 years.

Further analysis revealed that although Summit County is characterized by a disproportionately high population of White Americans—81.4% (Bureau of the Census, American FactFinder) and Oglala Lakota County has 92.9% Native Americans; socioeconomic factors combined with behavioral and disease-specific factors "explained" a far greater proportion of the difference in life expectancy than did race/ethnicity alone. In Union County, Florida, whose population consists of 70.7% White Americans, life expectancy was only 67.57 years. Owsley County, Kentucky, a population that consists of Americans who are 97.4% of European descent, had a life expectancy that was 16.09 years less than that of the residents of Summit County, Colorado. This research demonstrates the criticality of researchers asking different questions of the datasets that are available for the analysis of health disparities as scholars seek to advance the overall human condition.

Thus, healthcare administrators, public health professionals, and clinicians who deliver services in neighborhoods, zip codes, towns, cities, counties, and states with lower life expectancies must ask the following question: "Why are life expectancies so much lower and, critically, what can the component of the U.S. healthcare system that I serve do to reduce these disparities?"

Life expectancy disparities exist by the usually cited subgroups of race/ethnicity and sex. But, as a healthcare administrator, public health professional, or clinician, one should ask: "Have the numerous programs, policies, and interventions that have already been introduced been successful in reducing disparities in life expectancy?" The data listed in **TABLE 13.2** demonstrate that past efforts to reduce disparities in life expectancy by both race/ethnicity and sex have been effective. Table 13.2 reports data on disparities in life expectancy by race/ethnicity and sex as of 2014.

As Table 13.2 reveals, tremendous variance exists in life expectancy at birth in the United States by race/ethnicity and sex. Again, contrary to the thesis of "privilege" that is sometimes embedded in discussions of health disparities using the more traditional approach, health outcomes as measured by life expectancy (assuming the accuracy of the data) appear to be highest for Latino American women. This group can expect to live for 84.0 years from birth, or 2.9 years longer than females whose ancestry is primarily

TABLE 13.2 Life Expectancy Disparities by Race/Ethnicity and Sex: 2014

Sex and Race/Ethnicity	Life Expectancy (years)	Difference from Reference Group	% Difference from Reference Group
Female			
White, non-Hispanic Americans	81.1	Reference Group	Reference Group
Hispanic Americans	84.0	2.9 years higher	3.58% higher
African Americans, non-Hispanic	78.1	3.0 years lower	3.69% lower
Male			
Hispanic/Latino Americans	79.2	1.9 years lower	2.34% lower
White, non-Hispanic Americans	76.5	4.6 years less	5.67% lower
African Americans, non-Hispanic	72.0	9.1 years less	11.22% lower

Data from CDC/NCHS National Vital Statistics September, 2014: and in Health, United States, 2016, In Brief, (U.S. Department of Health and Human Services, CDC/NCHS, Hyattsville, MD 2016, pp. 19. Figure 18.7

TABLE 13.3 Life Expectancy by Race/Ethnicity and Sex: 1980 and 2014

Gap by Race/ Ethnicity and Sex*	1980	2014	Absolute Change	% Change
White males vs. African American males	6.9 years greater	4.2 years greater	2.7 years	39.13% decrease
White females vs. African American females	5.6 years greater	3.0 years greater	2.6 years	46.43% decrease

* Race/Ethnicity in this table includes Hispanic individuals
Calculated with data found in National Vital Statistics Reports, (2016). *65*(4), p. 34, Table 8.

European-based. However, American females of African descent have a life expectancy that is 3 years *lower* than that of American females of European descent.

As one reviews the data in Table 13.2, unexpectedly, Latino males lead the male category with a life expectancy of 79.2 years—a number that is 1.9 years lower (2.34% lower) than that for White American females. White American males rank relatively low in this racial/ethnic/gender hierarchy with a life expectancy of 76.5 years. White American males live, on average, 4.6 fewer years (5.67% fewer years) than their female counterparts. Finally, African American males, with a life expectancy of 72.0 years, can expect to live 9.1 fewer years (11.22% fewer years) than White American females. Thus, life expectancy rates are particularly adverse for African American males first and White American males second.

These disparities, despite their severity, improved from 1980 to 2014. **TABLE 13.3** demonstrates this point by comparing life expectancies for White Americans and African Americans for 1980 and 2014.

Table 13.3 demonstrates that disparities in life expectancy actually decreased over the 34-year period from 1980 to 2014. The gap in life expectancy between White males and African American males was 6.9 years in 1980 vs. 4.2 years in 2014. This represented a decrease of

39.13%. The life expectancy disparity between White American females and African American females decreased by 46.43%. By analyzing disparities in key healthcare institutions within the overall healthcare system, it may be possible for healthcare managers across subdisciplines to provide leadership in changes that can advance the closure of the disparity gap even more in the future. Additionally, the data suggest a need for sex-specific strategies to reduce the life expectancy gap between males and females. This process may require further disaggregation of the data so that intra- as well as intergroup disparities can be identified and targeted. Indeed, even this comparative data reveals the need for research and interventions to address the differences in life expectancy between White American males *and* African American males relative to Latino American males.

▶ Disparities in Death Rates by Age, Sex, and Race/Ethnicity

When death rates are analyzed by sex and race/ethnicity as well as age, even more unique areas of disparate outcomes can be identified. **TABLE 13.4** presents data on death rates per

TABLE 13.4 Death Rates per 100,000 by Age, Race/Ethnicity, and Sex, 2013

Age[d] (years)	All Races/Ethnicities		White Americans[a]		African Americans[a]		American Indian/Alaskan Native[a,b]		Asian/Pacific Islander Americans[a,c]	
	Male	Female	Male	Female	Male	Female	Male	Female	Male	Female
All ages[d]	839.1	804.4	899.1	879.4	739.3	651.1	416.5	348.2	347.4	297.4
<1[e]	650.5	536.1	566.4	456.8	1120.1	980.7	493.4	305.9	408.9	329.3
1–4	28.6	22.4	26.2	20.1	40.6	33.4	41.5	25.5	19.3	18.4
5–9	13.2	10.4	12.2	9.3	18.6	15.6	13.1	12.4	11.0	8.3
10–14	16.1	12.1	15.6	11.9	20.6	14.0	11.0	*	11.2	9.3
15–19	62.3	26.4	57.7	26.7	94.2	28.7	67.1	28.3	29.9	15.3
20–24	120.8	44.1	114.6	43.9	173.7	52.7	126.8	56.9	52.5	19.8
25–29	137.1	56.8	131.3	55.6	205.4	76.9	165.8	85.3	53.7	21.2
30–34	153.9	75.3	148.5	73.5	232.7	105.4	180.0	102.1	54.6	29.9
35–39	179.3	104.7	173.2	102.0	272.2	150.5	200.3	146.5	70.8	38.6
40–44	246.4	154.7	240.4	149.8	351.4	224.1	290.3	198.7	108.5	64.5
45–49	386.1	245.6	376.9	237.1	532.5	352.7	433.1	291.0	177.7	103.3

(continues)

TABLE 13.4 Death Rates per 100,000 by Age, Race/Ethnicity, and Sex, 2013 (continued)

Age[d] (years)	All Races/Ethnicities		White Americans[a]		African Americans[a]		American Indian/Alaskan Native[a,b]		Asian/Pacific Islander Americans[a,c]	
	Male	Female	Male	Female	Male	Female	Male	Female	Male	Female
50–54	609.4	378.0	598.7	363.9	824.0	554.3	582.8	377.9	266.9	154.6
55–59	914.1	540.5	883.7	518.6	1,347.6	810.9	805.2	541.3	413.7	226.7
60–64	1,295.0	770.7	1,245.4	742.8	1,995.1	1,150.1	1,115.7	715.8	644.5	358.5
65–69	1,798.4	1,171.9	1,760.0	1,155.8	2,608.4	1,584.1	1,529.2	1,095.1	913.5	560.6
70–74	2,734.7	1,858.0	2,702.7	1,849.4	3,751.2	2,362.4	2,347.9	1,645.7	1,429.4	909.8
75–79	4,311.2	3,058.8	4,304.0	3,072.5	5,409.0	3,532.3	3,494.4	2,730.2	2,473.7	1,738.2
80–84	7,137.6	5,253.1	7,194.3	5,309.9	7,949.2	5,669.5	5,515.2	3,983.7	4,484.4	3,196.3
≥85	14,911.6	13,021.6	15,220.4	13,316.1	13,657.1	11,929.2	9,034.3	8,008.4	10,142.8	8,240.4

* Figure does not meet standards of reliability or precision.

a   Race categories are consistent with the 1977 Office of Management and Budget (OMB) standards. In 2013, multiple-race data were reported by 42 states and the District of Columbia. The multiple-race data for these reporting areas were bridged to the single-race categories of the 1977 OMB standards for comparability with other reporting areas.

b   Includes Aleut and Eskimo persons.

c   Includes Chinese, Filipino, Hawaiian, Japanese, and other Asian or Pacific Islanders.

d   Figures for age not stated are included in "All ages" but not distributed among age groups.

e   Death rates for "<1 year" (based on population estimates) differ from infant mortality rates (based on live births).

Data from Xu, J., Murphy, S.L., Kochanek, K.D., & Bastian, B.A. (2016). Deaths: Final Data for 2013, National Vital Statistics Reports; 64:2. Table 3 Number of deaths and death rates, by age, race, and sex: United States, 2013.

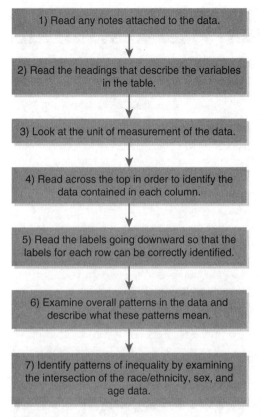

1) Read any notes attached to the data.

2) Read the headings that describe the variables in the table.

3) Look at the unit of measurement of the data.

4) Read across the top in order to identify the data contained in each column.

5) Read the labels going downward so that the labels for each row can be correctly identified.

6) Examine overall patterns in the data and describe what these patterns mean.

7) Identify patterns of inequality by examining the intersection of the race/ethnicity, sex, and age data.

FIGURE 13.1 How to interpret tabular data.

100,000 that have been disaggregated by age, sex, and race/ethnicity for 2013.

Table 13.4 contains data that can be used to identify disparities in death rates by age, race/ethnicity, and sex in 2013. Essential to using such data to uncover under-addressed disparities, one must first understand how to correctly *read* a data table.

How do we "read" the data?

FIGURE 13.1 outlines steps to apply in order to read secondary data from federal and other sources before attempting to use a dataset to extract information regarding disparities. **BOX 13.1** presents additional information that is key to interpreting the data in Table 13.4.

Before analyzing data for the presence of disparities, it is important to carefully study the dataset in order to understand the characteristics of the data. Once one has developed an understanding of the data, it becomes possible to ask, "What are some of the disparities in death rates by age and race/ethnicity based upon absolute differences in death rates per 100,000?" **BOX 13.2** presents a number of statements based on the data in Table 13.4. We now ask that you review the data in Table 13.4 and determine if each statement made in Box 13.2 is true or false.

One statement in Box 13.2 is intentionally false. Were you able to identify it? (The statement for the 75–79 age group is false. How much *is* that disparity?) This aspect of our case study clearly demonstrates how current definitions of health disparities have led to distorted responses. *Males are dying at a rate that is significantly (p < .05) higher than females.* Yet, healthcare professionals and providers are disproportionately focusing on females! The issue of health disparities and sex oftentimes includes the statement, "Yes, women have a lower death rate than men, but they are also sicker" (Apfel, 1982). Given that American culture tends to view length of life as the preferred outcome even when morbidity is present, the data suggest that, in some respects, *male health disparities have been subordinated to those of women.*

Stated differently, an implied conflict theoretical framework has been applied that has led to asymmetric interest in women's health. For example, Choy et al., (2015), in a study of America's top 50 highest-ranked hospitals, discovered that only 16 (32%) had established dedicated men's health centers, whereas 49 (98%) had a women's health center.

This case study clearly demonstrates the underlying framework of competitive and conflictual tribalism that undergirds the entirety of the health disparities "movement." Males and females live in common households as husbands and wives, uncles and aunts, sisters and brothers, fathers and mothers, and mothers and sons. Accordingly, it is in the mutual interest of males and females to understand the nature of their respective disparities and to

---

BOX 13.1 Identifying the Nature and Type of Information Presented in Table 13.4

What groups are included in Table 13.4? Table 13.4 presents data on death rates for all racial/ethnic groups: Whites without the exclusion of Latinos, African Americans without the exclusion of Latinos, Native Americans/Alaska Natives, and Asian/Pacific Islanders.

What type of data are presented by race/ethnicity? The data presented are death rates by age and sex.

What units are used to measure the death rates? Number of deaths per 100,000 persons.

Why are these units used rather than absolute numbers of deaths? Death rates per 100,000 are used rather than absolute death rates in order to standardize the data to account for the differences in the size of each population.

What does the note at the bottom of the table tell us about the data presented?

■ The note indicates that the data listed with an asterisk are not very reliable.
■ The notes inform us that data as reported in the table utilize the racial/ethnic classification used by the Office of Management in collecting the data but modified by the authors.

Why are the age data listed in 4-year intervals?
The age data listed in 4-year intervals are referred to as *age-specific data*. While the use of 4-year intervals can be considered as arbitrary, efforts are made to choose intervals that are neither too narrow nor too wide. The method used to construct these data is called *standardization*. Table 13.4 has 19 age groups, and mortality rates for the older groups are higher compared to the younger groups. Moreover, one can also divide the data based on race/ethnicity (i.e., *race-specific data*). By constructing the standardized data, we could eliminate the age, race/ethnicity, etc., difference so that comparisons of two populations can be made.

BOX 13.2 Disparities in Death Rates by Age and Race/Ethnicity: True or False?

True or False? Males have higher death rates than females in every single age group.

True or False? Males experience higher rates of death than their female counterparts across every single racial/ethnic group. Therefore, being a male in American society is hazardous to one's health.

True or False? In general, males of all races have a death rate (839.1 per 100,000) that is at least 4.31% higher than that of females (804.4 per 100,000).

In selected age groups, however, these disparities are much greater:

True or False? Males < 1 year have a death rate that is 21.26% higher than the rate for females.

True or False? Teen males aged 15–19 years have a death rate of 62.3 per 100,000, compared to 26.4 per 100,000 for females. The male death rate for this age group is 135.98% higher than for their female counterparts!

True or False? The disparity worsens for those 20–24 years, increasing to a 173.9% higher death rate for males than for females.

True or False? When males and females reach 25–29 years, the death rate disparity falls to 141.37%.

True or False? For the age range of 30–34 years, the differential by sex falls even more, to 71.58%.

True or False? For the age range of 35–39 years, males die 71.25% more often than their same-age female counterparts, a very slight drop from the age 30–34 interval.

True or False? At ages 40–44 years, a more significant change occurs. The disparity in death rates between males and females is only 59.27%.

True or False? At ages 45–49 years, the disparity drops even more, to 57.21%.

True or False? In the age range of 50–54 years, the disparity in male and female death rates reaches an even lower level—609.4 versus 245.6, or 48.13%.

True or False? Once the age range 55–59 is reached, however, the disparity ratio climbs to 69.12%.

True or False? In the 60–64 age group, the probability that a male will die declines slightly and is 68.83% higher than for females.

True or False? In the 65–69 age group, the disparity rate falls to a level that is only 53.46% higher for males than for females, as death more rapidly claims the lives of people of both sexes.

True or False? By the 70–74 age range, the disparity rate drops to 47.18%.

True or False? For the 75–79 age range, the death rate disparity for males and females drops even further, to 40.94%.

True or False? For males and females who reach the ages range of 80–84 years, the disparity in death rates drops to 35.87%.

True or False? Finally, in the range 85 and older, the death rate disparity drops to the lowest point in the life history of both sexes—14.51%. Thus, a male who reaches age 85 is only 14.51% more likely to die than his female counterpart and, for practical purposes, finally experiences equity in the probability of death.

be subject to *interventions that simultaneously target the causes of disparities in each respective group.*

Educational programs have been established to promote family literacy throughout the United States. Louie and Davis-Welton (2016) describe one strategy that is used by in-service and preservice teachers to deliver services that simultaneously elevate literacy across the whole family. Yet, because of the framework used in the field of health disparities, a similar model has not yet been exported from the field of education and applied as a design for reducing sex-based disparities. However, although the area of health disparities is more interdisciplinary, multidisciplinary, cross-disciplinary, and transdisciplinary than most fields, the noninclusion of education specialists has prevented the bilateral flow of information across these two disciplines.

What do you mean by "interdisciplinary," "multidisciplinary," "cross-disciplinary," and "transdisciplinary"?

These terms all refer to the way that a particular topic or problem is examined. An **interdisciplinary** approach to a subject involves two or more fields within the same discipline and/or two or more disciplines. **Multidisciplinary** refers to an assembly of a team of persons from a range of academic fields who apply their area

of expertise to a common problem. **Cross-disciplinary** generally describes an approach to knowledge in which one discipline and/or issues in one discipline are viewed from the perspective of another. **Transdisciplinary** suggests that theories, methods, and concepts of one discipline are neither viewed from the perspective of another discipline nor merged. Rather, issues are lifted from the arena of their kinship to a discipline and analyzed without the use of any disciplinary lenses.

A theme throughout this text is that health disparities are at a point in history when it is imperative to unshackle the subject matter from latent assumptions and timeworn frameworks. The objective in doing so is that of crafting interventions and solutions that will lead to win-win outcomes across all groups and subgroups. In the next part of our case study, the disparities data just presented will be used to demonstrate a very serious problem that is being under-addressed by healthcare administrators, public health professionals, clinicians, and the general public. *Specifically, as one reviews the data on death rate disparities by sex and age, it becomes clear that current frameworks have either masked and/or simply subordinated the fact that America's young males aged 15–20, 20–24, and 25–29 are dying at rates that are respectively 135.98%, 173.9%, and 141.37% higher than the death rates for females in the same age categories.* These differences are statistically significant ($p < .05$).

Sadly, public health personnel, healthcare administrators, policy analysts, parents, and the media have not been vocal regarding the existence of these disparities. No emergency measures have been implemented to identify and address the causes of these severe disparities, nor have approaches been designed, applied, or tested that will decrease both male *and* female death rates during this at-risk period of the life span.

▶ The Crisis of Early Death Disparities Among Young Males: An Analysis of the Data by Race/Ethnicity

Given the contemporary intensity of racial/ethnic conflict and the assignment of human interest among each group to the protection of their own current and future resources, it becomes necessary to ask, "Is the absence of a robust response to the crisis of the disproportionate early deaths of young men masked because the public is unaware that the problem intercuts all racial/ethnic groups?" Perhaps so, perhaps not. However, the data in **TABLE 13.5** indicate that males aged 15 to 29 years across all racial ethnic groups are at much higher risk of death than their female counterparts.

As Table 13.5 indicates, male/female disparity rates are extraordinarily high across every single ethnic group in the 15–19 age range; a White American male is 114.23% more likely to die than a White American female. This difference increases to 161.05% in the 20–24 age range, before dropping slightly to 136.15% for young adults aged 25–29.

African American youth and young adults have the highest overall death rates and the highest male/female disparities in death for each age bracket. Indeed, in the 15–19 age bracket, African American female death rates are only slightly higher than those of their White American counterparts. Because the

TABLE 13.5 Disaggregating the Disproportionate Risks of Early Deaths of Males Aged 15 to 29 Years

Age (years)	Males (death rates per 100,000)	Females (death rates per 100,000)	Disparity Rate
White			
15–19	57.7	26.7	116.10% higher for White American males than for White American females
20–24	114.6	43.9	161.05% higher for White American males than for White American females
25–29	131.3	55.6	136.15% higher for White American males than for White American females

African Americans			
15–19	94.2	28.7	228.22% higher for African American males than for African American females
20–24	173.7	52.7	229.60% higher for African American males than for African American females
25–29	205.4	76.9	167.1% higher for African American males than for African American females
American Indian/Alaskan Native Americans			
15–19	67.1	28.3	137.10% higher for American Indian/Alaskan Native males than for American Indian/Alaskan Native females
20–24	126.8	56.9	122.85% higher for American Indian/Alaskan Native males than for American Indian/Alaskan Native females
25–29	165.8	85.3	94.37% higher for American Indian/Alaskan Native males than for American Indian/Alaskan Native females
Asian/Pacific Islanders			
15–19	29.9	15.3	95.42% higher for Asian/Pacific Islander males than for Asian/Pacific Islander females
20–24	52.5	19.8	165.15% higher for Asian/Pacific Islander males than for Asian/Pacific Islander females
25–29	53.7	21.2	153.30% higher for Asian/Pacific Islander males than for Asian/Pacific Islander females

Disparity rates are calculated from data found in Table 13: Death Rates per 100,000 by Age, Race/Ethnicity, and Sex: 2013, using the difference analysis with a male reference point as the methodology.

Source: Constructed from data found in Xu, Jiaquan, Murphy, Sherry L, Kochanek, Kenneth D, and Bastian, Brigham A. (2016). *Deaths: Final Data for 2013, National Vital Statistics Reports*; 64:2. Table 3 Number of deaths and death rates, by age, race, and sex: United States, 2013.

death rate for African American males in the age group is 63.26% higher than that of White American males of the same age, the disparity by sex is 242.16% higher than for females. As African American females and males age, the racial/ethnic disparities with White Americans of the same sex widen. As a result, the sex-based disparity falls but remains extremely high—229.6% for African American males and

females aged 20 to 24 and 167.1% for those aged 25 to 29.

Native American/Alaskan Native females have death rates that are fairly close to both African American and White American females in the 15–19 bracket, 28.3%. In the 20–24 and 25–29 age brackets, death rates for Native American/Alaskan Native females remain fairly close to those of African American females.

As with White Americans and African American males, the male/female disparity rates for Native Americans/Alaskan Native Americans range from 137.10% higher for those aged 15 to 19, to 122.85% for those aged 20 to 24, and 94.37% higher for those aged 25 to 29.

If the data are fairly accurate on death rate disparities for male Asian American youth and adults, extremely high disparities also characterize this population group. In the 15–19 bracket, males die 95.4% more often than females. In the 20–24 bracket, the disparity rate is 165.15%. While it drops by ages 25 to 29, the disparity rate, nevertheless, remains extremely high—153.30%. The breadth of these disparities is extreme.

The data in Table 13.5 merge deaths for Latino and non-Latino American youth into one category—White Americans. It thus becomes instructive to disaggregate the data in order to identify sex-based disparities within this ethnic group (**TABLE 13.6**).

When the data are further stratified by Latino, non-white American ethnicity, the pattern of broad disparities by sex for this age group continues. For Latino Americans in the 15–19 age category, the male death rate is 146.57% higher than that for females. This disparity increases to

TABLE 13.6 Death Rate Disparities for Latino Youth by Sex			
Age (years)	Male Death Rates per 100,000	Female Death Rates per 100,000	Disparity Rate
Latinos			
15–19	50.3	20.4	146.57% higher for Latino American males than Latino female youth
20–24	94.6	30.9	206.15% higher for Latino American males than Latino female youth
25–29	96.6	35.5	172.11% higher for Latino American male youth than Latino female youth
White, non-Hispanic			
15–19	16.0	11.6	37.93% higher for White American male youth than White American female youth
20–24	58.6	28.2	107.80% higher for White American male youth than White female youth
25–29	118.3	47.0	151.70% higher for White American male youth than White female youth

Table constructed by the authors from data found in Table 13.4: per 100,000 Death Rates by Age, Race/Ethnicity, and Sex: 2013.
Source: Constructed from data found in Xu, Jiaquan, Murphy, Sherry L, Kochanek, Kenneth D, and Bastian, Brigham A. (2016). *Deaths: Final Data for 2013, National Vital Statistics Reports*; 64:2. Table 3 Number of deaths and death rates, by age, race, and sex: United States, 2013.

206.15% for the 20–24 age group before dropping to 172.11% for the 25–29 age group.

The table also disaggregates the data for White American youth alone. Although the disparity in death rates for males and females in the 15–19 interval is only 37.9%, the risk of death for the 20–24 age group increases so much that White American males are 107.8% more likely to die than White females. This disparity rate increases to 151.70% for the 25–29 age group.

▶ The Health Disparities of Young Males: An Underacknowledged Crisis

You may be familiar with the Save the Whales organization and the movement under way in the United States to protect all marine mammals, and this is a noble purpose. Rachel Carson, in the now classic book *Silent Spring* (1962), initiated a movement that successfully resulted in the reversal of the soaring disparities in death rates of brown pelicans relative to other birds. The Endangered Species Act has significantly supported the preservation of America's wildlife. However, a movement of similar magnitude has not been directed toward the reduction of disparities in the death rates of young males in American society. This is not to say that programs to reduce deaths due to accidents and injuries, violence, substance use, and other causes do not exist. **BOX 13.3** lists various federal initiatives that are designed to decrease death rates among youth and young adults in general. However, because males have higher risks than females in some of these areas, they may have some impact upon the disparate behaviors that result in young males losing their lives.

Yet, the data clearly reveal that more interventions are needed. At this point in history, a collective, unified movement is warranted that is designed to decrease avoidable death rates among males and females in these targeted age groups. These differential death rates have now altered the difference in sex ratios for the entire country in such a way that males are now 49.2% of the residents of the nation. Without aggressive intervention, this ratio will worsen. However, the design of such programs requires greater insight into causes of death rate disparities across various subgroups. Yet, the use of the current definitions of health disparities has not supported an aggressive campaign to address this issue.

BOX 13.3 Sample of Federal Programs That Seek to Reduce Early Death Rates Among Youth and Young Adults

National Tobacco Control Program (NTCP) – While the various NTCP programs are not specifically designed to address male/female disparities for youth and young adults, data from the Youth Risk Behavior Surveillance System (YRBSS) for 2015 revealed that 9.2% of male high school students smoked more than 10 cigarettes per day but only 5.9% of female high school students did so. Thus, tobacco interventions can reduce disparate young male/female death rates.
Striving To Reduce Youth Violence Everywhere (STRYVE) – Likewise, the same YRBSS dataset indicate that in 2015, 3.7% of males sustained injuries in a physical fight that were so severe that they required medical treatment but only 1.8% of females did the same.
National Centers for Excellence on Youth Violence Prevention (YVPCs) – Approximately 24.3% of males carried a weapon while in high school in 2015, but only 7.5% of females did so. (YRBSS, 2016)
Compendium of Evidence-Based Interventions and Best Practices for HIV Prevention – The YRBSS also reported that more than 14.1 males had sex with 4 or more persons but only 8.8% of females did so.

Chapter Summary

A wealth of data exists regarding disparities in life expectancy and death rates. A discussion of this full body of statistical information would necessarily overwhelm the reader. Accordingly, this chapter has introduced a minimum quantity of this body of statistics. All data included were carefully selected by asking the question, "What are some critical statistical information that current or future healthcare administrators, public health personnel, and clinicians need to address regarding ongoing health disparities in life expectancy at birth and overall disparities in death rates that have remained underaddressed due to definitional constraints in the field?" More important, this chapter focused on ensuring that current or future healthcare administrators and/or other personnel have the skills to properly read and interpret the data that serve as the basis for the calculation of disparities. This chapter also demonstrates that new questions can be asked of current data and under-acknowledged health disparities identified by using the simplest of statistical tools.

Review Questions and Problems

1. Locate life expectancy data for the year 2000, and cite the source. By how much has life expectancy changed since that time? To what degree did life expectancy disparities between males and females change between 2000 and 2017? Have those disparities improved or worsened?
2. Do you consider the disparities in life expectancy by states as being sufficiently wide so as to motivate you to consider living and working as a healthcare administrator, public health professional, or clinician in one state as opposed to another? Why or why not?

3. Write a short story (250 to 350 words) about a female "gold digger" who wants to marry a wealthy man in order to inherit his wealth. Be sure to include a statistical rationale for the age range and ethnicity she should choose if she wishes to minimize the number of years she must live with her targeted prey.
4. Write a blog entry of at least 500 words that informs readers about the severe disparities that exist in death rates between young males aged 15 to 29 years.
5. How do the definitions of life expectancy presented in the chapter differ?
6. List at least three federal programs to reduce health disparities.
7. Differentiate among interdisciplinary, multidisciplinary, cross-disciplinary, and transdisciplinary.

Key Terms and Concepts

cross-disciplinary An approach to knowledge in which one discipline and/or issues in one discipline are viewed from the perspective of another.

interdisciplinary Approach to a subject that involves two or more fields within the same discipline and/or two or more disciplines.

life expectancy The number of years that an individual can expect to live at birth.

multidisciplinary An assembly of a team of persons from a range of academic fields who apply their area of expertise to a common problem.

transdisciplinary Theories, methods, and concepts of one discipline are neither viewed from the perspective of another discipline nor merged. Rather, issues are lifted from the arena of their kinship to a discipline and analyzed without the use of any disciplinary lenses.

References

Apfel, R. J. (1982). How are women sicker than men? An overview of psychosomatic problems in women. *Psychotherapy and Psychosomatics, 37*(2), 106–118.

Arias, E., Heron, M., & Xu, J. (2017). United States life tables, 2014, National Vital Statistics reports; vol. 66, no. 4, Hyattsville, MD: National Center for Health Statistics.

Carson, R. (1962). *Silent spring*. Greenwich, CT: Houghton Mifflin.

Choy, J., Kashanian, J. A., Sharma, V., Masson, P., Dupree, J., Le, B., & Brannigan, R. E. (2015). The men's health center: Disparities in gender specific health services among the top 50 "best hospitals" in America. *Asian Journal of Urology, 2*(3), 170–174.

Collins Dictionary. (n.d.). Life expectancy. Retrieved from https://www.collinsdictionary.com/us/dictionary/english/life-expectancy

Dictionary.com. (n.d.). Life expectancy. Retrieved from http://www.dictionary.com/browse/life-expectancy

Dwyer-Lindgren, L., Bertozzi-Villa, A., Stubbs, R. W., Morozoff, C., Mackenbach, J. P., van Lenthe, F. J., . . . Murray, C. J. L. (2017). Inequalities in life expectancy among U.S. counties, 1980 to 2014: Temporal trends and key drivers. *JAMA Internal Medicine, 177*(7), 1003–1011.

Kann, L., McManus, T., Harris, W. A., Shanklin, S. L., Flint, K. H., Hawkins, J., ... & Whittle, L. (2016). Youth Risk Behavior Surveillance–United States, 2015. Morbidity and Mortality Weekly Report. Surveillance Summaries. 65(6). Centers for Disease Control and Prevention.

Kochanek, K. D., Murphy, S. L., Xu, J. & Tejada-Vera, B. (2016) National Vital Statistics Reports 65(4). P. 34.

Table 8: Live expectancy at birth, by race, Hispanic origin, race for non-Hispanic population, and sex: United States, 1940, 1950, 1960, 1970 and 1975–2014. https://www.cdc.gov/nchs/data/nvsr/nvsr65/nvsr65_04.pdf

Kochanek, K. D., Murphy, S. L., Xu, J. Q., & Arias, E. Mortality in the United States, 2016. NCHS Data Brief, no. 293. Hyattsville, MD: National Center for Health Statistics, 2017.

Louie, B., & Davis-Welton, K. (2016). Family Literacy Project. *The Reading Teacher, 69*(6), 597–606.

Merriam Webster's Learner's Dictionary. (n.d.). Life expectancy. Retrieved from http://www.learnersdictionary.com/definition/life%20expectancy

National Center for Health Statistics. Health, United States, 2015: With Special Feature on Racial and Ethnic Health Disparities. Hyattsville, MD. 2016. Table 15, pg. 95

National Center for Health Statistics. Health, United States, 2015: With Special Feature on Racial and Ethnic Health Disparities. Hyattsville, MD. 2016. Table 18, pg. 38

U.S. Census Bureau. American FactFinder. Community Facts. 2016 American Community Survey. Demographic and Housing Estimates for 2014. American Community Survey 5-Year Estimates. https://factfinder.census.gov/faces/nav/jsf/pages/community_facts.xhtml

Xu, J., Murphy, S. L., Kochanek, K. D., & Bastian, B. A. (2016). *Deaths: Final Data for 2013, National Vital Statistics Reports*; 64:2. Table 3 Number of deaths and death rates, by age, race, and sex: United States, 2013.

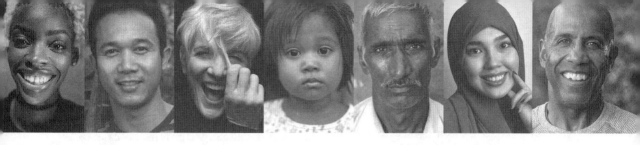

CHAPTER 14

Uncovering Health Disparities: A Case Study on Adverse Childhood Experiences and Unintentional Injuries

"Safety and security don't just happen, they are the result of collective consensus and public investment. We owe our children, the most vulnerable citizens in our society, a life free of violence and fear."

—**Nelson Mandela**, Former President of South Africa

Michelle Sotero, MPH, PhD

CHAPTER OBJECTIVES

After completing this chapter, each learner will be able to:

- Describe the importance of statistical analyses to the field of health disparities.
- Outline a step-by-step case study of how sophisticated statistical tools can be used to identify previously unidentified disparities.
- Interpret findings from a more sophisticated health disparity study that demonstrates the need to address all subgroup differences in health disparities.
- Demonstrate understanding of the disparity chain via an original statistical exercise that reveals the impact of adverse childhood experiences (ACEs) on injury disparities among persons aged 24 to 32 years.

▶ Introduction

In some respects, the field of health disparities has, itself, contributed to asymmetric analyses of the distribution of health problems that require the application of public health prevention and intervention strategies. For example, based on the facts that white males die earlier but females experience greater illnesses, the number of women's health clinics is now significantly higher than the number of men's health clinics. Similarly, declining life expectancy of lower-income, less-educated White Americans has only recently been identified as a health problem. Public health interventions to address the issue have yet to be developed. In this chapter, we seek to reverse this trend in disparity-based research by applying logistic regression to data from Wave I (1994) and Wave IV (2007–2008) of the National Longitudinal Study of Adolescent and Adult Health in order to test the hypothesis that adverse childhood experiences (ACEs) are associated with unintentional and intentional injuries among young adults aged 24 to 32 years. Data will be stratified by race/ethnicity, sex, and socioeconomics in order to identify interventions that can target all subgroups with disparate outcomes. The goal of this case study is to add to current knowledge by initiating a repositioning of the field of health disparities away from its current implicit adoption of a "comparative victimology" approach. Accordingly, this chapter uses empirical findings to advance alterations in the health disparities conceptual framework that currently dominates the field of health disparities.

Empirically speaking, this research, when extracted from health disparities, adds to current knowledge regarding the impact of ACEs as a variable in the disparity chain. Specifically, it uses data from the only nationally representative longitudinal study of adolescent and adult health in the United States. Additionally, it adds to current knowledge in this unique area because the trend in epidemiologic and injury prevention research is to focus upon the proximate causes of injury.

Proximate causes are the last set of causes in the disparity chain. In this case, we argue that currently public health prevention and intervention strategies are directed toward risk factors that immediately precede an injury. This same pattern is also evident in dialogues regarding health disparities. The results in this case study indicate an extreme need for interventions based on the chain of risk to complement current approaches.

How does this case study address health disparities?

Patterned asymmetries in morbidity and mortality in American society have been firmly substantiated (Desai, Zhang, & Hennessy, 1999). Accordingly, it is less than surprising that in November 2000 U.S. Public Law 106-525 was passed by the 106th Congress as an amendment to the Public Health Act. Based on the unequal distribution of adverse health outcomes among "African Americans, Hispanics, Native Americans, Alaska Natives, and Asian/Pacific Islanders, compared to the United States population as a whole" the Minority Health and Health Disparities Research and Education Act of 2000 was passed. Paragraph (2) of this act also acknowledges that "the largest numbers of the medically underserved are white individuals, and many of them have the same health care access problems as members of minority groups." Yet, health disparities has developed as a field that has largely excluded medically underserved whites. Moreover, despite the language of the initial legislation, health disparities as a health area has not emerged as a transethnic, transracial, transgender field of inquiry that seeks to identify and diminish modifiable differentials in morbidity and mortality across all subgroups within the society. As a result, the current opioid crisis, a health disparity that systematically affects low-income whites, was not identified until it reached crisis proportion (Hansen & Netherland, 2016). Similarly, the decline in life expectancy of undereducated whites has only recently been detected (Case & Deaton, 2015).

Accordingly, this chapter demonstrates the urgent need to more inclusively define health disparities so that strategies to strengthen healthcare outcomes can be developed that address areas of need across America's combinations and permutations of underserved subgroups. This chapter applies techniques of causal analysis to illustrate the usefulness of both simple and more sophisticated tools of analysis in the area of health disparities.

▶ ACEs, Injuries, and Health Disparities

Adverse childhood experiences (ACEs) are highly stressful and often traumatic events that occur during childhood and adolescence; they are also termed *developmental trauma* or *complex trauma*. The presence of ACEs as a potential threat to the health of children is now widely acknowledged (Courtois, 2004; Courtois & Ford, 2009; Felitti et al., 1998; Van der Kolk, 2005).

ACEs can include (1) child maltreatment (physical, emotional, or sexual abuse; neglect); (2) exposure to substance abuse and/or domestic violence in the home; (3) parents and/or household members with physical and/or mental disabilities; (4) interpersonal loss such as the death of a parent or friend; or (5) parental transitions such as divorce, entry into foster care, or the incarceration of a parent. ACEs are often chronic, but can also be acute, such as in the sudden dramatic death of a parent or close friend (Giovanelli, Reynolds, Mondi, & Ou, 2016).

ACEs may have lasting developmental and neurobiological effects on the individual (Brodsky & Biggs, 2012; Danese & McEwen, 2012; Heim, Newport, Bonsall, Miller, & Nemeroff, 2001; Shonkoff, Bryce, & McEwen, 2009). Childhood and adolescence are crucial

stages of life for cognitive, emotional, and psychological development. As a result, adverse or traumatic experiences during these critical stages can have lifelong effects on identity development, self-esteem, trust and intimacy, mental health, and physical health (Dolgin, 2011).

Approximately 80% of ACEs are centered within the family (Van der Kolk, 2005). However, research has shown that children in non-parental care (e.g., foster care) are almost three times more likely to report ACEs compared to children living with their biological parents (Bramlett & Radel, 2014).

A number of other childhood experiences have been identified that qualify as ACEs, such as household dysfunction (Anda et al., 2002; Beautrais, 2003; Dube et al., 2003; Felitti et al., 1998; Fergusson, Boden, & Horwood, 2000; Rothman, Edwards, Heeren, & Hingson, 2008). Household dysfunction includes events such as witnessing domestic violence (English et al., 2009; La Noue, Graeber, Helitzer, & Fawcett, 2013), residential transitions or divorce (Beautrais, Joyce, & Mulder, 1996; Reavis, Looman, Franco, & Rojas, 2013; Springer, Sheridan, Kuo, & Carnes, 2007), parental substance abuse (Hussong et al., 2008), and parental criminality (Sprinkle, 2007). Other studies have examined parental illness or disability, interpersonal loss such as the death of a parent or close friend, or experiencing street violence (Bruffaerts et al., 2010; Fried, Williams, Cabral, & Hacker, 2013; Johnson et al., 2002; Kaplow, Gipson, Horwitz, Burch, & King, 2014; Pilowsky, Keyes, & Hasin, 2009; Ramstad, Russo, & Zatzick, 2004; Turner & Lloyd, 2003). Some studies have also included experiences with war or natural disasters (O'Donnell et al., 2009).

How prevalent are ACEs?

ACEs are common in the general population. The most studied type of ACE is child maltreatment. In 2012 in the United States, child protective services at state and local agencies responded to approximately 3.8 million reports of child maltreatment. More recent data indicate that in 2016 this number had decreased to 3.15 million (Child Trends Databank, 2016).

In 2012, the rate of substantiated reports of child maltreatment was 9.2 per 1,000 children aged 0 to 17 years. Nationally, 78.3% of victims were neglected, 18.3% were physically abused, 9.3% were sexually abused, and 8.5% were psychologically maltreated (Child Trends Databank, 2014). Epidemiological surveys of adolescents have reported a lifetime prevalence rate of 8% for sexual abuse, 17% for physical abuse, and 40% for witnessing violence (Costello, Erkanli, Fairbank, & Angold, 2002). Among adults, the ACE study found that over 30% of participants had reported physical abuse as a child, 24% reported being exposed to family alcohol abuse, 20% reported being sexually abused, and 13% had witnessed domestic violence (Felitti et al., 1998; Van der Kolk, 2005). Duke, Pettingell, McMorris, and Borowsky (2010) reported that the most prevalent type of ACE in their 3-year longitudinal study of adolescents was alcohol abuse by a household member (14.5%). Moreover, Hamby et al., (2018) contend that such estimates may actually be underestimates because they do not measure the occurrence of ACEs in multiple environments.

Are there disparities in exposure to ACEs?

Both current and classic research suggests that exposure to ACEs is differentially distributed by both race/ethnicity and sex. For example, the incidence of child maltreatment differs by race/ethnicity (Elliott & Urquiza, 2006). In 2012, African American and American Indian/ Alaska Native children had the highest substantiated rates of reported maltreatment at 14.2 and 12.4 per 1,000, respectively. Exposure in Latino/Hispanic (8.4 per 1,000) and White children (8.0 per 1,000) held a ranking that was significantly lower than their listed counterparts. More recent data also confirm such patterns.

Which group had the lowest rate of ACEs?

The subgroup with the lowest risk of ACEs nationwide was Asian Americans (1.7 per 1,000).

Thus, African American children were 731.9% more likely to experience an ACE than Asian children, and Latinos/Hispanic children had an ACE risk factor that was 629.4% higher than for Asian American children. Similarly, White American children (8.0 per 1,000) were 370.58% more likely to experience an ACE than Asian American children (Child Trends Databank, 2014).

Are you saying that almost every single racial/ ethnic group needs interventions to reduce ACEs?

Yes. Moreover, when we "mine" the data, we see that many Asian subpopulations also have ACE problems. Therefore, the goal of the healthcare system must be direct interventions toward Asian Americans as well as other groups so that as few children as possible are exposed to ACEs. This is important because intersectoral factors are operative in producing these disparate outcomes. For example, being taken out of a home or placed in foster care can cause significant trauma for children and adolescents (Bramlett & Radel, 2014; Finkelhor, Shattuck, Turner, & Hamby, 2013; Whitfield, 1998). Some experts have suggested that nonorganic variables create the racial/ethnic disparities that are observable in the referrals of children of color into the child welfare system (Bullock, 2003; Dixon, 2008; Dorch, 2010; Drake et al., 2011; Morton, 1999). This claim is supported by data from the National Incidence Study of Abuse and Neglect (NIS) that indicate that *actual rates of maltreatment have never been statistically different across racial groups* (Dixon, 2008). Research on child maltreatment rates among Native American/Alaskan Native populations also indicate the criticality of data disaggregation beyond the larger group. For example, studies reveal that rates of adverse childhood experiences are lower or similar to the general U.S. population among Navajo and San Carlos Apache children. However, studies have documented ACE rates that are as high as 26 per 1,000 among Lakota children on the Cheyenne River Reservation (DeBruyn, Chino, Serna, & Fullerton-Gleason, 2001).

This rate per thousand is 300% higher than for White children in the aggregate. However, disaggregating data on White females reveals broad variations by income and rural status.

Could a disparity chain that begins in childhood result in negative health outcomes in adulthood?

Despite the acknowledgment of the existence of ACEs, the effect of ACEs on physical health was not really considered until 1995 (Finkelhor et al., 2013) when the CDC funded one of the largest investigations into this area. This chapter examines only one adverse outcome—unintentional injury. While the body of literature on ACEs is growing, an extensive literature review of various health databases only produced a few studies that examined ACEs and unintentional injury. Most of the studies used the number of ACEs (i.e., an ACE score) as the independent variable. For example, one ACE study found a significant association between having four or more ACEs and ever having skeletal fractures, with an odds ratio of 1.6 (confidence interval, CI = 1.3 to 2.0) (Felitti et al., 1998). This means that children with four or more ACEs had a 60% higher rate of skeletal fractures as adults compared to adults who experienced no ACEs.

In an Australian study on the prevalence of trauma exposure, O'Donnell et al. (2009) found that of those respondents admitted to trauma services for unintentional injury, 86% had experienced at least one traumatic event prior to the current injury. The most frequent traumatic events were seeing a dead body, excluding funerals and anatomy studies (39%), being threatened or harassed by someone without a weapon (38%), and witnessing domestic abuse (31%). In a representative sample of injured acute care inpatients in the United States, Ramstad et al. (2004) found that unintentionally injured patients were 400% more likely to have been exposed to four or more lifetime traumas before their admission to the hospital.

At the time of this research, no studies could be identified that assessed the association of ACEs with motor vehicle collisions.

Interestingly, however, in an overview of the literature of motor vehicle crashes, Pompili et al. (2012) estimated that more than 2% of traffic collisions were the result of suicide behaviors and that 50% of driver suicides were males between the ages of 15 and 34 years. Another study in Pompili's review found that participants who were deemed suicidal averaged 2.7 motor vehicle collisions, compared to 1.3 for those who were nonsuicidal. Although none of the reviewed studies directly measured ACEs, many ACE-associated outcomes were identified as risk factors associated with traffic collisions. These studies did not address ACEs, unintentional injuries, and racial/ethnic and sex disparities. Accordingly, this chapter reports original research that was designed to answer two key questions. First, is there a relationship between ACEs and unintentional injuries in young adulthood, and if so do disparities exist by race/ethnicity and sex? Second, what are the implications of the empirical results for the area of health disparities?

▶ Determination of Relationships Between ACEs and Unintentional Injuries in Young Adulthood

Data from the National Longitudinal Study of Adolescent to Adult Health (Add Health) were analyzed to determine the relationship between ACEs and unintentional injuries in young adulthood. Add Health is the only nationally representative study in the United States that follows participants from adolescence into young adulthood (Harris, 2013). Add Health is a school-based study. Study participants consist of a nationally representative, probability-based sample of U.S. middle and high school students (Chen & Chantala, 2014).

Adolescents were initially interviewed when they were in grades 7 through 12 (13 to 17 years) and then followed into young adulthood (24 to 32 years). Four survey waves were conducted: Wave I, 1994–1995; Wave II, 1996; Wave III, 2001–2002; and Wave IV, 2007–2008. The primary goal of the Add Health study is to "examine the developmental and health trajectories across the life course of adolescence into young adulthood using an integrative approach that combines social, behavioral, and biomedical sciences in its research objectives, design, data collection, and analysis" (Harris, 2013).

The full restricted dataset was used for this study. To answer the research questions, a subset of variables was drawn from the full dataset. The subset of data included questions on ACEs and injury occurrence, as well as the demographic information needed to assess disparities. Information on how to obtain the Add Health data files is available on the *Add Health* web site (http://www.cpc.unc.edu/addhealth). The data included students from diverse racial/ethnic backgrounds, including Native American, Cuban, Puerto Rican, and Chinese students, as well as African American students with highly educated parents. Additionally, parental household incomes varied from low income to high income.

Did you use an online statistical calculator?

No, online calculators cannot be used for a study of this nature. Instead, we used IBM SPSS Sample Power software to perform logistic regression analyses to answer the research questions. Analyses were performed using SPSS v22. Findings that were statistically significant ($p < .05$) are presented in the results section.

Data on the prevalence of injury in young adulthood were analyzed for unintentional injuries. Prevalence rates were calculated by sex and by race/ethnicity. The mean number of all injuries experienced in young adulthood by sex and race/ethnicity were calculated from the data. These data were later matched with the mean ACE scores listed in **TABLE 14.1**.

TABLE 14.1 Mean Score of Adverse Childhood Experiences by Sex and Race/Ethnicity			
		Mean ACE Score	**Standard Error (S.E.)**
Sex		*2.99*	*0.026*
	Male	2.91	0.04
	Female	3.04	0.036
Race/Ethnicity		*2.98*	*0.026*
	White	2.78	0.036
	Black	3.42	0.061
	Hispanic	3.17	0.079

	American Indian/Alaska Native	3.67	0.305
	Asian/Pacific Islander	2.59	0.092
Males		*2.91*	*0.039*
	White	2.68	0.047
	Black	3.44	0.104
	Hispanic	3.19	0.100
	American Indian/Alaska Native	3.80	0.611
	Asian/Pacific Islander	2.47	0.127
Female		*3.04*	*0.035*
	White	2.86	0.052
	Black	3.40	0.072
	Hispanic	3.14	0.115
	American Indian/Alaska Native	3.55	0.261
	Asian/Pacific Islander	2.72	0.138

Reflects the representative proportion of the target U.S. population.
Taken from Sotero, Michelle M., "The Effects of Adverse Childhood Experiences on Subsequent Injury in Young Adulthood: Findings from the National Longitudinal Study of Adolescent and Adult Health" (2015). UNLV Theses, Dissertations, Professional Papers, and Capstones. 2432. https://digitalscholarship.unlv.edu/thesesdissertations/2432

Results

Table 14.1 presents differentials in exposure to ACEs by race/ethnicity and sex. As the data in Table 14.1 reveal, the mean ACE score for males and females combined was 2.99. Thus, on average, all participants in Wave I of the study had nearly three adverse childhood experiences. When analyzed separately, the ACE score for females was 4.46% higher than that for males at 3.04 versus 2.91, respectively.

Intergroup variations in exposure to ACEs were higher by race/ethnicity than by sex. While the mean number of exposures by race/ethnicity was 2.98, Asian/Pacific Islanders had the lowest mean exposures (2.59) and

American Indian/Alaska Natives had the highest number of exposures (3.67). Thus, American Indian/Alaska Natives had mean ACE scores that were 41.69% higher than Asian Americans, the least exposed groups. African Americans in the sample had mean exposure rates (3.42) that were 32% higher than Asian Americans. The percentage difference for Latinos (3.19) was 23.2% higher than Asian Americans, and White Americans (2.78) had mean ACE scores that were 8.5% higher than those of Asian Americans.

When intersectoral analysis is applied, the data revealed that the highest absolute mean ACE scores were for American Indian/Alaska Native males (3.80). American Indian/Alaska Native females ranked second (3.55), African American males ranked third (3.44), African American females (3.40) ranked fourth, Latino males (3.19) ranked fifth, Latino females (3.14) ranked sixth, Caucasian females (2.86) ranked seventh, White males (2.68) ranked eighth, Asian/Pacific Islander females (2.72) ranked ninth. Asian/Pacific Islander males (2.47) had the lowest mean number of ACEs of any other racial/ethnic/sex group in the study.

What percentage of the participants also experienced unintentional injuries?

TABLE 14.2 summarizes data regarding the number and percentage of the participants who experienced unintentional injury based

TABLE 14.2 Prevalence Rates of Unintentional Injury by Demographic and Psychosocial Characteristics at Wave IV

	Serious Injury[a]		Motor Vehicle Accident	
	No. of Participants[b]	Weighted Percentage[c]	No. of Participants[b]	Weighted Percentage[c]
Sex				
Male	881	17.3%	548	10.4%
Female	560	9.8%	559	9.7%
Race/Ethnicity				
White	880	15.5%	594	9.8%
African American	242	10.4%	259	11.0%
Hispanic/Latino	224	11.3%	177	9.5%
Native American/Alaska Native	d	23.2%	d	13.7%
Asian American	66	8.8%	51	8.6%

Age (years)				
24–25	66	12.5%	72	14.4%
26–27	380	12.6%	322	11.6%
28–29	554	14.2%	393	9.4%
30–32[e]	441	12.9%	320	8.9%
Education				
Less than high school	158	18.1%	98	11.1%
High school diploma or equivalent	245	13.8%	149	7.3%
Some college/ vocational training	685	14%	516	11.4%
College graduate or higher	353	10.7%	344	9.4%
Depression				
Yes	372	19.1%	241	12.6%
No	1069	12.0%	866	9.5%
Anger/Hostility				
Yes	683	15.9%	489	10.9%
No	756	11.4%	618	9.5%
Nicotine Dependence				
Yes	251	23.1%	142	12.4%
No	1156	12.0%	942	9.7%

(continues)

TABLE 14.2 Prevalence Rates of Unintentional Injury by Demographic and Psychosocial Characteristics at Wave IV *(continued)*

	Serious Injury[a]		Motor Vehicle Accident	
	No. of Participants[b]	Weighted Percentage[c]	No. of Participants[b]	Weighted Percentage[c]
Alcohol Dependence/Abuse				
Yes	507	18.8%	314	10.9%
No	934	11.4%	793	9.8%
Illegal Drug Dependence/Abuse				
Yes	186	25.6%	105	13.1%
No	1255	12.3%	1002	9.8%

[a] Injury was defined as occurring in the past 12 months in Wave IV of the Add Health study when participants were 24 to 32 years of age.
[b] Represents the number of participants who endorsed the injury as having occurred versus not occurred.
[c] Reflects the representative proportion of the target U.S. population.
[d] Due to small sample sizes, the number of participants are not reported to protect participants from deductive disclosures. Weighted prevalence should be interpreted with caution.
[e] 34 participants were 33 to 34 years old.
Sotero, M.M. "Experiences on Subsequent Injury in Young Adulthood: Findings from the National Longitudinal Study of Adolescent and Adult Health" (2015). UNLV Theses, Dissertations, Professional Papers, and Capstones. 2432. https://digitalscholarship.unlv.edu/thesesdissertations/2432 64

upon race/ethnicity, sex, education, and key psychosocial characteristics that may have intermediated the relationship between unintentional injuries and ACEs.

The data in Table 14.2 can be used to determine how unintentional injury in Wave IV participants varied by sex, race/ethnicity, and key psychosocial characteristics. The data indicate that American Indian/Alaska Natives (23.2%) had the highest prevalence rates of serious injury. This rate was 163.64% greater than that for Asian Americans (8.8%). White American participants in the sample (15.5%) had weighted prevalence rates of injury that were 76.14% higher than Asian Americans (8.8%), the group with the lowest rates of serious injuries. Latino Americans, with a serious injury prevalence rate of 11.3%, had a rate that was 28.4% higher than that for Asian/Pacific Islanders. Finally, African American Wave IV participants had the second lowest serious injury rate, 10.4%. This rate was 18.1% higher than that for Asian Americans.

Disparities in serious injury rates also existed by sex. Males (17.3%) had a serious injury rate that was 76.5% higher than that for females (9.8%). Serious injury differentials also existed by education and adverse psychosocial characteristics as young adults (24 to 32 years).

With regard to motor vehicle accidents, Asian Americans (8.6%) and Latinos (9.5%) had the lowest prevalence rates. American Indian/Alaska Natives (13.7%) and African

Americans (11.0%) had the highest prevalence rates for motor vehicle accidents; White young adults were in the middle (9.8%). While persons with higher prevalence rates of adverse psychosocial characteristics also had higher prevalence rates of motor vehicle accidents, age was inversely related with motor vehicle prevalence rates.

Analysis of disparities for serious injury and motor vehicle accidents by highest level of education showed a nonlinear relationship. Specifically, persons with some college/vocational training had the highest number of motor vehicle accidents and the second highest rate of serious injury. Interestingly, college graduates or higher had the lowest risk of serious injury but a rate of motor vehicle accidents that was 28.7% higher than Wave IV participants with a high school diploma and/or equivalent.

Given that the mean number of ACEs were higher by minority status and by female sex, multiple logistic regression was used to answer the following question: Did the association between the higher number of ACEs by ACE type increase the odds of a serious injury? **TABLE 14.3** reveals that the odds of serious injury were higher based on a range of different ACE types. As Table 14.3 indicates, the odds of serious injury were 24% to 35% higher based on ACE type. Moreover, these relationships were significant ($p < .05$).

The multiple logistic regression also revealed that sex, depression, drug use, and other covariates were significant in mediating the relationship between ACEs during Wave I and reports of serious injury by these Wave I participants in Wave IV. Although the key psychosocial covariates increased the odds of injury, the focus of this study was upon differential outcomes by sex and race/ethnicity. As Table 14.3 illustrates, male sex more than doubled the odds that exposure to ACEs was associated with a serious unintentional injury as a young adult. Interestingly, the odds of serious injury were actually lower for African American, Hispanic/Latino, and Asian/Pacific Islander Americans than for their White American counterparts. These findings definitely suggest that interventions are needed across all categories of children

TABLE 14.3 Final Model: Association Between Exposure to ACEs and the Adjusted Odds of Unintentional Injury in Young Adulthood at Wave IV

Dependent Variable - Unintentional Injury (serious injury)			
Independent Variable[a]	**(A)OR**[b]	**95% CI**	***p*-Value**
ACE type			
Community violence (shot/stabbed/jumped)	1.35	1.072–1.697	0.01
Child maltreatment	1.33	1.068–1.654	0.01
Emotional neglect	1.27	1.059–1.530	0.01
Interpersonal loss (past year friend attempted suicide) (Wave I)	1.24	1.018–1.504	0.03

(continues)

TABLE 14.3 Final Model: Association Between Exposure to ACEs and the Adjusted Odds of Unintentional Injury in Young Adulthood at Wave IV *(continued)*

Dependent Variable - Unintentional Injury (serious injury)			
Independent Variable[a]	**(A)OR**[b]	**95% CI**	***p*-Value**
Covariates			
Sex (male)	2.06	1.737–2.439	< 0.001
Depression (Wave IV)	1.50	1.23–1.819	< 0.001
DSM-4 lifetime diagnosis of drug abuse/ dependence (Wave IV)	1.49	1.135–1.957	0.003
Nicotine dependence (Wave IV)	1.44	1.162–1.775	< 0.001
DSM-4 lifetime diagnosis of alcohol abuse/ dependence (Wave IV)	1.30	1.101–1.538	0.001
Angry/hostile personality trait	1.26	1.083–1.474	0.004
Race/ethnicity			0.007
White	(Reference)		
African American	0.74	0.601–0.917	
Hispanic/Latino	0.79	0.627–1.002	
American Indian/Alaskan Native/Native American	1.78	0.851–3.737	
Asian American/Pacific Islander	0.62	(0.426-0.91)	

[a] Final model tests significant ACE types from model 2 and significant demographic and psychosocial correlates
[b] (A)OR = (Adjusted) Odds Ratio; CI, Confidence Interval
Taken from Sotero, Michelle M., "The Effects of Adverse Childhood Experiences on Subsequent Injury in Young Adulthood: Findings from the National Longitudinal Study of Adolescent and Adult Health" (2015). UNLV Theses, Dissertations, Professional Papers, and Capstones. 2432. https://digitalscholarship.unlv.edu/thesesdissertations/2432

who are exposed to ACEs. Moreover, it suggests that it is urgent for pediatricians, schools, and other institutions to educate parents beginning before conception regarding the potential impact of ACEs upon the lives of their children as adults. This analysis also demonstrates the importance of broadening the concept of health disparities so that it is more inclusive.

Chapter Summary

The purpose of this chapter was to provide an example of the Disparity Chain by examining racial/ethnic and sex differentials in the long-term impact of ACEs associated with nonintentional injuries among young adults aged 24 to 32 years. In doing so, this case study demonstrates the operation of a Disparity Chain that leads from childhood into adulthood. Although this chapter only focused on disparities in ACEs and unintentional injuries, the implications are much broader. It suggests that whenever health disparities are identified, it is critical to address not merely health care, but every single determinant of health outcomes.

Reliable data were obtained from Wave I and Wave IV of the Add Health study, a longitudinal database. Logistic regression using complex samples was performed to determine whether a relationship existed between ACEs and unintentional injuries in the initial participants between ages 24 and 32 years. Logistic regression was used to determine the probability of injuries by injury type. Logistic regression was used to assess the differential impact of ACEs upon the odds of unintentional injuries by race/ethnicity and sex.

Using this multivariate tool of regression analysis, the analysis identified a significant relationship between community violence ($p < .01$), child maltreatment physical abuse ($p < .01$), child maltreatment emotional neglect ($p < .01$), and interpersonal loss measured by past year friend attempted suicide

($p < .03$) in Wave I, and the adjusted odds of unintentional serious injury in young adulthood in Wave IV. Based on White Americans as the reference group, the analysis revealed that whereas the odds of serious injury were 78% higher for American Indian/Alaskan Native/Native Americans (1.78), African Americans (0.74), Latino Americans (0.79) and Asian/Pacific Islander Americans (0.62) had lower odds of unintentional injury than did the White American participants in this longitudinal dataset. In addition, males were 106% more likely to have a relationship between the described ACE types and serious injuries than were females. Approximately 15.5% of White participants experienced serious injury in Wave IV relative to 23.2% of American Indians/Alaska Natives. However, only 10.4%, 11.3%, and 8.8% of African Americans, Latinos, and Asian/Pacific Islanders, respectively, experienced serious injury.

As mentioned, in a 2008 publication by the CDC's Community Health and Program Services (CHAPS) entitled "Health Disparities Among Racial/Ethnic Populations," health disparities are defined as "*preventable differences in the burden of disease, injury, violence, or opportunities to optimal health that are experienced by socially disadvantaged populations.*" This chapter used empirical data on ACEs and unintentional injuries to demonstrate the critical need for broadening this definition so that overall disparate health outcomes can be addressed.

Review Questions and Problems

1. What are the key findings of this chapter that can be used to explain the Disparity Chain Model?
2. Discuss the roles that healthcare administrators, public health officials, and clinicians can play in the disparity chain in response to the incidence of ACEs.

Key Terms and Concepts

adverse childhood experiences (ACEs)
Highly stressful and often traumatic events
that occur during childhood and adolescence,
also termed *developmental trauma* or *complex
trauma*.

proximate cause An event that is closest to,
or immediately responsible for causing, some
observed result.

References

Anda, R. F., Whitfield, C. L., Felitti, V. J., Chapman, D.,
Edwards, V. J., Dube, S. R., & Williamson, D. F. (2002).
Adverse childhood experiences, alcoholic parents, and
later risk of alcoholism and depression. *Psychiatric
Services (Washington, D.C.), 53*(8), 1001–1009.

Beautrais, A. L. (2003). Life course factors associated
with suicidal behaviors in young people. *American
Behavioral Scientist, 46*(9), 1137–1156.

Beautrais, A. L., Joyce, P. R., & Mulder, R. T. (1996). Risk
factors for serious suicide attempts among youths aged
13 through 24 years. *Journal of the American Academy
of Child & Adolescent Psychiatry, 35*(9), 1174–1182.

Bramlett, M. D., & Radel, L. F. (2014). Adverse family
experiences among children in nonparental care,
2011–2012. *National Health Statistics Report, 74*, 1–9.

Brodsky, B. S., & Biggs, E. (2012). Adverse childhood
experiences and suicidal behavior. *Suicidologi, 17*(3),
16–21.

Bruffaerts, R., Demyttenaere, K., Borges, G., Haro, H.,
Chiu, W., Hwaing, I., . . . Nock, M. K. (2010).
Childhood adversities as risk factors for onset and
persistence of suicidal behavior. *British Journal of
Psychiatry, 197*, 20–27.

Bullock, C. (2003). Low-income parents victimized by
child protective services. *American University Journal
of Gender Social Policy and Law, 11*(2), 1023–1053.

Case, A., & Deaton, A. (2015). Rising morbidity and mortality
in midlife among white non-Hispanic Americans in the
21st century. *Proceedings of the National Academy of
Sciences USA, 112*(49), 15078–15083.

Centers for Disease Control and Prevention (CDC).
(2008). *Community Health and Program Services
(CHAPS): Health disparities among racial/ethnic
populations*. Atlanta, GA: U.S. Department of Health
and Human Services.

Chen, P., & Chantala, K. (2014). *Guidelines for analyzing
Add Health data*. Carolina Population Center
University of North Carolina at Chapel Hill.

Child Trends Databank. (2014). Child maltreatment:
Indicators on children and youth. Retrieved from
http://www.childtrends.org/wp-content
/uploads/2014/07/40_Child_Maltreatment.pdf

Costello, E. J., Erkanli, A., Fairbank, J. A, & Angold, A.
(2002). The prevalence of potentially traumatic events

in childhood and adolescence. *Journal of Traumatic
Stress, 15*(2), 99–112.

Courtois, C. A. (2004). Complex trauma, complex
reactions: Assessment and treatment. *Psychotherapy:
Theory, Research, Practice, Training, 41*(4), 412–425.

Courtois, C. A., & Ford, J. D. (Eds.). (2009). *Treating
complex traumatic stress disorders: An evidence-based
guide*. New York, NY: Guilford.

Danese, A., & McEwen, B. S. (2012). Adverse childhood
experiences, allostasis, allostatic load, and age-related
disease. *Physiology & Behavior, 106*(1), 29–39.

DeBruyn, L., Chino, M., Serna, P., & Fullerton-Gleason,
L. (2001). Child maltreatment in American Indian
and Alaska Native communities: Integrating culture,
history, and public health for intervention and
prevention. *Child Maltreatment, 6*(2), 89–102.

Desai, M., Zhang, P., & Hennessy, C. (1999). Surveillance
for morbidity and mortality among older adults—
United States, 1995–1996. *Morbidity and Mortality
Weekly Report: Surveillance Summaries, 48*(SS-8), 7–25.
Retrieved from http://www.jstor.org/stable/24676724

Dixon, J. (2008). The African American Child Welfare
Act: A legal redress for African American dispro-
portionality in child protection cases. *Berkeley Journal
of African American Law and Policy*, 109–145.

Dolgin, K. (2011). *The adolescent: Development, relationships,
and culture*. Boston, MA: Pearson Education.

Dorch, E. (2010). Social service availability and the
over-representation of minority children in child
welfare. *Journal of the Health and Human Services
Administration, 33*(3), 277–320.

Drake, B., Jolley, J., Lanier, P., Fluke, J., Barth, R. P.,
& Jonson-Reid, M. (2011). Racial bias in child
protection? A comparison of competing explanations
using national data. *Pediatrics, 127*(3), 471–478.

Dube, S. R., Felitti, V. J., Dong, M., Chapman, D. P., Giles,
W. H., & Anda, R. F. (2003). Childhood abuse, neglect,
and household dysfunction and the risk of illicit drug
use: The Adverse Childhood Experiences study.
Pediatrics, 111(3), 564–572.

Duke, N. N., Pettingell, S. L., McMorris, B. J., & Borowsky,
I. W. (2010). Adolescent violence perpetration:
Associations with multiple types of adverse childhood
experiences. *Pediatrics, 125*(4), e778–e786.

Elliott, K., & Urquiza, A. (2006). Ethnicity, culture, and child maltreatment. *Journal of Social Issues*, *62*(4), 787–809.

English, D. J., Graham, J., Newton, R. R., Lewis, T. L., Thompson, R., Kotch, J. B., & Weisbart, C. (2009). At-risk and maltreated children exposed to intimate partner aggression/violence: What the conflict looks like and its relationship to child outcomes. *Child Maltreatment*, *14*(2), 157–171.

Felitti, M. D., Vincent, J., Anda, M. D., Robert, F., Nordenberg, M. D., Williamson, M. S., & James, S. (1998). Relationship of childhood abuse and household dysfunction to many of the leading causes of death in adults: The Adverse Childhood Experiences (ACE) study. *American Journal of Preventive Medicine*, *14*(4), 245–258.

Fergusson, D. M., Boden, J. M., & Horwood, L. J. (2008). Exposure to childhood sexual and physical abuse and adjustment in early adulthood. *Child Abuse & Neglect*, *32*, 607–619.

Finkelhor, D., Shattuck, A., Turner, H., & Hamby, S. (2013). Improving the adverse childhood experiences study scale. *JAMA Pediatrics*, *167*(1), 70–75.

Fried, L. E., Williams, S., Cabral, H., & Hacker, K. (2013). Differences in risk factors for suicide attempts among 9th and 11th grade youth: A longitudinal perspective. *Journal of School Nursing*, *29*(2), 113–122.

Giovanelli, A., Reynolds, A. J., Mondi, C. F., & Ou, S. R. (2016). Adverse childhood experiences and adult well-being in a low-income, urban cohort. *Pediatrics*, peds-2015.

Hamby, S., Taylor, E., Jones, L., Mitchell, K. J., Turner, H. A., & Newlin, C. (2018). From poly-victimization to poly-strengths: understanding the web of violence can transform research on youth violence and illuminate the path to prevention and resilience. *Journal of interpersonal violence*, *33*(5), 719–739.

Hansen, H., & Netherland, J. (2016). Is the prescription opioid epidemic a white problem? *American Journal of Public Health*, *106*(12), 2127–2129.

Harris, K. (2013). *The Add Health study: Design and accomplishments*. Carolina Population Center University of North Carolina at Chapel Hill.

Heim, C., Newport, D. J., Bonsall, R., Miller, A. H., & Nemeroff, C. B. (2001). Altered pituitary-adrenal axis responses to provocative challenge tests in adult survivors of childhood abuse. *American Journal of Psychiatry*, *158*(4), 575–581.

Hussong, A. M., Bauer, D. J., Huang, W., Chassin, L., Sher, K. J., & Zucker, R. A. (2008). Characterizing the life stressors of children of alcoholic parents. *Journal of Family Psychology*, *22*(6), 819.

Johnson, J. G., Cohen, P., Gould, M. S., Kasen, S., Brown, J., & Brook, J. S. (2002). Childhood adversities, interpersonal difficulties, and risk for suicide attempts during late adolescence and early adulthood. *Archives of General Psychiatry*, *59*(8), 741–749.

Kaplow, J. B., Gipson, P. Y., Horwitz, A. G., Burch, B. N., & King, C. A. (2014). Emotional suppression mediates the relation between adverse life events and adolescent suicide: Implications for prevention. *Prevention Science*, *15*(2), 177–185.

La Noue, M., Graeber, D. A., Helitzer, D. L., & Fawcett, J. (2013). Negative affect predicts adults' ratings of the current, but not childhood, impact of adverse childhood events. *Community Mental Health Journal*, *49*(5), 560–566.

Morton, T. D. (1999). The increasing colorization of America's child welfare system: The overrepresentation of African American children. *Policy & Practice of Public Human Services*, *57*(4), 23–29.

O'Donnell, M. L., Creamer, M., Elliott, P., Bryant, R., McFarlane, A., & Silove, D. (2009). Prior trauma and psychiatric history as risk factors for intentional and unintentional injury in Australia. *Journal of Trauma*, *66*(2), 470–476.

Pilowsky, D. J., Keyes, K. M., & Hasin, D. S. (2009). Adverse childhood events and lifetime alcohol dependence. *American Journal of Public Health*, *99*(2), 258–263.

Pompili, M., Serafini, G., Innamorati, M., Montebovi, F., Palermo, M., Campi, S, & Girardi, P. (2012). Car accidents as a method of suicide: A comprehensive overview. *Forensic Science International*, *223*(1), 1–9.

Ramstad, S. M., Russo, J., & Zatzick, D. F. (2004). Is it an accident? Recurrent traumatic life events in level I trauma center patients compared to the general population. *Journal of Traumatic Stress*, *17*(6), 529–534.

Reavis, J. A., Looman, J., Franco, K. A., & Rojas, B. (2013). Adverse childhood experiences and adult criminality: How long must we live before we possess our own lives? *The Permanente Journal*, *17*(2), 44–48.

Rothman, E. F., Edwards, E. M., Heeren, T., Hingson, R. W. (2008). Adverse childhood experiences predict earlier age of drinking onset: Results from a representative US sample of current or former drinkers. *Pediatrics*, *122*, e298–e304.

Shonkoff, J. P., Boyce, W. T., & McEwen, B. S. (2009). Neuroscience, molecular biology, and the childhood roots of health disparities: Building a new framework for health promotion and disease prevention. *JAMA*, *301*(21), 2252–2259.

Sotero, M. M. (2015). The effects of adverse childhood experiences on subsequent injury in young adulthood: Findings from the National Longitudinal Study of Adolescent and Adult Health. *UNLV Theses, Dissertations, Professional Papers, and Capstones*. 2432. Retrieved from https://digitalscholarship.unlv.edu/thesesdissertations/2432

Springer, K. W., Sheridan, J., Kuo, D., & Carnes, M. (2007). Long-term physical and mental health consequences of childhood physical abuse: Results from a large population-based sample of men and women. *Child Abuse & Neglect*, *31*(5), 517–530.

Sprinkle, J. E. (2007). Domestic violence, gun ownership, and parental educational attainment: How do they affect the aggressive beliefs and behaviors of children? *Child and Adolescent Social Work Journal, 24*(2), 133–151.

Turner, R. J., & Lloyd, D. A. (2003). Cumulative adversity and drug dependence in young adults: Racial/ethnic contrasts. *Addiction (Abingdon, England), 98*(3), 305–315.

U.S. Public Law 106–525. Minority Health and Health Disparities Research and Education Act of 2000. 106th Congress 2d session, November 22, 2000. 114 STAT. 2496, paragraph (2).

Van der Kolk, B. A. (2005). Developmental trauma disorder. *Psychiatric Annals, 35*(5), 401–408.

Whitfield, C. L. (1998). Adverse childhood experiences and trauma. *American Journal of Preventive Medicine, 14*(4), 361–364.

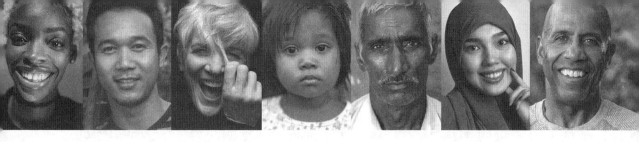

CHAPTER 15

Health and Healthcare Disparities: Where Do We Go from Here?

"The Earth is the cradle of humanity, but mankind cannot stay in the cradle forever."

—**Konstantin Tsiolkovsky (1857–1935)**, Russian-Soviet rocket scientist

LEARNING OBJECTIVES

After completing this chapter, each learner will be able to:

- Compile an extended inventory of various disparity-reducing strategies that have been proposed and considered.
- List new subgroups with disparity needs.
- Compare, contrast, and assess alternative recommendations for disparities reductions.
- Evaluate the probability that the comprehensive disparity chain model will be implemented.

▶ Introduction

Once obscured by the absence of systematically collected data and, consequently relegated to the realm of the anecdotal and the mythological, subgroup asymmetries in health or healthcare outcomes were largely undocumented. Over the past 25 years, however, the introduction of information systems into healthcare services has lent itself to the collection, editing, storage, retrieval, and analysis of data regarding the diagnostic, therapeutic, and rehabilitative subsystems that comprise patient care. Likewise, a growing body of data are now available on the support systems and community relations systems that interact with patient care. Medically generated data have also been supplemented by improved data collection by healthcare administrators, public health researchers, and other practitioners. As a result, a body of scientific evidence now confirms statistically significant differences in health outcomes exist by race/ethnicity, income status, sex, gender preference, age, urban/rural status, education, income, environment, and even by spiritual beliefs, support group status, marital status, and an array of other variables.

These subgroup differences frequently conjoin to create disparate outcomes in both mortality and morbidity, access to health care, and, more importantly, the quality of health care received. Current data also confirm improvements in many areas of both health and healthcare disparities. Nevertheless, increases in comorbidities such as diabetes

mellitus, uncontrolled hypertension, glomerular disease, and other illnesses continue to complicate efforts to identify and remedy remediable differences in morbidity and mortality. Thus, even more must be known regarding disparities reduction.

▶ Efforts to Reduce Health and Healthcare Disparities

The current gains have not been generated spontaneously. Numerous organizations have collaborated in the effort to research and seek solutions to improve health and healthcare differentials. **BOX 15.1** lists just a few of these efforts by federal agencies. A number of

---

BOX 15.1 Sample of Federal Programs, Policies, and Initiatives to Reduce Health and Healthcare Disparities

Office of Civil Rights
- Investigates whether healthcare institutions such as managed care organizations, home health agencies, and others violate civil rights laws in their healthcare access and service provision practices.
- Urges healthcare administrators and providers to engage in self-assessment of data from their institutions in order to determine whether remediable disparities can be identified.
- Analyzes location decisions of healthcare organizations in order to determine whether a process of healthcare "redlining" is occurring or has occurred.
- Provides other supports to the country's effort to improve health and health care for all of its residents.

For additional information on other services, visit Office of Civil Rights, https://www.hhs.gov/ocr/index.html

Office of Management and Budget
- Supports the quality of the data collected by healthcare organizations by ensuring that the race/ethnicity terminology/classifications are standardized and, as a result, can be compared across healthcare organizations that choose to disaggregate their data in terms of racial/ethnic subgroups.

For additional information, visit HHS.gov's Minority Health OMB's browser.

Agency for Healthcare Research and Quality
- Funds projects to identify and remediate disparities in health care. While the focus areas for this federal agency change depending on the public's needs, at one point, this agency funded Centers of Excellence that:

- Sought to analyze and design healthcare disparity–reducing innovations.
- Examined how general health improvements programs and initiatives could be cost-effectively customized to increase their effectiveness.
- Used measures designed to pinpoint specific areas of the disparity chain that were characterized by significant disparities and implement measures for their education.

For more information, visit Agency for Healthcare Research and Quality at https://www.ahrq.gov/research/findings/nhqrdr/nhqdr16/index.html

Centers for Disease Control and Prevention

- Partners with community organizations to implement promising and evidence-based interventions with various groups and subgroups in communities characterized by disparities.
- Has expanded the use of healthcare registries and improved the quality of the data collected for various subgroups through a systematic process of providing training and technical assistance to staff.
- Partners with organizations from various subgroup communities in order to better understand how differential behavior, values, etc., contribute to subgroup health differences.
- Designs public health initiatives to market preventive behaviors to groups with disparate health outcomes.
- Develops clinical training initiatives to improve patient–provider communication.
- Implements programs to improve bidirectional communication between providers and their partners.
- Provides funds for new tools and training programs to promote cultural competence and to assess their effectiveness within healthcare organizations.
- Develops and disseminates videos, films, print materials, etc., to enhance knowledge about how to reduce disparities.
- Designs and executes many other programs, policies, and initiatives.

For more information, visit Centers for Disease Control and Prevention at https://www.cdc.gov/minorityhealth/index.html

National Institutes of Health

- Develops and updates strategic research agendas.
- Supports programs to increase the representation of subgroups among the ranks of healthcare professionals.
- Added new organizational divisions to serve as a managerial "hub" for disparity-reducing activities.

For more information, visit National Institutes of Health at https://www.nimhd.nih.gov

Substance Abuse and Mental Health Services Administration

- Expanded inclusion of underrepresented groups in behavioral and mental health initiatives.
- Translates materials to support behavioral and mental health so they are accessible to language minorities.
- Funds services for substance abuse and mental health programs.
- Partners with state, regional, and local organizations to combat substance abuse and promote mental health.

For further information, visit https://www.samhsa.gov/health-disparities

Department of Veterans Affairs

- National action plans have been developed to address the differential representation of various subgroups within the military and the need for services to reach these various categories of veterans.

BOX 15.2 State-Level Strategies for Addressing Health and Healthcare Disparities

- State laws are now being assessed in a search for solutions that can reduce the 100% to 600% higher rates of suicide that exist for youth who are members of sexual minority subgroups. However, some states have already taken action in this direction. For example, in 2016, California, Assembly Bill 2246 was passed to mandate local educational agencies (LEAs) serving youth in grades 7–12 to provide suicide prevention. Each educational agency must create suicide prevention/intervention and post-intervention policies and procedures that focus upon the needs of LGBT youth, homeless youth, youth with mental health issues, those with substance use disorders, those who have disabilities, and those who have lost someone to suicide (California Legislative Information, 2016). A survey of over 30,000 high school students found that anti-bullying policies that included all sexual orientations and genders also had lower rates of suicide attempts by lesbian and gay youth (Hatzebuehler et al., 2014). Currently, 19 U.S. States (and the nation's capital) have current anti-bullying laws that seek to protect LGBT and other students. However, the remainder do not (Williams Institute, 2018). Selected states are funding research to uncover factors that reduce the enrollment and retention of socioeconomic subgroups in public health programs that are assigned to assist them.
- Public policy reconfigurations that can strengthen the use of the Civil Rights Act of 1964 to address health and healthcare disparities are being examined in some states.
- Interventions are being considered for reducing health disparities that are magnified by external and internal stigma.
- The possibility of intersectional relationships between state-based immigration laws and patterns are being examined. For example, Martinez et al. (2016) evaluated the impact of immigration policies in America and other countries on the health status among undocumented immigrants. These researchers found that there is a need for collaboration between healthcare professionals, government officials, and other stakeholders in these countries to work together in an effort to adequately address the health needs of all immigrants.

Other disparity-related initiatives are listed in Box 15.3.

initiatives are also taking place at the state level to address health and healthcare disparities (**BOX 15.2**). Numerous other programs, policies, and initiatives are being conceived and/or tested (**BOX 15.3**).

A number of books and articles have been written with the goal of educating the public in general regarding this new field of health and healthcare disparities. We have included a small listing of books on health disparities in **TABLE 15.1**.

Likewise, systematic initiatives have been launched to decrease the prevalence and incidence of documented differentials in the treatment of primary morbidities (i.e., hypertension, diabetes mellitus, and other diseases). Similarly, informal activities by public and private partnering organizations continue to seek to improve equity in access to the limited pool of available health resources.

Despite such efforts, disparities in health outcomes and health care continue to climb in selected areas, decrease in other areas of need, and remain masked for some groups because of the use of a paradigm that has, in the past, been limited in focus. As a result, the differentials in health outcomes for some subgroups have grown while other areas have improved. Thus, approaches to supplement and complement these ongoing approaches are needed. Indeed, efforts to reduce health and healthcare disparities can possibly benefit by the introduction of a comprehensive framework that can support the identification and remediation of individual, infrastructure-related, and systemic factors that affect health outcomes.

BOX 15.3 Other Disparity-Related Initiatives

- To ensure the inclusion of cultural, gender, and other types of concordance opportunities between clinicians and patients, efforts are being made to restructure the National Residency Match Program in order to ensure that 100% of medical school graduates find residencies.
- Prison health systems and policies that create disparities between the "imprisoned" and the "free" are being revised. Efforts are being made to examine such disparities to determine how these intermediate health outcomes occur across and within subgroups.
- Research is being conducted to determine whether the existence of healthcare stereotype threat (i.e., a phenomenon that emerges simply because one is a member of a health disparity subgroup) increases the probability of healthcare disparities.
- E-health opportunities are being considered as tools for reducing health disparities.
- Greenways are being introduced into selected neighborhoods in order to reduce environment-related disparities in health behavior and outcomes.
- New tobacco-control interventions are being considered to reduce disparities in this very important problem area.
- Development of electronic communities has been proposed to reduce geographically related health and healthcare disparities.
- Some researchers are advocating the use of simulation models to train clinicians to better communicate with various subgroups.

TABLE 15.1 Sample Books on Health Disparities

- *Health Disparities, Diversity, and Inclusion: Contexts, Controversies and Solutions*, by Patti R. Rose, Jones & Bartlett Learning (February 14, 2017).

- *Essentials of Health Justice: A Primer*, by Elizabeth Tobin-Tyler and Joel B. Teitelbaum, Jones & Bartlett Learning (August 15, 2018).

- *Just Medicine: A Cure for Racial Inequality in American Health Care*, by Dayna Bowen Matthew, NYU Press; First edition (December 11, 2015).

- *Health Disparities in the United States: Social Class, Race, Ethnicity, and Health*, by Donald A. Barr, Johns Hopkins University Press; Second edition (August 20, 2014).

- *Health Care Disparities and the LGBT Population*, by Vickie L. Harvey, Lexington Books; Reprint edition (March 14, 2016).

- *Reducing Health Disparities: Communication Interventions*, by Mohan J. Dutta and Gary L. Kreps, Peter Lang Inc., International Academic Publishers; First edition (September 30, 2013).

- *Health Disparities: Epidemiology, Racial/Ethnic and Socioeconomic Risk Factors and Strategies for Elimination*, by Owen T. Jackson and Kathleen A. Evans. Nova Science Pub Inc; UK ed. edition (August 8, 2013).

- *Essentials of Health, Culture, and Diversity: Understanding People, Reducing Disparities (Essential Public Health)*, by Mark Edberg. Jones & Bartlett Learning; First edition (February 8, 2012).

- *Minority Populations and Health: An Introduction to Health Disparities in the United States*, by Thomas A. LaVeist. Jossey-Bass; First edition (April 11, 2005).

The recurring theme in this text is that health and healthcare disparities improvements cannot be analyzed or proposed without contextualizing recommendations against the overall backdrop of *the role of health and health care as contributors to the human experience*. When positioned within this framework, stagnation and/or slow growth in health and healthcare disparities reduction becomes easy to understand. Bowen and Casadevall (2015) argue that if biomedical research outcomes for the past 5 years are measured relative to their contributions to life expectancy via new foods and/or drugs, *a state of constancy rather than improvement* in the human condition has occurred. This is despite the fact that many dollars have been spent and the quantity of new knowledge as measured by the number of published articles and books has increased exponentially. The impact of this "new knowledge" has had only an incremental net impact upon the magnitude and/or quality of life.

However, when the arena of new knowledge is extended beyond that of the area of biomedical research, other areas of research have generated extreme gains for the human experience. For example, the International Space Exploration Coordination Group (2013) argues that through a multiplicity of pathways, the research completed by their agency provides an extraordinary model of collaboration and promise because multiple human entities are partnering toward the goal of addressing *the use of research for improvements in the human condition*.

All behaviors are the outcome of each individual's behavior guidance system. The objective of the partnership between governments, scientists and other researchers, and global businesses who have come together as part of the International Space Exploration Coordination Group (2013) is to ready humankind for an expansion beyond our current life "cradle." While many humans cling to their unique subtribes in a singular and/or intersectoral fashion, some contend that in the near and/or distant future, humans will be joined by robotic entities and/or by humans intricately joined with technology in the introduction of new ways of life within and under new conditions (International Space Exploration Coordinating Group, 2013).

What does all of this have to do with health disparities?

Health care is, has been, and will continue to be the beneficiary of these extraordinary efforts by exceptional partners who have selected to subordinate subgroup differences in order to harvest the benefits that accrue from a unified humanity. New robotic technologies are being tested in the treatment of many cancers (Ryan et al., 2018). The benefits associated with the provision of remotely deliverable medical care must be available to all. Relatedly, newly discovered processes for the removal of impurities from water that have been developed for space travel can address water needs in rural areas both in the United States and worldwide. Numerous other futuristic health-related technologies and therapies are also emerging from various areas in which an increasingly better future for humankind is the explicit gain to be obtained. In this regard, this chapter borrows from this area of science by using an alternative conceptual framework to "house" current and proposed efforts to reduce remediable disparities in health.

What type of framework do you propose to support further improvements in health and health care across all subgroups?

One framework that has become dominant in the area of healthcare disparities has come to be called *cultural competency*. Whether in the area of health care and/or education, numerous colleges and universities not only offer courses in cultural competency as a remedy for disparities, but many now offer certificate programs. The **cultural competency framework** is viewed as a tool for changing the worldview of humans in healthcare settings toward key subgroups. Renzaho, Romios, Crock, and Sønderland (2013) examined 1,450 articles on cultural competence training in health care. Analyzing 13 studies that met their selection criteria, they found that cultural competence training did elevate knowledge and awareness of healthcare disparities. *However, no benefits could be identified relative to decreases in healthcare disparities.* Truong, Paradies, and Priest (2014) also completed a systematic literature review of research regarding the concept of cultural competency. This study, too, found that some benefits did accrue in terms of provider-based outcomes, access, and utilization of healthcare resources. Again, however, very little improvement occurred in patient outcomes. Thus, it is less than surprising that some analysts are suggesting that alternate frameworks may be needed to support the embracing of a behavioral code that disallows actions that are not supportive of the optimal outcomes for humanity (Nadan, 2014).

▶ Ontological Reconfiguration as a Framework for Health Disparities Interventions

The concept of ontological reconfiguration is related to ontological change. An **ontological change** is traceable to religion. It suggests a moment in time when a profound alteration occurs within the "spirit" and "soul" of the priest. It has come to mean a change in the basic premises and conclusions that one draws regarding the nature of existence. The concept of **ontological reconfiguration** can be found in modular manufacturing. In manufacturing engineering, the term is used to describe an automated, internal process of change that occurs through self-automation. Stated differently, whether religious-based or otherwise catalyzed, it can be argued that the behavioral

changes that are required within each member of humankind to generate humanity-supportive actions cannot be legislated but must occur from within each individual.

How can this process of change be started? Are new policies needed?

Ontological reconfiguration differs from the types of changes that public health professionals seek to trigger through the use of evidence-based interventions. It does not include the type of behavioral change that clinicians seek to initiate when they have candid conversations with their patients regarding the mortality impacts of continued health-related behaviors. It is not the type of change that healthcare administrators seek to generate when they craft policies and procedures to direct the operation of the organizations that they manage. And, it is absolutely not the type of change that new policies, regulations, and governmental initiatives can affect.

Are you saying that these other levels of change are not important?

Absolutely not! All efforts to create life-affirming changes are critical. However, we are introducing the theoretical concept that **ontological transformation**, an individual level of change that sprouts and blossoms within, is the platform upon which other levels of change must occur. Michie, Van Stralen, and West (2011) introduce the concept of the "behavior change wheel." Based on a comprehensive review of the literature, Michie et al. argue that behavior is not singularly determined; rather, it is a causal system with a multiplicity of related components. Changes in the system at all levels are dependent upon capability, opportunity, and motivation. However, as one analyzes such a thoroughly developed model of change, we see that even this is not equivalent to the concept of ontological transformation.

In philosophy, *ontology* refers to beliefs regarding the nature of reality. When philosophy is combined with science, the nature of reality can be defined at two levels. At the first level, the nature of reality is that which we can see, touch, hear, or otherwise perceive through our physical senses. But, as we observe the difference between a mountain of rocks and living things, we see that reality has a second level, which philosophers and scientists call *consciousness*. The concept of ontological reconfiguration suggests that change must begin by individuals reorganizing their consciousness in order for remediable changes in all aspects of the human condition to experience the continued positive change that has characterized the known presence of humankind upon the earth. Moreover, this framework suggests that ontological transformation must be based upon an individualized behavioral system that leads to the conclusion that actions, thoughts, and beliefs that support continual improvements in the human condition are "good" and those that are aligned with a deterioration in the human condition are "bad." To the degree that this ontological transformation takes

place, it becomes possible to not merely remediate positive changes in health outcomes, but in other areas of the human condition as well.

But, health isn't everything!

We disagree. Health is at the root of everything. If we adopt the ontology from science that the nature of existence is composed of material and consciousness, our bodies become the "houses" in which consciousness lives. Healthy behaviors and health care become the tools for maintaining and improving our body—the material aspect of human reality. Education, knowledge, and original thinking become the tools to improve consciousness so that we can support the maximization of the human experience. Thus, the measure that guides all human behavior becomes, "What will be the impact of my individualized way of thinking or behaving upon the future of humankind?" **BOX 15.4** provides an opportunity for readers to better understand their own ontological beliefs.

BOX 15.4 Changing Health and Other Human Behaviors Through Ontological Transformation

1. Do you believe that one component of reality is that which we can perceive through our physical senses (i.e., sight, hearing, sound, taste, and touch)?
   Yes ☐ No ☐ Unsure ☐
   Comment: _____
   _____

2. Do you believe that a second component of reality is consciousness?
   Yes ☐ No ☐ Unsure ☐
   Comment: _____
   _____

3. Do you believe that by supporting your own physical, emotional, or mental survival you are contributing to the survival and growth of humankind?
   Yes ☐ No ☐ Unsure ☐
   Comment: _____
   _____

4. Do you believe that human differences may be needed to contribute to the survival and growth of humankind?
   Yes ☐ No ☐ Unsure ☐
   Comment: _____
   _____

5. Do you believe that seeing other individuals' differences as equal, and not as inferior and/or superior, contributes to the survival and growth of humankind?
Yes ☐   No ☐   Unsure ☐
Comment: _____

6. Do you believe that the adoption of negative views regarding various subgroups of humanity supports the survival and growth of humankind?
Yes ☐   No ☐   Unsure ☐
Comment: _____

7. Do you believe that potential threats to humankind from changing weather, meteors, and/or other projectiles from outer space, food shortages, etc., can be best managed by "each person sticking to their own kind"?
Yes ☐   No ☐   Unsure ☐
Comment: _____

8. Do you believe that you will be better prepared to contribute to the task of improving the overall survival and growth of humankind if you develop a chronic disease such as diabetes mellitus, obesity, hypertension, substance abuse disorder, HIV/AIDS, etc.?
Yes ☐   No ☐   Unsure ☐
Comment: _____

9. Do you believe that other humans will be better able to support the growth and development of human beings if they have lower life expectances, a greater number of chronic diseases, and poorer health?
Yes ☐   No ☐   Unsure ☐
Comment: _____

10. Are you ready to commit to a lifetime of choices that support the survival and growth of humankind?
Yes ☐   No ☐   Unsure ☐
Comment: _____

If you answered "yes" to questions 1–5 and 10, and "no" to questions 6–9, you have already undergone the ontological transformation necessary and are now ready to change humankind's outcomes by intervening at key points in the disparity chain.

▶ Reducing Remediable Health and Healthcare Disparities by Reengineering the Disparity Chain

Consider the following definitions of **reengineering**:

- To engineer again or anew; to redesign; to reorganize the operations of (an organization) so as to improve efficiency (*Merriam-Webster*, n.d.a)
- To engineer anew (Dictionary.com, n.d.)
- To restructure a company or part of its operations by utilizing information technology (TheFreeDictionary.com, n.d.a)

The disparity chain can be reengineered in order to address remediable differences in health and healthcare outcomes.

Are you advocating for social engineering?

No, we are not advocating for social engineering. **Social engineering** can mean the following:

- Management of human beings in accordance with their place and function in society (*Merriam-Webster*, n.d.a)
- The practical application of sociological principles to social problems (The FreeDictionary.com, n.d.b)

Based on these definitions, you can see that the concept of social engineering is diametrically opposed to all premises of change discussed herein. Rather, disparity chain reengineering is based on micro rather than macro levels of change.

The concept of ontological transformation references a process that occurs *within* the individual. As these changes occur, individuals lay claim to their power to "reengineer" various elements of their own life structure by no longer allowing choices and decisions to be made by default. Thus, when the concept of reengineering the disparity chain is introduced, it references each individual consciously exercising informed choice behavior rather than choices by defaults and/or merely active choices.

What do you mean by "informed choices" versus "choices by default"?

Choices by default are those actions taken by an individual without actively thinking about the choice. **Active choices** are decisions made by an individual to select one option over another. **Informed choices** occur when individuals know and understand their options; have knowledge of the benefits and costs of each option; assess the benefits and costs; and then make a decision based on their ontology (beliefs about the world) and axiology (values).

Are these concepts a part of health and health care?

Yes, these concepts are absolutely a part of the field of health and health care. Hart and Halpern (2014) discuss decisions by default in clinical care. They argue that although default

options are widely used by staff in intensive care units in order to decrease errors and increase efficiency in urgent care units of hospitals, such decision-making sometimes harms patients. Blumenthal-Barby and Burroughs (2012) describe the shift in public health efforts to change behavior from a more dominant and intrusive approach to one that simply seeks to "nudge" individuals to exercise active choices that support positive health outcomes. More important, they extricate the ethical implications of alternative forms of nudging. Kosters and Van der Heijden (2015) seek to shift the debate around nudging from the arena of ethics to the domain of practicality by in effect answering the question, "Does the use of 'nudging' by healthcare administrators, public health professionals, clinicians, and others generate more active choice behavior?" In contrast, Voyer (2015) argues that the systematic effort to generate active choice behavior via nudging is superior to attempting to legislate change.

The shift from *choice by default* to *active choice* to *informed choice* has now been under way for more than a decade. Within the United States, consumers can now access "knowledge" through Hospital Compare, Nursing Home Compare, and other quality measurement datasets. Accordingly, a body of literature has emerged regarding consumer use of these tools to support informed choice. Yet, researchers such as Radha et al. (2012) pose questions regarding the competency of consumers to make informed choices. Ghanouni, Renzi, Meisel, and Waller (2016) emphasize the critical need for healthcare administrators, public policy professionals, clinicians, and policy makers to ensure the availability of easy-to-read and accurate information to healthcare consumers so that they can make informed choices.

What does all of this have to do with your argument that remediating healthcare disparities in a way that is win-win for everyone requires a reengineering of the health disparity chain?

Understanding the different types of choice behaviors is critical to reengineering the health disparity chain. To move humankind forward, individuals must commit to foregoing choices by default and/or active choices alone. *The pathways that will lead to improved health outcomes in the future requires individuals to make an absolute commitment to informed choice behavior as a nonnegotiable aspect of their day-to-day life.*

Does an informed choice mean a research-driven choice?

That is an excellent question, because it shifts the focus from the philosophical concepts of ontology (assumptions regarding the nature of reality), axiology (values), and ethics (standards of right and wrong) to epistemology (theories of knowledge). Although there are numerous theories of knowing, we are restricting our comments to the area of research-driven knowledge.

Do you mean research-driven knowledge in the area of health care?

Absolutely not! Health outcomes are determined by numerous variables outside of health care. As a result, interdisciplinary, cross-disciplinary, and transdisciplinary knowledge is needed to know how to intervene in the health disparity chain.

How do we begin reengineering the health disparity chain? Is this something that the government does, or is this something that we, as current and future healthcare administrators, public health professionals, and clinicians, do?

Every single individual can play a role in reengineering the health disparity chain.

▶ Steps in Reengineering the Health Disparity Chain

The process of reengineering the health disparity chain requires the use of interventions such as those previously outlined in this chapter. However, our argument is that three types

of change at the individual level will exponentially increase the effectiveness of current initiatives to reduce health disparities.

Step 1: Ontological Reconfiguration

Our behavior is related to our beliefs regarding the nature of reality. Thus, it is important that individuals clarify their own beliefs in this area, because every aspect of our behavior is, in some respect, driven by our individual understanding of the nature of reality and our axiological beliefs.

Step 2: Adopt an Informed Choice Framework to Guide Decision Making

The adoption of an informed choice framework enables individuals to harness their inner power to transform reality by foregoing choice by default and refusing to engage in active choices that result in error because of too little information.

Step 3: Adopt Self-Learning as a Way of Life

If one were to complete research on the first "books" that were used to transmit knowledge, one would find an array of scrolls, papyrus, and tablets dating back more than 2,400 years (Suarez & Woudhuysen, 2013). In earlier eras, however, knowledge was largely inaccessible to the general public. Therefore, the inaccessibility of knowledge and information itself was a key link in a disparity chain that was characterized by vast differentials in virtually every social institution. However, in the contemporary United States, the Internet allows most individuals to access information on a continuous basis. Accordingly, individuals are no longer reliant upon teachers and professors nor their ability to purchase "books"; rather, information is readily available. Individuals can electronically "harvest" data and information and then process it into *knowledge*. In 2017, more than half of the world's population has access to the Internet (Internet World States, 2018). Accordingly, through electronic and/or non-electronic information sources, most individuals can obtain the information needed to guide choices that will support the reengineering of the disparity chain that has operated within their lives, the lives of their families, and/or subtribes.

Step 4: Reengineering the Health Disparity Chain Begins by Introducing Data on the Intergenerational Transfer of Social Position

The healthcare community continually analyzes the intergenerational impact of genetics upon health outcomes and health needs (McCormick & Calzone, 2016). However, less attention has been directed to nonphysiological impacts of intergenerational influences upon the disparities chain. Larson et al. (2018) emphasize the criticality of health disparities researchers shifting from a present-focused framework that analyzes health disparities and outcomes that are sourced within the human life span. Rather, they recommend the adoption of a developmental perspective, which is sometimes described as a "life course health development framework," that is reliant on findings and discoveries that traverse multiple disciplines. This research is then harnessed and critical components extracted in order to understand health disparities across generations.

What are some of the factors that directly and/or indirectly influence intergenerationally transferred health outcomes?

Income and wealth are causally and associationally linked with health disparities. Income and wealth are intergenerationally transferred. Carr, Chrisman, Chua, and Steier (2016) describe challenges that may affect this process. Ganzeboom,

Treiman, and Ultee (1991) demonstrate that the intergenerational transfer of outcomes is inclusive of areas beyond economics. Swartz (2008) specifically discusses the transfer of privilege over *three generations*. Mortimer, Zhang, Wu, Hussemann, & Johnson, (2017) in an analysis of three generations of 422 families found that intergenerational aspects of the disparity chain are so powerful that even children's current perceptions of their intellectual and academic possibilities and future educational pathways are shaped by the experiences of their families going back for at least three generations.

Are you saying that each individual reading this text at this moment has been shaped by very powerful intergenerational forces?

An abundance of research suggests that this is, indeed, the case.

What are the implications of intergenerational forces for the disparity chain?

The body of research on the intergenerational transfer process for position is common knowledge among academics. However, the general public only has a vague notion that this process is operative, and even fewer persons have an informed understanding of the power that intergenerational forces have in creating, sustaining, and reinforcing future disparities in key life outcomes. Accordingly, the reengineering of the disparities chain requires that research on the intergenerational transfer of position be lifted from the pages of academic journals, translated into a form that is comprehensible by all, and made a part of the general knowledge pool. This process will support informed choices and behavioral change as individuals contemplating future parenthood make decisions within their own lives.

What makes you think that this concrete knowledge will drive change?

Immigrants comprise a case study that firm knowledge of the intergenerational transfer of position generates change. Feliciano and Lanuza (2017) describe how immigrant parents, a group who arrive in a country for the sole purpose of releasing their families from past disparities chains and generating a reengineered process of intergenerational transition, are, on average, successful in doing so. The children of immigrants, whether from India, China, Ghana, Australia, Haiti, or another country, on average, exceed the level of educational attainment of the children of Americans of European descent who embody multiple generations of residency in the United States, according to these and other authors. The work of Waithaka (2014), when analyzed, suggests that a conscious decision to build "family capital" can reengineer the disparities chain.

Are you suggesting that current and future healthcare administrators, public health personnel, and clinicians "educate" the public on how to reengineer the disparities chain?

The importance of informing potential parents regarding this possibility includes but extends far beyond those who inhabit the realm of health and health care. Educators, media, community organizations, those who are currently parents, and all who endorse the need to advance humankind may choose to participate in the effort to inform future parents of the possibility of initiating actions to reengineer the disparities chain.

Based upon an understanding of the role of family in the disparities chain, we anticipate that the current generation of future parents will more intensely prepare themselves educationally, socially, emotionally, and occupationally for assuming the role of reengineering the disparities chain for future generations. But, another nonnegotiable step is also necessary.

Step 5: Use Current Research to Create a Family Context That Maximizes the Possibilities for Children as Part of Reengineering the Disparity Chain

Adverse childhood experiences (ACEs) can impact the health of individuals once they reach adulthood. Thus, not only must future parents make a conscious decision to reengineer the disparities chain, they must make informed choices about direct and indirect child-rearing practices that will positively impact the overall health and other outcomes of their children's lives. A large body of research can assist parents in making informed choices regarding childrearing practices (Sotero, 2015). Chapter 14 in this text provides original data on the impact of adverse childhood experiences. House (2018) describes a few child-rearing practices that are positive for child development.

However, a few general recommendations can be made. At the first level, research suggests that "family planning" is more than a formalized synonym for the controlling of the fertility process given the fact that the experiences of each child born can be intergenerationally transferred. Tsui, McDonald-Mosley, and Burke (2010) focus on family planning as a framework that is less focused on preventing pregnancy. Rather, it is an area of health that allows future parents to situate pregnancies within a framework of what the authors call "intendedness". If this concept is borrowed, it becomes clear that family initiation as an "intended action" is required if one is seeking to reengineer the disparities chain. However, Dehlendorf, Rodriquez, Levy, Borrero, and Steinauer (2010) identify subgroup disparities in intentionalities of family initiation. Such differences cannot, based upon the intergenerational transfer of position, multiplicatively strengthen the disparities chain unless greater intentionality is introduced into reproduction decisions. Williams, Sassler, Frech, Addo, and Cooksey (2013), utilizing data from the National Longitudinal Survey of Youth, confirmed adverse health outcomes for children whose presence occurred as a result of less intentionality in the family initiation and structuring process. Again, public health professionals, pediatricians and gynecologists, and researchers can strengthen intentionality in the family initiation process by making research-based, objective data available to young adults regarding the circumstances and behaviors that support improvements in the disparities chain if they make parenting an intentional decision.

What types of behaviors can support relationships with children that can help reengineer the disparity chain?

The familial structure in which the intentional childbearing and childrearing process occurs supports the reengineering of the disparities chain. A large body of research suggests that if informed choices lead individuals to ensure that the familial structure includes above poverty–level income (Lerman & Wilcox, 2013), values and behaviors that reduce conflict and maximize positive interactions (Straus, Gelles, & Steinmetz, 2006), and levels of education (Dickson, Gregg, & Robinson, 2016) that assist the parents in having the knowledge base needed to advance within the given society, the resulting intergenerational transfer of position will generate a reengineered disparities chain.

Step 6: Reengineering the Health Disparity Chain Through Family Health

The steps described thus far are designed to reengineer experiences that affect broader aspects of the disparity chain. Within this context, the neighborhood selected by the family unit can have direct impacts on the disparities chain because, independent of family structure, neighborhood selection can have an impact on the outcomes of children and youth. Jocson and McLoyd (2015), utilizing a sample of low-income families of all ethnicities with children aged 6 to 16 years, determined that there was a relatively linear relationship between neighborhoods and the health of children. Specifically, neighborhoods with high levels of noise, poor sanitation, crime, and other such characteristics cannot

be characterized as "desirable" neighborhoods. The circumstances that exist in such environments subsequently lead to "housing disorder," parental psychological distress, and a subsequent search for relief from the psychological distress. These activities may lead to dysfunctional parenting responses and, as a result, less than optimal outcomes for youth. Again, such factors are not benign. Assari, Caldwell, and Zimmerman (2015) found that girls aged 13 to 14 years who perceived their neighborhood to be unsafe experienced significant declines in their assessment of health over a period of the next 18 years.

Wouldn't this suggest the need for healthcare providers to implement additional screening for such families and referral to treatment?

Yes, it would. Indeed, it indicates a need for primary care providers of pediatric health to routinely not only capture data on the physical health status of children and youth from high-poverty neighborhoods but to also employ case management services to identify special needs that may emerge from their unique circumstances.

What other steps are needed to reduce the disparities chain?

As the discussion thus far indicates, the reengineering of the disparities chain is complex. This discussion has also revealed that this process of disassemblement can make tremendous progress in as little as one generation. The purpose of this discussion is not, of course, to outline a detailed plan for every single point of causation that generates an intricately linked social system that results in socioeconomic, environmental, and behavioral disparities (that then result in health disparities). Such a task would be beyond the scope of this text. Nevertheless, this chapter has emphasized the fact that neither social policy, nor educational policy, nor economic policy, nor healthcare policy can legislate a world of individuals behaving in a collective fashion to address all remediable factors that reduce the progress of humankind.

Rather, policy change must co-occur with change that begins at the individual level, and subsequently extends to various institutions.

Yet, because individuals shape and are shaped by sociocultural forces, healthcare administrators, public policy professionals, and clinicians are positioned to support alterations in the health disparities chain by partnering with researchers, policy makers, and personnel from key disciplines such as education and employment specialists. But, before remedial health disparities can be addressed, their presence must be identified through descriptive statistics, and their correlates and causes analyzed through causal analyses. This text has sought to introduce future healthcare administrators, public health specialists, and clinicians to some of the research methods and data analysis strategies that can be used in this process. Ultimately, information transformed into new knowledge becomes a primary tool for improving the state of humankind.

Chapter Summary

This chapter began by seeking to untangle some of the multiple factors that coalesce to sustain health and healthcare disparities. This chapter first reviewed the many efforts of the public sector to reduce health and healthcare disparities. It then reiterated the extreme need for individuals to assess behavioral choices by using the ultimate guide, "How will a specific choice affect my life as a member of humankind and, via my relationship with individuals, groups, and social institutions, the overall future of humankind?" Since such a question suggests that there is a need for behavioral change, the concept of an ontological transformation was introduced as the core process that can ignite change. Subsequently, the concept of change was related to family status and behavior, the decision to become a parent and parenting circumstances. The recommendations made are by no means exhaustive. Rather, the objective of not merely this chapter, but the whole of the text, is that of triggering new and expanded thought regarding a subject matter that does, indeed, relate to the overall survival and growth of humankind.

Key Terms and Concepts

active choices Decisions made by an individual to select one option over another.

choices by default Those actions taken by an individual without actively thinking about the choice.

cultural competency framework A tool used to inform and educate persons about cultural competency in healthcare settings.

informed choices Occur when individuals know and understand their options; have knowledge of the benefits and costs of each option; assess the benefit and costs; and then make a decision based on their ontology (beliefs about the world) and axiology (values).

ontological change In religious practices, a moment in time when a profound alteration occurs within the "spirit" and "soul" of the priest. It has come to mean a change in the basic premises and conclusions that one draws regarding the nature of existence.

ontological reconfiguration In manufacturing engineering, an automated, internal process of change that occurs through self-automation.

ontological transformation An individual level of change that sprouts and blossoms within, is the platform upon which other levels of change must occur.

reengineering To redesign or to reorganize the operations of an organization in order to improve its efficiency.

social engineering The use of centralized planning or macro levels of change to manage social change among human beings. The idea is first to establish a theory and then gradually resolve various complex social issues using natural, social, and functional approaches.

References

Assari, S., Caldwell, C. H., & Zimmerman, M. A. (2015). Perceived neighborhood safety during adolescence predicts subsequent deterioration of subjective health two decades later; gender differences in a racially-diverse sample. *International Journal of Preventive Medicine, 6*, 117.

Blumenthal-Barby, J. S., & Burroughs, H. (2012). Seeking better health care outcomes: The ethics of using the "nudge." *American Journal of Bioethics, 12*(2), 1–10.

Bowen, A., & Casadevall, A. (2015). Increasing disparities between resource inputs and outcomes, as measured by certain health deliverables, in biomedical research. *Proceedings of the National Academy of Sciences USA, 112*(36), 11335–11340.

California Legislative Information. AB-2246 pupil suicide prevention policies. (2015-2016). Retrieved from https://leginfo.legislature.ca.gov/faces/billNavClient.xhtml?bill_id=201520160AB2246

Carr, J. C., Chrisman, J. J., Chua, J. H., & Steier, L. P. (2016). Family firm challenges in intergenerational wealth transfer. *Entrepreneurship Theory and Practice, 40*(6), 1197-1208.

Dehlendorf, C., Rodriguez, M. I., Levy, K., Borrero, S., & Steinauer, J. (2010). Disparities in family planning. *American Journal of Obstetrics & Gynecology, 202*(3), 214–220.

Dickson, M., Gregg, P. & Robinson, H. (2016). Early, late, or never? When does parental education impact child outcomes. *Economic Journal (London)* F184–F231, doi:10.1111/ccbj.2356.

Dictionary.com. (n.d.). Reengineering. Retrieved from http://www.dictionary.com/browse/reengineer?s=t

Feliciano, C., & Lanuza, Y. R. (2017). An immigrant paradox? Contextual attainment and intergenerational educational mobility. *American Sociological Review, 82*(1), 211–241.

Ganzeboom, H. B., Treiman, D. J., & Ultee, W. C. (1991). Comparative intergenerational stratification research: Three generations and beyond. *Annual Review of Sociology, 17*(1), 277–302.

Ghanouni, A., Renzi, C., Meisel, S. F., & Waller, J. (2016). Common methods of measuring 'informed choice' in screening participation: Challenges and future directions. *Preventive Medicine Reports, 4*, 601–607.

Hart, J., & Halpern, S. D. (2014). Default options in the ICU: Widely used but insufficiently understood. *Current Opinion in Critical Care, 20*(6), 662.

Hatzenbuehler, M. L., & Keyes, K. M. (2013). Inclusive anti-bullying policies and reduced risk of suicide attempts in lesbian and gay youth. *Journal of Adolescent Health. 51*(1_0). S21-S26. 10.1016/j.jadohealth.2012.08.010

House, R. (2018). Childhood, well-being and a therapeutic ethos, 1st ed. (Routledge: London) ISBN 9780429897634.

International Space Exploration Coordination Group. (2013). Benefits stemming from space exploration, pp. 1–22. Retrieved from https://www.nasa.gov/sites/default/files/files/Benefits-Stemming-from-Space-Exploration-2013-TAGGED.pdf

Internet World Stats (2018). World Internet usage and population statistics, Dec. 31, 2017 – Update. https://www.internetworldstats.com/stats.htm. Accessed July 20, 2018.

Jocson, R. M., & McLoyd, V. C. (2015). Neighborhood and housing disorder, parenting, and youth adjustment in low-income urban families. *American Journal of Community Psychology, 55*(3–4), 304–313.

Kosters, M., & Van der Heijden, J. (2015). From mechanism to virtue: Evaluating nudge theory. *Evaluation, 21*(3), 276–291.

Larson, K., Russ, S. A., Kahn, R. S., Flores, G., Goodman, E., Cheng, T. L., & Halfon, N. (2018). Health disparities: A life course health development perspective and future research directions. In N. Halfon, C. B. Forrest, R. M. Lerner, & E. M. Faustman. (Eds.), *Handbook of life course health development* (pp. 499–520). New York: Springer.

Lerman, R. I., & Wilcox, W. B. (2014). For richer, for poorer: How family structures economic success in America. *AEI and Institute for Family Studies.* Retrieved from http://www.aei.org/publication/for-richer-for-poorer-how-family-structures-economic-success-in-america/

McCormick, K. A., & Calzone, K. A. (2016). The impact of genomics on health outcomes, quality, and safety. *Nursing Management, 47*(4), 23.

Merriam-Webster. (n.d.a). Reengineer. Retrieved from https://www.merriam-webster.com/dictionary/reengineer

Merriam-Webster. (n.d.b). Social engineering. Retrieved from https://www.merriam-webster.com/dictionary/social engineering

Michie, S., Van Stralen, M. M., & West, R. (2011). The behaviour change wheel: A new method for characterising and designing behaviour change interventions. *Implementation Science, 6*(1), 42.

Mortimer, J. T., Zhang, L., Wu, C. Y., Hussemann, J., & Johnson, M. K. (2017). Familial transmission of educational plans and the academic self-concept: A three-generation longitudinal study. *Social Psychology Quarterly, 80*(1), 85–107.

Nadan, Y. (2014). Rethinking 'cultural competence' in international social work. *International Social Work, 60*(1), 74–83.

Radha, S. S., Caplan, N., St. Clair Gibson, A., Shenouda, M., Konan, S., & Kader, D. (2012). Can patients really make an informed choice? An evaluation of the availability of online information about consultant surgeons in the United Kingdom. *BMJ Open, 2*(4), e001203.

Renzaho, A. M. N., Romios, P., Crock, C., & Sønderlund, A. L. (2013). The effectiveness of cultural competence programs in ethnic minority patient-centered health care—a systematic review of the literature. *International Journal for Quality in Health Care, 25*(3), 261–269.

Ryan, S., Murphy, A., Tameron, A., Hussain, L. Teng, A., Dunki-Jacobs, E.M., & Yee, D. (2018). Robotic versus laparoscopic gastrectomy for gastric adenocarcinoma: Propensity matched analysis of the National Cancer Database. *Journal of Clinical Oncology, 36* (H-Suppl), 104.

Sotero, M. M. (2015). The Effects of Adverse Childhood Experiences on Subsequent Injury in Young Adulthood: Findings from the National Longitudinal Study of Adolescent and Adult Health. UNLV Dissertation. Retrieved from https://digitalscholarship.unlv.edu /thesesdissertations/2432/

Straus, M. A., Gelles, R. J., & Steinmetz, S. K. (2006). Behind closed doors: Violence in the American family. New York: Routledge Taylor and Francis Group.

Suarez, M. F., & Woudhuysen, H. R. (Eds.). (2013). *The book: A global history.* New York: Oxford University Press.

Swartz, T. T. (2008). Family capital and the invisible transfer of privilege: Intergenerational support and social class in early adulthood. *New Directions for Child and Adolescent Development, 119,* 11–24.

TheFreeDictionary.com. (n.d.a). Reengineer. Retrieved from https://www.thefreedictionary.com/reengineer

TheFreeDictionary.com. (n.d.b). Social engineering. Retrieved from https://www.thefreedictionary.com /socialengineering

Truong, M., Paradies, Y., & Priest, N. (2014). Interventions to improve cultural competency in healthcare: A systematic review of reviews. *BMC Health Services Research, 14*(1), 99.

Tsui, A. O., McDonald-Mosley, R., & Burke, A. E. (2010). Family planning and the burden of unintended pregnancies. *Epidemiologic Reviews, 32*(1), 152–174.

Voyer, B. (2015). 'Nudging' behaviours in healthcare: Insights from behavioural economics. *British Journal of Healthcare Management, 21*(3), 130–135.

Waithaka, E. N. (2014). Family capital: Conceptual model to unpack the intergenerational transfer of advantage in transitions to adulthood. *Journal of Research on Adolescence, 24*(3), 471–484.

Williams Institute. (2018). LGBT youth experiences with discrimination, harassment, and bullying in school. Fact Sheet. Retrieved from https://williamsinstitute .law.ucla.edu/press/lgbt-youth-bullying-press-release/

Williams, K., Sassler, S., Frech, A., Addo, F., & Cooksey, E. (2013). Mothers' union histories and the mental and physical health of adolescents born to unmarried mothers. *Journal of Health and Social Behavior, 54*(3), 278–295.

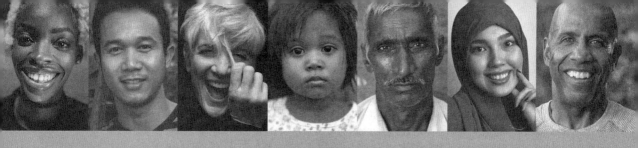

Glossary

accountable care health community model Care model that seeks to link patients not only with physicians, hospitals, and other types of clinical care but with the broad range of community services that will allow other health-related needs to be addressed.

active choices Decisions made by an individual to select one option over another.

adjusted rate A type of "refined" rate that can be used to make comparisons more accurately.

adjuvant hormonal therapy Breast cancer treatment that specifically targets the hormones that are associated with the growth of breast tumors in order to decrease their size.

adverse childhood experiences (ACEs) Highly stressful and often traumatic events that occur during childhood and adolescence, also termed *developmental trauma* or *complex trauma*.

affective level Responses that occur at the level of emotions and/or feelings.

Affordable Care Act (ACA) Nicknamed "Obamacare," this statute was signed into law by President Barack Obama in 2010. It was the first major overhaul of the U.S. healthcare system and expansion of coverage since the passage of Medicare and Medicaid in 1965. Among its many goals, it seeks to reduce the number of uninsured Americans.

ambulance diversion A process in which an emergency department at one hospital refers the patient to another hospital. Although most often capacity based, it also occurs for other reasons, such as a consumer's need for services outside of the hospital's area of expertise.

analysis of variance (ANOVA) A statistical method that tests general differences among two or more means. That is, it is used to test if there exists a significant degree of difference between two or more means (variables, observations, etc.). While the possible variances are being measured, the means are tested to identify significant differences.

atrial fibrillation Condition whereby irregularities in heart rate distort the flow of blood in the body.

axiology The study of the nature of value and valuation and of the kinds of things that are valuable (Oxford Dictionary).

behavioral change contract A patient-centered process of change whereby the patient agrees to adhere or not adhere to certain behaviors and the benefits or repercussions of doing so.

bivariate analysis The process of analyzing data across two or more variables in order to determine whether there is a relationship among those factors.

cancer registry Registry established in 1992 as part of the National Program of Cancer Registry Amendment Act to collect and manage data on cancer nationwide.

causal research Research conducted in order to identify the extent and nature of cause-and-effect relationships.

census Collection of data from every single individual, household, and/or other entity that is the defined unit of analysis for the data collection effort.

chi-square test A statistical tool that is used to determine whether differences between two categories of variables are significantly associated.

choices by default Those actions taken by an individual without actively thinking about the choice.

coefficient of determination (R^2) A statistical tool that is used to determine the proportion of the variance in the dependent variable that can be predicted from the independent variable.

community hospital Public institution that provides acute or short-term care. May provide general services and/or treatment for highly specialized illnesses and diseases.

conflict theory Assumes that competition and conflict over scarce resources are natural forces between groups and subgroups.

confounding variables Unforeseen "extraneous" variables that affect the dependent and independent variables. Thus, a confounding variable distorts or renders the study inaccurate by its presence.

contemporary subtribalism The emergence of values, beliefs, and attitudes that develop in defense and protection of any subgroup, whether defined by race/ethnicity, sex, sexual preference, religion, geographic area, occupation, and/or any other grouping when such feelings of loyalty become so intense as to mask solutions and strategies that generate win-win outcomes for all subgroups.

correlation analysis Statistical evaluation of the association and strength of the connection that exists between two variables.

count The simplest way to measure disease frequency in epidemiology. It is the number of how many cases (individuals) meet a particular definition (have a disease or health issue).

cross-disciplinary An approach to knowledge in which one discipline and/or issues in one discipline are viewed from the perspective of another.

cross-sectional datasets Datasets that examine a unique set of variables at a particular point in time.

crude rate A summary rate that expresses how many cases existed in a population during a given time period.

cultural competency framework A tool used to inform and educate persons about cultural competency in healthcare settings.

cultural competency model Based upon the belief that educating individuals and groups regarding quality of life of different subgroups will allow them to reduce bias and discrimination.

data validation and verification The process of carefully checking that data that have been copied, typed, or otherwise imported to ensure that the data are accurate and consistent.

degrees of freedom The abbreviation is "df," which tells us by how much a value can vary given the number of values that are fixed in a statistical calculation.

disparities chain Refers to the historic and contemporary factors that interactively affect current and future outcomes.

empirical Information and knowledge that transcend theory. Data generated by statistical observation of real-life experiences and/or via experiment or data analysis.

equivalence Relationships between numbers that, although different, are equal in value, effect, force, and/or significance.

ethnocentrism Tendency of people to view their own subgroup as superior and to reject subgroups with different physical, cultural, behavioral, and/or other characteristics.

factor analysis A statistical method by which a larger set of variables are reduced in order to reveal the cause and effect relationship between variables and/or to support a hypothesis.

fixed-dose, low-dose combination therapy The use of two or more complementary agents in lower doses to manage hypertension.

full-text Access to the complete text of an article in a database.

gross domestic product (GDP) per capita An economic concept that is used to measure the amount of dollars each resident would have based on the market value of all goods and services produced in a country.

HbA(1c) test A glycated hemoglobin test that determines a person's blood glucose level. The test is designed to show the average level of blood glucose over the previous 3 months. High blood glucose levels are an indicator of diabetes mellitus.

health disparities Population and subpopulation differences in health outcomes.

health disparities research Emerging field that seeks to identify those areas of health that are characterized by sustained differences in mortality and morbidity across subgroups.

health disparity measure A measure that summarizes the width of differentials in health outcomes between populations and/or subpopulations relative to one another.

health insurance Component of the American healthcare system that assists Americans in purchasing the protection needed to prevent them from having to pay out-of-pocket costs for the full range of services and products needed in case of illness and disease treatment or illness and disease prevention.

healthcare disparities The differential processes and outcomes that occur within the operation of various components of the healthcare system.

hierarchical linear modeling or multilevel modeling is used to analyze hierarchical data.

hypertension A chronic disease in persons with a blood pressure greater than 130/80 mm Hg.

implicit bias Beliefs, attitudes, and values regarding various subgroups that are operative at a subconscious level.

in site search Google search strategy that enables the user to limit a search to a particular website.

incidence rate The number of new cases of diseases or deaths per defined unit. The unit may be 1,000 persons, 10,000 persons, or 100,000 persons a year.

index A single number that utilizes weights and other statistical processes to develop a single summary measure.

informed choices Occur when individuals know and understand their options; have knowledge of the benefits and costs of each option; assess the benefit and costs; and then make a decision based on their ontology (beliefs about the world) and axiology (values).

in-group Any group with which an individual identifies; identification is not necessarily based upon race/ethnicity, culture, gender, etc.

interdisciplinary Approach to a subject that involves two or more fields within the same discipline and/or two or more disciplines.

interval data Quantitative data that do not have a true "zero" but are numerical.

lag variable A lag variable is used when the relationship between the independent and dependent variables did not occur within the same time period.

legacy Older documents on health disparity topics.

life expectancy The number of years that an individual can expect to live at birth.

lipid metabolism The process by which fats in the body are converted into energy.

logistic regression A statistical method that is used to identify an outcome from the analysis of one or more independent variables.

longitudinal datasets Datasets that contain information from the same individuals and/or families at different points in time.

long-term care Medical and nonmedical services that are provided in order to help people with age-related limitations and/or disabilities to maximize their physical, social, mental, psychological, and spiritual outcomes despite the irreversibility and progression of their disabling physical and/or cognitive status.

maximal rate difference A method that is used by the federal government for calculating disparities. This method is simply based upon subtracting the lower value from the higher value.

Medicaid Analytic eXtract (MAX) A set of person-level data files on Medicaid eligibility, service utilization, and payments. The MAX data are created to support research and policy analysis.

Medical Subject Headings (MeSH) Syntax by which PubMed indexes articles to aid in the discovery of their content.

MEDLINE The underlying database that "seeds" PubMed. MEDLINE data are freely available from the National Library of Medicine for developers to create different applications using the data.

multicollinearity Defined as one or more significantly high correlations between two or more (independent) variables. When multicollinearity occurs it may indicate that there is too much correlation between variables to be able to support reliability of the regression.

multidisciplinary An assembly of a team of persons from a range of academic fields who apply their area of expertise to a common problem.

multilevel regression is also known as a hierarchical linear model or multilevel model. This statistical model may have variances at one or more levels.

multiple regression A statistical tool that allows causation to be identified and measured. It is used to identify relationships between two or more independent variables and one dependent variable.

multivariate analysis A statistical approach that allows the statistician to simultaneously assess the impact of multiple variables upon a dependent variable.

National Healthcare Quality and Disparities Report Annual report produced by the U.S. Department of Health and Human Services that documents health and healthcare measures for the U.S. population.

National Library of Medicine The federal agency responsible for many of the free tools that health and healthcare disparities researchers can use in their research efforts. Among its many offerings, is MEDLINE/PubMed.

National Vital Statistics System Part of the Centers for Disease Control and Prevention's National Center for Health Statistics, this agency is the most reliable primary source of secondary data on deaths, death rates, life expectancy, and infant mortality by race/ethnicity, gender, age, geographic area, and cause of deaths.

nominal data Data that are distinguished by name or category, such as sex, race/ethnicity, rural/urban status, or sexual preference.

nonequivalent inequalities This term references relationships that are mathematically different that do not equate to the same sum. For example, if an individual with hypertension had the same life expectancy as one with diabetes, it would be an equivalent inequality. If these differences are associated with different life expectancies, it becomes a nonequivalent inequality.

nonlinear There is not a straight-line causal relationship between two variables.

normal curve A bell-shaped curve that shows the probability distribution of a continuous random variable.

ontological change In religious practices, a moment in time when a profound alteration occurs within the "spirit" and "soul" of the priest. It has come to mean a change in the basic premises and conclusions that one draws regarding the nature of existence.

ontological reconfiguration In manufacturing engineering, an automated, internal process of change that occurs through self-automation.

ontological transformation An individual level of change that sprouts and blossoms within, it is the platform upon which other levels of change must occur.

ontology The study of the nature of existence, including the nature of things in relationship to each other.

ordinal data Data that are based upon order.

outgroup A group with which an individual does not identify; often accompanied by hostility toward that group.

panel size The total number of patients who see a physician on a regular basis.

parameter A number based upon the entirety of the target population.

path analysis A statistical analysis tool used to assess relationships that exist between variables.

patient mix The characteristics of the patients served by a healthcare facility, including the severity of the patients' health needs. May also incorporate patient demographics and socioeconomic characteristics.

patient self-management Provision of services and/or support so that a patient can manage a chronic disease.

patient-centered care A collaborative form of health care and decision-making that involves healthcare providers, patients, and their families wherein the main goal is to strategize a customized and comprehensive healthcare plan.

patriarchy Traditionally, a power structure within a social system or family dominated by the patriarch or other privileged elder men. In modern context, it is a power structure within a social system that is dominated by males.

paywall When access to the full text of an article requires a paid subscription.

Pearson correlation coefficient (r) Statistical tool used to assess whether two or more variables are associated.

percentage difference The difference, categorized in percent format, between two variables. The calculation of the percentage difference can be accomplished by taking the difference between the two values and dividing it by the average of the two values.

philosophical anthropology Controversial area of study that uses philosophy (which focuses on the nature of all that is in existence) to study humankind, including intrapersonal and interpersonal relationships and all aspects of people as humans.

population health The study of nonclinical and clinical variables that determine the health outcomes of various groups or subgroups of individuals.

power The ability to exercise control over human and/or non-human resources with a physical and/or human environment.

prevalence rate The percentage of the total population or subpopulation affected by a condition in a specified time period.

preventive screenings Examinations and tests designed to detect certain diseases in their early stages when a cure is more likely.

primary data Data collected by a researcher through a direct process of observation or experimental design, in order to answer one or more research questions.

primary prevention Activities that involve the prevention of illness and disease.

probability theory The branch of mathematics concerned with the random distribution of quantities.

proportion A measure in the form of ratio in which the numerator is also included as part of the denominator. It can be calculated by dividing the number of interested cases [A] by the total cases [B].

prospective payment Payment system for healthcare services where services are first delivered, and the provider is then reimbursed based on a predetermined, fixed amount.

proximate cause An event that is closest to, or immediately responsible for causing, some observed result.

PubMed The free search engine supported by the National Library of Medicine that is based on the MEDLINE database of references and abstracts on life sciences and biomedical topics.

range check A check to make sure that the data all fall within a certain range.

rate A type of proportion that incorporates a given time period into the denominator. The numerator represents the cases that met the definition, and the denominator includes all cases that may or may not meet the definition.

ratio A fractional relationship between the numerator and denominator. You divide one quantity by another, but the two quantities do not belong to each other.

ratio data Numbers that have a true zero and can be expressed as fractions.

reengineering To redesign or to reorganize the operations of an organization in order to improve its efficiency.

registered hospital A hospital that has listed itself with the American Hospital Association (AHA), has met all accreditation standards of the Joint Commission on the Accreditation of Healthcare Organizations (JCAHO), and is certified under Titles 18 and 19 of the Social Security Act.

reliable Data measurements that produce the same values independently of user, time, or place.

renin-angiotensin-aldosterone system The hormone system that regulates blood pressure and fluid balance. If this system is overactive, blood pressure will be too high.

respite care Short-term, temporary caregiving for an elderly, ill, incapacitated, or handicapped person provided by a secondary caregiver. Primary caregivers are given time away from their duties for a brief period in order to rest. Respite care is provided in a variety of settings, including homes and institutionally based sites.

retrospective payment A system in existence until 1983 whereby hospital services were not pre-priced. Hospitals delivered the service, decided on a price, and then billed Medicare after services were delivered.

sample A set of data collected and/or selected from a statistical population.

scatterplot A scatter graph or scatterplot consists of a series of plots that outline the connection between two sets of variables (or data).

secondary data Data that were not collected by the end user. This includes data that is public information that was originally collected by other entities such as government and quasi-government agencies, public and private companies, and other entities.

secondary prevention Activities that prevent the recurrence of illness and disease.

self-management The adoption of behaviors that maximize treatment outcomes and minimize the progression of a disease.

self-management supports Tools, materials, and training provided by healthcare institutions to assist the individual in the maximization of their self-management activities.

sleep architecture Patterns of sleep as an individual moves through different aspects of the sleep cycle.

social engineering The use of centralized planning or macro levels of change to manage social change among human beings. The idea is first to establish a theory and then gradually resolve various complex social issues using natural, social, and functional approaches.

social stratification Basis for a caste or class society in which specific subgroups of people are grouped into categories based on certain characteristics.

specific rate A type of "refined" rate that can be used to make comparisons more accurately.

standard error Based on statistics, the standard error measures spread between the observed data value and mean data values.

statistic A number that is derived from a sample taken from a total of the target population.

structural functionalism A highly partisan approach to systems of social stratification that is supportive of the status quo.

subtribe A subset or subdivision of a larger tribe.

systemic lupus erythematosus (SLE) Chronic disease of the immune system where the body misreads healthy tissue as being infected and begins attacking itself.

systems of social stratification Societal mechanisms whereby people are positioned in a hierarchy based on their wealth, status, power, prestige, gender, race/ethnicity, and other identifying characteristics.

telehealth Remote provision of nonclinical services through electronic means to provide health education and training for end users and/or medical personnel, surveillance, caregiver support, and other areas.

telemedicine Use of telecommunications technologies to provide remote diagnosis and treatment of patients.

tertiary care A third level of care by providers. It can be viewed as the last segment of care that is available to the patient. Accordingly, it is the most complex level of care that can be provided.

transdisciplinary Theories, methods, and concepts of one discipline are neither viewed from the perspective of another discipline nor merged. Rather, issues are lifted from the arena of their kinship to a discipline and analyzed without the use of any disciplinary lenses.

tribe "A group of people who are linked by physical and societal factors such as place of residency or birth, ancestry, culture and customs, religious beliefs, economics, blood relations, common language, or other social constructs, who may or may not have a common ancestor or common leader."

t-test A statistical tool that is used to assess whether the means of two or more populations are equal or not sufficiently different as to be considered unequal.

unit of analysis The major entity that is being analyzed in a study, such as individuals, groups, social organizations, etc.

univariate analysis The process of organizing, describing, and summarizing data along one dimension.

valid Data that measure that which it purports to measure.

Variance Inflation Factor (VIF) A VIF is used in regression analysis to determine the existence of multicollinearity. The VIF, after being applied to all of the model's variables will result in the R-square values.

workload The total sum of time associated with all activities completed as part of the delivery of health care. Includes time spent with patients, as well as time spent reviewing patient files, writing prescriptions, communicating with labs, completing referrals, managing the clinical and administrative team, and completing other tasks.

zero-sum game Situations in which resources are fixed and gains or losses experienced by one group are exactly balanced by the gains or losses of the other group.

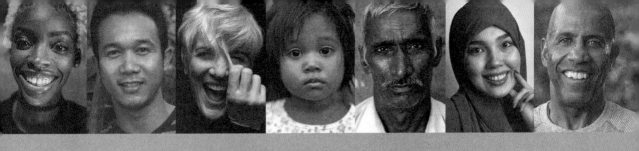

Index

Note: Page numbers followed by b, f, or t indicate material in boxes, figures, or tables, respectively.

H